APPLIED ANGIOGRAPHY FOR RADIOGRAPHERS

► **PAUL LAUDICINA, M.A., R.T. (R.)**
Professor, Radiological Sciences
College of DuPage
Glen Ellyn, Illinois

► **DOUGLAS WEAN, A.A.S., R.T. (R.)**
Assistant Supervisor and Clinical Instructor
Special Procedures and Imaging
Edward Hines Jr. Veterans Administration Hospital
Hines, Illinois

APPLIED ANGIOGRAPHY FOR RADIOGRAPHERS

W.B. SAUNDERS COMPANY
A Division of Harcourt Brace & Company
Philadelphia London Toronto Montreal Sydney Tokyo

W.B. SAUNDERS COMPANY
A Division of Harcourt Brace & Company

The Curtis Center
Independence Square West
Philadelphia, Pennsylvania 19106

Library of Congress Cataloging-in-Publication Data

Laudicina, Paul F.
   Applied angiography for radiographers   /   Paul Laudicina, Douglas
Wean.—1st ed.
      p.   cm.
   ISBN 0-7216-3283-1
   1. Angiography.   I. Wean, Douglas.   II. Title.
   [DNLM: 1. Angiography.   WG 500 L371a 1994]
RC691.6.A53L38   1994
616.1'3'07572—dc20
DNLM/DLC   93-27002

Applied angiography for radiographers   ISBN 0–7216–3283–1

Printed in the United States of America.

Last digit is the print number: 9   8   7   6   5   4   3   2   1

In memory of my mother and father,
and to my wife Vicki,
and our sons
Dan and Jeff

DLW

To my parents,
my wife Rita,
and our sons
Anthony and Michael

PFL

► ACKNOWLEDGMENTS

Writing a textbook is a monumental task. When one views a finished product the degree of commitment and the amount of time expended are not always apparent. The completion of *Applied Angiography for Radiographers* could not have been achieved without the invaluable assistance, support, and encouragement of numerous individuals. We are grateful to many people and apologize to those who may have been inadvertently omitted.

First of all, we are grateful to our families, who have had to put up with many late nights of our seclusion and dedication to this project.

A great deal of our support and resources came from physicians, co-workers, and vendors. We would like to acknowledge the following individuals from Edward Hines Jr. Veterans Administration Hospital: Mark Van Drunen, M.D., Chief of Diagnostic Radiology; Subramanian Ramamurthy, M.D., Section Chief, Angiography, Interventional Radiology; M.H. Naheedy, M.D.; Rao-Malyala, M.D.; Marcy McIntosh, M.D.; and the angiography team—Huey Metts, R.T. (R), Charles Jones, R.T. (R), Steve Fletcher, R.T. (R); Dan Martellota, R.T. (R); and Benard Robinson, R.T. (R). We appreciate the fine efforts of our illustrator, Martha J. Dane, R.T. (R). The vendors were also an invaluable resource to us. We wish to acknowledge the following: Agfa Technical Imaging Systems, a division of Miles Incorporated; Cook Incorporated; Elema Schonander; Eastman Kodak Co.; Phillips Medical Systems, North America; Picker International; Medrad Corporation; Liebel-Plarsheim Incorporated; Medi-Tech Corporation; Mallinckrodt Pharmaceutical Co.; Squibb Diagnostics; Winthrop Laboratories; Cordis Corporation; and Datel Incorporated.

▶ PREFACE

In 1972 Paul Laudicina became employed in the radiography program at College of DuPage in Glen Ellyn, Illinois. His first assignment was to teach a second-year-student course in radiologic special procedures. Eventually this course was offered for continuing education for graduate radiographers. Some of the first enrollees were radiographers from Edward Hines Jr. Veterans Administration Hospital. As a result of this course and their mutual interest in special procedures, Paul Laudicina and Douglas Wean developed a dedicated clinical rotation component in special procedures at Hines Hospital for College of DuPage radiologic technology students. This was the only program in the state of Illinois at that time that combined classroom theory and dedicated clinical education in special procedures. Since 1981, this cooperative venture has been refined, improved, and expanded. We have had over 600 students complete this rotation in the last 13 years.

A 20-year friendship and a shared love of special procedures provided Paul Laudicina and Douglas Wean the impetus to develop *Applied Angiography for Radiographers.*

The text is prepared in four sections: Introduction to Angiography, Equipment and Image Enhancement Techniques, Procedural Angiography, and Interventional Procedures. The relationship of technology to the patient is emphasized throughout this text.

Cardiovascular/interventional procedures are performed in many different types of clinical environments. Many factors influence how procedures are performed and how images are produced. We have tried to describe some of the accepted, established techniques we have worked with. We do not mean to suggest that "our way" is the only way.

Section One (Chapters 1 through 4) discusses the beginning of special procedures, what we now call cardiovascular/interventional technology. Topics such as the history of angiography, the medical and legal implications, pharmaceuticals and contrast agents, and patient care procedures are discussed.

Section Two (Chapters 5 and 6) discusses equipment and image enhancement techniques.

In Sections Three and Four, the focus is on the procedural aspects of clinical angiography. Again, the procedural methods are used at the discretion of the physician, whether he is a radiologist or a cardiologist. In Chapters 7 through 12, the discussions include the topics of normal vascular and nonvascular anatomy, equipment and accessories, procedural approaches, and pathology. Each chapter includes numerous case studies for further information and correlation.

Chapter 13 focuses on the continuing emergence of cardiovascular/interventional technology as an integral and advancing component of diagnostic and therapeutic radiologic procedures. We have merely scratched the surface and can only speculate where our specialty may lead us.

DOUGLAS WEAN
Villa Park,
Illinois

PAUL LAUDICINA
Wheaton, Illinois

► CONTENTS

▶ SECTION FOUR
INTERVENTIONAL PROCEDURES 223

CHAPTER ELEVEN
Vascular Interventional
Procedures 225

CHAPTER TWELVE
Nonvascular Interventional
Procedures 247

CHAPTER THIRTEEN
The Future of Cardiovascular/
Interventional Technology 265

▶ SECTION ONE

▶ **INTRODUCTION TO ANGIOGRAPHY**

► CHAPTER ONE

► HISTORY OF ANGIOGRAPHY

► CHAPTER OBJECTIVES

Upon completion of Chapter 1 the technologist will be able to:

1. Explain the significance of the work of William Harvey, Christopher Wren, and Claude Bernard
2. Describe the technical limitations of the early x-ray tubes
3. Describe the work of five pioneers who made significant contributions in the evolution of equipment for special procedures
4. Describe the work of five pioneers who developed injection techniques for the heart and vascular system
5. Describe the work of three pioneers who are responsible for the emerging field of interventional radiography

The history of angiography predates the discovery of x-rays. Physicians and practitioners have long been fascinated by the mysteries of the anatomy and physiology of the vascular system. During those early years, numerous scientists and physicians conducted research and contributed greatly to the field of medicine and radiologic special procedures. To include all of these pioneers is beyond the scope of this text; however, some of these pioneers and their work are highlighted in this chapter.

Autopsies were the earliest and foremost procedures used to study the organs, their functions, and their blood flow. William Harvey (1578–1657), in his pioneer work on circulation of the blood, proved that blood was continually circulated around the body within a contained system. This contribution by Harvey is considered to be one of the most important in the history of medicine.

Christopher Wren (1632–1723) was an English scientist who created detailed illustrations of the vascular system. He developed a technique using reeds and vegetable dyes to outline superficial veins in both corpses and live humans. Wren illustrated the work of Thomas Willis (1621–1675), whose name is used in connection with the circle of arteries at the base of the brain called the circle of Willis.

Claude Bernard (1813–1878), who was a French physiologist, developed the principle of homeostasis, which stated that the "internal environment" is constant in warm-blooded organisms and that physiologic mechanisms resist any external factors that tend to alter this internal state. Bernard also described the multiple functions of the liver and conducted research on digestive activity of the pancreatic secretions and their relationship with diabetes. In 1865 Bernard published *Introduction to the Study of Experimental Medicine* and set down the standards for future experimentalists. In 1869, using arteriovenous cut-down techniques, Bernard was able to sample both arterial and venous blood flow from the jugular veins, inferior vena cava, and the femoral arterial system using a catheter system. For these reasons, Bernard is considered to be the founder of experimental physiology.

Wilhelm Conrad Roentgen (1845–1923), who was a German physicist, revolutionized the field of medicine when he presented a paper to the Wurzburg Physical Medical Society on December 28, 1895, concerning his discovery of x-rays. Less than 1 month later, in January 1896, Edward Haschek and Otto Lindenthal of Vienna (both physicians) had duplicated Roentgen's radiographic results and began to envision and develop an intravascular contrast media.

The first contrast agent was *Teichmanns' paste,* which was a mixture of petroleum jelly, cinnebar, and chalk. Haschek and Lindenthal injected this mixture into an amputated hand, using an exposure time of 57 minutes.

From the 1890s to 1910, studies on cadavers were performed using mixtures of bismuth subnitrate, lead oxide, and metallic mercury as contrast agents. The problem with these substances was their chemotoxicity.

In addition to the chemotoxicity of contrast media, a major problem during the early 1900s was the lack of technology in radiographic tube development. Roentgen had used a partially vacuumed Hittorf-Crookes tube and an induction coil to create x-rays. These tubes suffered from a condition that was commonly referred to as a "gassy" tube effect. This effect was caused by overheating the metal electrodes and by the resultant emissions of gas ions into the glass envelope.

In 1913, William D. Coolidge, who was an American chemist and inventor, produced a high vacuum, hot cathode, x-ray tube with a pure tungsten filament. For the first time this allowed for a predetermined, controlled electron output. This contributed to the longer life of the tube, increased radiographic detail, and a decrease in exposure factors. In 1929 the rotating anode was introduced and provided for more efficient heat dissipation.

Interest in vascular angiography was hampered during this time frame with the continued search for a nontoxic viable contrast agent. In 1923, Edmund Osborne used sodium iodine for direct cystography and pyelography. The real turning point in the development of contrast media was when Barney Brooks, who was a physician, used sodium iodide for lower limb arteriography. Brooks' experiments used iodine for the first time on humans for intravascular opacification in 1924.

Egas Moniz, in 1927, introduced cerebral arteriography by injecting solutions of sodium bromide and sodium iodide into the exposed carotid arteries of the neck. Many violent reactions to these chemicals took place. The exposure of the carotids and the potential reactions resulted in an inconvenient and dangerous procedure.

The pioneering progress of Brooks in femoral arteriography, of Moniz (1928) in carotid arteriography, and of Reybaldo dos Santos (1929) in translumbar aortography rapidly brought angiography to a new threshold.

The 1930s and 1940s proceeded with developments in catheter placement technique, contrast agents, rapid serial film changers, improved imaging techniques, and double-coated film emulsions on a polyester base.

Early arteriography was accomplished by single film and injection. This entailed ligation of vessels in order to control flow and often required multiple injections. The first roll-film changer was developed by Howard Ruggles in 1925. This changer transported an 8"-wide, 30 ft-long roll of x-ray film between two intensifying screens. The x-ray exposures were triggered each time that a film was secured or compressed between the screens. In 1932, Moniz and Pereira Caldas built a rudimentary serial changer. This serial changer, which had a capacity of three films, allowed for examination of all three circulatory phases: arterial, capillary, and venous.

During the late 1940s, Jesus Sanchez-Perez developed a serial changer that utilized film cassettes and a motorized chain-driven system (Fig. 1–1). This was followed by the development of a roll-film changer in 1949 and by further refinement of both the serial changer and the roll-film changer in the early 1950s.

The first widely used film changer, which was developed in the United States, was built at the University of Minnesota by Rigler and Watson in 1953. Roll film was pulled through intensifying screens by a Geneva drive cam that pierced and pulled the film through the receiving bin. The maximum film rate was six films per second.

In 1956, Gidlund developed an injector that operated on the principle of compressed gas. In 1960, Kurt Amplatz described a cardiovascular injector that operated with carbon dioxide cartridges. These cartridges could deliver several low-pressure injections or a single injection of 240 lb/in^2.

The development of electrically powered, mechanical drive injectors represented the birth of a new generation of injectors. Cordis, Viamonte-Hobbs, and Medrad were the proponents of this new birth. It did not take long for these injectors to include optional features that enhanced vascular angiography. Cordis developed a means of timing an injection to correspond with a specific phase of the cardiac cycle. Viamonte-Hobbs and Medrad designed safeguards against the hazard of ventricular fibrillation (Fig. 1–2).

Other pioneers included physicians Loman and Myerson, who in 1936 made the first successful injection of a radiopaque contrast agent into the carotid artery by percutaneous needle puncture and without any surgical exposure of the carotid arteries.

In Japan in 1940, S. Takahasi developed a percutaneous technique of injecting the vertebral artery just before its entry into the costotransversal foramen of the sixth cervical vertebra. This is the first percutaneous technique developed for direct puncture of the vertebral artery.

The first application of the catheter technique on the vertebral artery was introduced by Radner in 1947. S. I. Seldinger in 1953 presented his technique for percutaneous introduction of a catheter. The transfemoral catheter technique was first performed by Lindgren in 1956 and was refined by Bonte and associates in 1958 and by Cronquist in 1961.

In 1959, Rastelli and associates were the first to investigate the therapeutic applications of angiography for active gastrointestinal hemorrhage. In 1960, Lussenhop and Spence developed a technique of artificial embolization of a cerebral arteriovenous malformation. Margulis, in that same year, described the application of intraoperative mesenteric arteriography to show cecal arteriovenous malformation.

In 1963, W. Hanafee and T. H. Newton developed a method of selective catheter vertebral angiography by a transaxillary catheter. This method was most successful in patients with marked atherosclerosis of the iliac arteries and thoracic aorta. These selective catheter approaches are now considered to be a most reliable, easy method of obtaining a consistently excellent delineation of the vessels.

Nusbaum and Baum in 1963 described an angio-

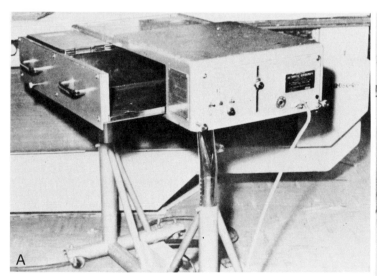
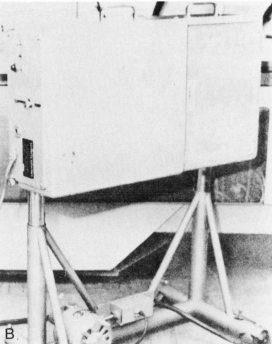

▶ Figure 1–1

A, Sanchez-Perez cassette film changer in the film-loading position. The open drawer reveals several 11 × 14″ cassettes in the storage chamber. Upon exposure, cassettes are sent to the receiving chamber by the chain-driven mechanism. B, The cassette film changer is adjusted in the vertical position for lateral projection. The exposure surface with the grid is on the right.

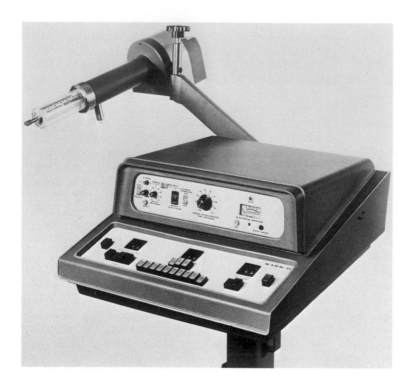

▶ **Figure 1–2**
Medrad Mark II pressure injector with electrocardiogram trigger. (Courtesy of Medrad, Inc., Pittsburgh, PA.)

▶ **Table 1-1**
CHRONOLOGIC SUMMARY—EVOLUTION OF ANGIOGRAPHY

Date	Pioneer	Contribution	Date	Pioneer	Contribution
	Harvey	Circulation of the blood	1956	Rigler and Watson	First roll-film changer used in the United States
	Willis	Circle of Willis			
	Wren	Detailed illustrations of the vascular system	1956	Lindgren	Transfemoral catheter technique
1895	Roentgen	Discovery of x-rays	1956	Gidlund	Compressed gas injector
1896	Coolidge	Hot cathode x-ray tube			
1896	Edison	Fluoroscope	1959	Rastelli et al	Therapeutic angiography for active gastrointestinal hemorrhage
1896	Haschek and Lindenthal	Application of contrast media to angiography			
1913	Coolidge	Tungsten filament x-ray tube	1960	Lussenhop and Spence	Artificial embolization of cerebral arteriovenous malformation
1918	Dandy	Air as a contrast agent injected into cerebral ventricles			
1921–22	Osborne and Roundtree	Sodium iodide used for direct cystography and pyelography	1960	Margulis	Intraoperative mesenteric arteriography
1924	Brooks	Femoral arteriography	1960	Amplatz	Cardiovascular injector using CO_2 cartridges
1925	Ruggles	First roll-film changer	1963	Hanafee and Newton	Selective catheterization of the vertebral artery using the transaxillary approach
1927	Moniz	Carotid arteriography			
1929	dos Santos	Translumbar artography			
1932	Moniz and Caldas	Serial film changer	1963	Nusbaum and Baum	Technique for determining the site of a gastrointestinal hemorrhage
1936	Loman and Myerson	First direct injection of contrast media into the carotid arteries			
1940	Takahasi	Percutaneous puncture of the vertebral artery	1964	Dotter and Judkins	Recanalization of stenosed arteries with a coaxial catheter system
1947	Radner	Catheterization of the vertebral artery			
1948	Sanchez-Perez	Serial film changer	1969	Nusbaum	Use of vasopressin for a variceal hemorrhage
1953	Seldinger	Percutaneous needle puncture and catheterization	1965–1970s	Cordis and Viamonte-Hobbs	Electromechanical injector

► **Table 1-1**

CHRONOLOGIC SUMMARY—EVOLUTION OF ANGIOGRAPHY *Continued*

1972	Rösch	Transcatheter embolization for treatment of gastrointestinal hemorrhage
1974	Gruntzig and Hopff	Double-lumen balloon sheath dilatation catheter

1976	Wallace	Coined the term *interventional procedures*
1980s–1990s		Evolution of interventional procedures

graphic technique for demonstrating unknown sites of gastrointestinal bleeding. This contribution by Nusbaum and Baum was the prototype technique that led to the specialty of vascular interventional procedures.

In 1964, Charles Dotter and M. P. Judkins devised a new catheter technique for percutaneous transluminal angioplasty, which was a treatment designed to relieve arteriosclerotic obstructions.

Other significant milestones in angiography include the use by Nusbaum and associates of vasopressin for variceal and also visceral hemorrhage in 1969. In 1972, J. Rösch and associates developed a technique of transcatheter embolization for treatment of gastrointestinal bleeding.

Margolis and associates created a transcatheter embolization technique that could be utilized in trauma situations. In 1974, Gruntzig and Hopff created the balloon dilatation catheter.

The term *interventional procedures* was first coined in 1976 by S. Wallace, who described percutaneous catheterization for therapeutic purposes.

Many electrical improvements coincided with the progress in tubes, changers, and contrast media. Generators, rectifiers, and transformers with higher load characteristics were produced. Cooling systems for x-ray tubes were developed and refined. These improvements combined and vastly improved the quality of the x-ray source and the resultant radiograph.

The use of digital subtraction angiography and the relatively new interventional procedures became common in most angiographic suites in the early to mid-1980s. Digital venous imaging was introduced and had the advantage of permitting angiograms to be done on an outpatient basis. Despite the advantages, the venous study did not provide the opacification that was found with the arterial study. Thus, in most cases, digital venous angiography is performed only on patients in whom intra-arterial angiography is not possible.

In the middle to late 1970s, the applications of ultrasound and computed tomography increased in diagnostic radiology. About that time therapeutic angiography began to emerge. Significant advances in equipment and procedures were noted in cardiac catheterization and angiography as well as in neurologic, visceral, and peripheral angiography. Magnetic resonance imaging only further enhanced the capabilities of angiography.

Table 1–1 provides a chronologic record of some of the pioneers whose research produced many milestones in the evolution and progress of angiography and interventional procedures. The work of many of these pioneers is discussed further throughout this text.

► **BIBLIOGRAPHY**

Abrams L: Abrams Angiography, Vol 1, 3rd ed. Boston, Little, Brown, 1983.

Athanasoulis CA: Therapeutic Angiography: Its Scope and Basic Principles. Philadelphia, WB Saunders, 1982.

Bordley J III and McGehee HA: Two Centuries of American Medicine. Philadelphia, WB Saunders, 1978.

Davidoff LM, et al: Neuroradiology Workshop, Vol 1. New York, Grune & Stratton, 1961.

Fuchs AW: Principles of Radiographic Exposure and Processing, 2nd ed. Springfield, IL, Charles C Thomas, 1979.

Grigg E: The Trail of the Invisible Light. Springfield, IL, Charles C Thomas, 1965.

Grollman JH, Rösch J, and Steckel RJ: Selective Angiography: Golden's Diagnostic Radiology. Baltimore, Williams & Wilkins, 1972.

Lyons AS and Petrucelli RJ II: Medicine: An Illustrated History. New York, Harry N. Abrams, 1978.

Parvez Z, Moncada R, and Sovak M: Contrast Media: Biologic Effects and Clinical Application, Vol 1. Boca Raton, CRC Press, 1987.

Radiographics. Monograph Issue: The Technical History of Radiology. Radiological Society of North America 9(6):1095–1269, 1989.

Skucas J: Radiographic Contrast Agents. Rockville, MD, Aspen Publications, 1989.

Takahashi M: Atlas of Vertebral Angiography. Baltimore, MD, University Park Press, 1974.

Tortorici M: Fundamentals of Angiography. St Louis, CV Mosby, 1982.

► **SELF-ASSESSMENT QUIZ**

1. Christopher Wren is best known for
   a. the development of the fluoroscope
   b. using reeds and vegetable dyes to outline superficial veins
   c. being the founder of experimental physiology
   d. the development of the first serial changer

2. What is the major contribution of William Harvey?
   a. his ability to illustrate human vascular anatomy
   b. performance of the first carotid arteriogram
   c. the coaxial catheter system
   d. his pioneer work on blood circulation

3. Who is known as the founder of experimental physiology?
   a. Bernard
   b. Wren
   c. Edison
   d. Harvey

4. Who first used sodium iodine for direct cystography and pyelography?
   a. Willis
   b. Osborne
   c. Brooks
   d. Moniz

5. Who was the first man to inject iodine into humans?
   a. Moniz
   b. Brooks
   c. Osborne
   d. Loman and Myerson

6. Who is noted for injecting solutions of sodium bromide and sodium iodide into the exposed carotid arteries of the neck?
   a. Moniz
   b. Takahasi
   c. Cronquist
   d. Radner

7. Who made the first successful injection of a radiopaque contrast into the carotid artery by percutaneous needle puncture?
   a. Loman and Myerson
   b. Moniz
   c. Takahasi
   d. Lindgren and Bonte

8. Who made the first percutaneous injection into the vertebral artery?
   a. Loman and Myerson
   b. Cronquist
   c. Radner
   d. Takahasi

9. Who devised the first application of the catheter technique on the vertebral artery?
   a. Loman and Myerson
   b. Cronquist
   c. Radner
   d. Lindgren

10. The transfemoral catheter technique was first performed by
    a. Bonte
    b. Lindgren
    c. Radner
    d. Hanafee

11. Hanafee and Newton developed a method of
    a. transfemoral catheterization
    b. percutaneous direct-stick injection
    c. direct puncture of the vertebral artery
    d. selective catheter vertebral angiography by a transaxillary catheter

12. What are Moniz and Caldas best known for?
    a. the first serial film changer
    b. the first three-phase generator
    c. the stepping-table
    d. the first power injector

13. Who first developed the roll-film changer?
    a. Sanchez-Perez
    b. Cordis
    c. Caldas
    d. Ruggles

14. Who first developed a chain-driven, motorized film changer?
    a. Sanchez-Perez
    b. Ruggles
    c. Gidlund
    d. Amplatz

15. Who developed the automatic injector that operated on the principle of compressed gas?
    a. Cordis
    b. Medrad
    c. Gidlund
    d. Amplatz

16. Amplatz described a(n)
    a. electromechanical injector
    b. roll-film changer
    c. cardiovascular injector that operated by carbon dioxide cartridges
    d. reciprocating high-speed bucky diaphragm

17. Which of the following individuals developed an electromechanical injector?
    1. Cordis
    2. Viamonte-Hobbs
    3. Medrad
       a. 1 only
       b. 1 and 2
       c. 2 and 3
       d. 1, 2, and 3

18. Who first developed a method of timing an injection to correspond with a specific phase in the cardiac cycle?
    a. Cordis
    b. Medrad
    c. Viamonte-Hobbs
    d. Amplatz

▶ STUDY QUESTIONS

1. Explain the significance of the work of William Harvey.

2. Describe the relationship between Christopher Wren and Thomas Willis.

3. Why is Claude Bernard considered to be the founder of experimental physiology?

4. What were the limitations of the contrast media that were used in the early 1900s?

5. List five pioneers and describe their work in the area of equipment that led to the present application in angiography.

6. List five pioneers and their contributions to the development of percutaneous needle and arteriovenous puncture techniques.

7. Describe the contributions of the individuals who furthered the efforts of therapeutic interventional procedures.

► CHAPTER TWO

► MEDICAL AND LEGAL IMPLICATIONS OF ANGIOGRAPHY

► **CHAPTER OUTLINE**

Malpractice
Job Description
Informed Consent
    Informed Consent Form

Responsibilities of the Technologist
Contrast Media

► **CHAPTER OBJECTIVES**

Upon completion of Chapter 2 the technologist will be able to:

1. Define the terms malpractice, negligence, assault, battery, reasonable care, and standard practice
2. Describe the content of an informed consent form
3. Complete a medical record
4. List the duties of an invasive procedures technologist that should be included in a job description
5. Describe some of the considerations regarding the selection criteria of contrast agents for invasive procedures

The earliest recorded decision against a physician and surgeon was in 1374 in England. In fact, this case probably is the landmark case in the establishment of the doctrine of due diligence and care.

In 1957, a landmark decision was handed down in the California Court of Appeals in the case of *Salgo versus (vs) Leland Stanford, Jr., University Board of Trustees*. This case centered on an angiographic procedure. The question was whether the patient was paralyzed following the procedure and whether the patient was adequately informed by the physician with regard to the risks and dangers of the angiogram. Was the dialogue between the physician and the patient sufficient to constitute informed consent? Did the patient consent to the procedure? The court stated that "A physician violates his duty to his patient and subjects himself to liability if he withholds any facts which are necessary to form the basis of an intelligent consent by the patient to the proposed treatment." The court decided in favor of the plaintiff, based on the premise that the patient did not receive sufficient information to grant appropriate informed consent. Ten years prior to this decision, the Kansas Supreme Court made the decision that properly informing the patient of risks was an expected facet of the practice of medicine and was necessary for procurement of the patient's consent to a procedure. Furthermore, the court stated that failure to adequately disclose information constituted professional negligence.[5] In order to understand the full implications of informed consent one must first possess an understanding of assault, battery, and negligence. Assault is defined as an implied attempt or threat to do harm to another. Battery is performance of the harmful act. Negligence may be defined as behavior that does not conform to expected standards of care. The *Salgo vs Leland Stanford, Jr., University Board of Trustees* decision was argued successfully by the plaintiff on this basis. In this case, the deviation from standard was represented by the lack of adequate disclosure resulting in appropriate consent.[5]

Adequate documentation of the discussion of informed consent between the patient and the surgeon is very important. Even a surgeon who is completely aware of all the requirements for a full informed consent and actually carries out the necessary documents with the patient but does not adequately document the consent process may easily be found liable for damages in court.[3]

Historically, it has always been the law that unlawful touching of the body of one person by another constitutes assault and battery, for which the person committing the offense is liable without proof of negligence and without proof of damages. This has long been applied to acts of the physician for which the consent of the patient was not obtained.

Another legal doctrine, the law of contracts, states that anyone who is induced to sign a document is not bound by such signature unless he or she is made aware of what he or she was signing and that his or her act of signing (which is an agreement to be bound to whatever the document states) is not binding on him or her as a consent unless his or her consent was informed consent and unless he or she understood what it was he or she was agreeing to. As an example, when an untoward result followed a gynecologic surgical procedure, the patient would testify that although she consented to the procedure, her consent was not an informed one because she had not been told by the surgeon of the possible recurrence of the untoward result, which did occur in her case (vesicovaginal fistula following hysterectomy). If she had been given complete information, she would never have consented to surgery.[4]

► MALPRACTICE

In order for a radiologist to be legally proven guilty of malpractice, four requirements must be met: (1) there has to be a duty that the radiologist has to the patient; (2) the radiologist has to commit a negligent act; (3) that negligent act has to be shown to have caused an injury to the patient; and (4) the patient must have sustained an injury.[2]

Legally, there is no absolute liability for negligence. The doctrine of liability for fault states that a person can be held liable for a negligent act when he or she has failed to observe the standard of care that the law requires in the performance of his or her duty to the injured person. If a patient is injured during treatment, he or she is required by the American system of jurisprudence to file a lawsuit and prove that his or her physician was negligent.[4]

One study by an independent risk-management firm found that 70% of losses related to radiology from closed claims involved invasive diagnostic procedures. This study indicated many different reasons for the lawsuits. Specific invasive procedures accounted for only 17% of the filed suits, but that 17% accounted for 71% of the total radiology losses. The numbers may be small, but most losses were significant, and the injuries were devastating. Amputation, paralysis, brain damage, nerve injury, and death were among some of the causes for these lawsuits. Other reasons for these lawsuits included contrast media reaction, vascular damage by a catheter, nerve injury during cardiac catheterization, lack of informed consent, misdiagnosis, failure to diagnose, equipment-related injuries, mislabeled x-rays, and a failure to contact the patient or attending physicians regarding a change in diagnosis.

In December, 1986, Berlin published an article in the American Journal of Radiology entitled *Malpractice and radiologists, update: An 11.5-year perspective*.[1] This article described in detail the numbers and types of various lawsuits that were filed in Cook County, Illinois. Of particular interest in this journal article is Table 6: Suits Alleging Complication from Radiologic Procedures, 1980 to 1986. Of a total number of 193 lawsuits, 69, or 35.75%, involved angiography. This category represented 21% of all radiology-related lawsuits. Although the 69 angiographic complications were not broken down further, we presume that a large majority were related to contrast media or to complications of the procedure itself.[2]

► JOB DESCRIPTION

Written job descriptions should be established for all cardiovascular/interventional technologists. The job description serves to encompass the "scope of practice." The technologist should possess the proper qualifications to function within the confines of the job description. If a technologist passes the advanced level examination for cardiovascular/interventional technology, the American Registry of Radiologic Technologists issues a certificate that implies competency. The wage scale for technologists holding advanced level certificates should reflect their level of knowledge and skills. The administration of intravenous injections by technologists under the supervision of a radiologist has been a common practice for a long time. Although considered legal when the technologist is "supervised" by a radiologist, patients are often given injections without a radiologist being present. Without making a judgment regarding this practice, it goes without saying that if a radiologist requires a technologist to give an injection to a patient, it only makes sense that the technologist should be qualified to do so. Since this would constitute a required skill, injecting patients with contrast media or medications should be included within the written job description for the technologist. It would also be reasonable for technologists to receive adequate compensation for this additional skill. The technologist may consider legal advice with regard to whether malpractice or liability insurance should be purchased in addition to the coverage provided by his or her employer.

► INFORMED CONSENT

"Every human being of adult years and sound mind has a right to determine what shall be done with his own body." The courts therefore are stating that the patient has the right to determine his or her own submission to health care procedures.

In radiology, when invasive procedures are a common practice, informed consent is generally obtained. Invasive procedures are generally perceived as having a "surgery-like" quality. In *Salgo vs Leland Stanford, Jr., University Board of Trustees,* (1957), a decision was rendered that stated the following: "A physician violates his duty to his patient and subjects himself to liability if he withholds any facts which are necessary to form the basis of an intelligent consent by the patient to the proposed treatment."[5]

The case of *Natanson vs Kline* (1957) stated "that a failure to perform adequate disclosure represents professional negligence, and the performance of such disclosure must conform to the standard of care practiced by other doctors under similar circumstances."[4] Most patients undergoing computed tomography scanning are not routinely informed in writing that they will receive contrast media. The same holds true for routine procedures in which patients receive contrast media such as intravenous urography. However, in all examinations utilizing contrast media, a history of allergies must be documented.

Informed Consent Form

The type of informed consent varies from one hospital to another as well as from one procedure to another. There are standard types of informed consent as well as consent forms for specific or unique procedures. For example, one consent form may simply indicate that the physician has verbally related information to the patient regarding that procedure. Other consent forms may also contain a written list of risks and complications, along with a description of the procedure. At the bottom of the consent form there is listed the "Patient's Acknowledgment and Consent," which states that the physician discussed the need for the procedure and the implications involved if the patient chooses not to have the procedure performed. The patient attests to the fact that all questions have been answered, and the patient then gives the physician authorization to perform the procedure and to utilize resources and staff as the physician deems appropriate. This permission includes any further care that may become necessary during the procedure. Figure 2–1 is an example of a consent form that could be utilized in a cardiovascular/interventional (special) procedure imaging department.

► RESPONSIBILITIES OF THE TECHNOLOGIST

The role of the technologist cannot be overstated in regard to getting the patient prepared for an invasive procedure. The patient may have been premedicated and may have had his or her laboratory work completed; however, the patient may still be apprehensive. The technologist should prepare the patient mentally as well as physically for the invasive procedure. The role of the cardiovascular/interventional technologist varies from one hospital to another. Because of the increased sophistication of equipment and complexity of procedures, the technologist is becoming more actively involved as a participant and "team member" in a procedure. The days are past when the technologist simply positioned the patient, made the exposure, and otherwise just stayed out of the way. The ever-increasing computerized sophistication of equipment requires a "thinking" technologist—one whose duties include decision-making.

CONSENT OF RADIOLOGIC SPECIAL PROCEDURES

Patient's Name_____

Date_____Time_____ A.M.—P.M.

A. Physician_____

B. Operation or Procedure_____

C. Statement of Request
   The nature and purpose of the operation or procedure, possible alternative methods of treatment, the risks involved, and the possibility of complications have been fully explained to me. I acknowledge that no guarantees have been made to me concerning the results of the operation or procedure.

D. Statement of Consent
   I hereby consent to the performance upon me of the radiological special procedures and to the administration of premedication and anesthetics as may be considered necessary for this service. I also consent to any measures necessary to correct complications which may occur. I assume all risks and harmful effects in connection with the radiological special procedures indicated above.

Signed _____
           Patient or Person Authorized to Consent for Patient

_____

WITNESS

_____

Date

_____
Relationship to Patient

I have explained the radiologic special procedure indicated above and its attendant risks and consequences to the patient, who has indicated understanding thereof and has consented to its performance.

_____   _____
Date   Physician

► Figure 2–1

Sample consent form for a cardiovascular/interventional (special) imaging department.

In many hospitals, there is a "team concept" methodology and attitude, and the technologist is now taking a more active role with regard to invasive interventional procedures. The patient care role in many facilities has also expanded for the technologist. Two technologists or more are often required to assist the radiologist with a cardiovascular/interventional procedure. Even when a radiologic nurse is present, the technologist assists the radiologist with operation of equipment, technique selection, film sequencing, film processing, and so forth. Technologists often assist the radiologist within the sterile field. A staff of technologists working with the same radiologists on a regular basis can enhance the quality and efficiency of the overall effort of the department. It is important to maintain a professional attitude within the working environment. All members of the interventional team should respect one another.

   The technologist is usually the first person to greet the patient. Even though the physician spoke to the patient about the procedure and obtained an informed consent, the patient is usually quite apprehensive and will have additional questions. Thus, the technologist continually reassures the skeptical patient and attempts to answer the patient's questions. The technologist should thoroughly review the patient's chart to ensure that all is in order. Table 2–1 shows an example of the type of information contained within a patient's chart that would be important to the technologist.

Many of the technologist's duties occur before the procedure takes place. The angiographic suite must be made ready for the procedure. Sterile trays must be prepared. All equipment must be tested to ensure that it operates correctly. Serial film changers must be loaded, and contrast media must be prepared for loading within the automatic injector. The patient's chart should arrive with the patient, and a film file jacket should be available so that prior radiographic studies can be examined. The technologist greets the patient and prepares the patient for the procedure. The specific duties and responsibilities related to patient care are described in Chapter 4.

One of the ways to avoid complications is to make all preparations in advance of the procedure. An established protocol should be followed for all procedures, and the angiographic suite should be prepared prior to the arrival of the patient.

► CONTRAST MEDIA

For an invasive procedure, one of the most important considerations concerns the selection of a contrast medium. The medical community is divided with regard to which approach is most appropriate. The merits of one type of contrast agent compared with another are not discussed here.

The relative cost of ionic versus nonionic contrast media is a very controversial issue. Regardless of the criteria used to make a decision, most agree that, because of the cost differential, the patient should be informed of the choices. Although some believe that nonionic contrast media (low osmolar) are much safer to inject, nonionic agents are at least 10 times the cost of the ionic agents. What if the patient is not at high risk? Who decides which contrast agent to use? Perhaps the decision is easier to make when the patient is at high risk. In this case, the physician's choice may be based on established criteria for the high-risk patient. In either event, it would be wise to develop an information sheet that explains the basic differences between the two classes of contrast agents. A reasonable patient would want to know relative risk information in order to make a decision. Choice of contrast medium is an integral part of informed consent.

From the patient's perspective, the most exasperating aspect of his or her radiologic experience is coping with anxiety. The technologist plays a most important role in helping the patient to deal with anxiety.

► REFERENCES

1. Berlin L: Malpractice and radiologists, update: An 11.5-year perspective. Am J Radiol 147:1291–1298, 1986.
2. James AE Jr: Medical/Legal Issues for Radiologists. Chicago, Precept Press and The American College of Radiology, 1987.
3. Meaney TF, Lalli AF, and Alfidi RJ: Complications of Radiologic Special Procedures. St. Louis, CV Mosby, 1973.
4. *Natanson vs Kline.* 187 Kan 186, 354p 2nd 170, 1957.
5. *Salgo vs Leland Stanford, Jr., University Board of Trustees,* 154 Cal Apl 2nd 560, 317p 2nd 170, 1957.

► BIBLIOGRAPHY

Becker V Jr: The informed consent for the surgical procedure: Documentation of the consent. Contemp Orthoped 17:193, 1989.

Reuter SR: The use of conventional vs low-osmolar contrast agents: A legal analysis. Am J Radiol 21:429–433, 1988.

Schloendorff vs Society of New York Hospital, 211 N.Y. 125, 105 N.E. 92, 1914.

Tortorici MR: Fundamentals of Angiography. St. Louis, CV Mosby, 1982, pp 7–12.

Zaremski MJ and Goldstein JD: Medical and Hospital Negligence, Vol 4. Deerfield, IL, Callagan & Co., 1988.

► SELF-ASSESSMENT QUIZ

1. In which year was the earliest recorded decision in English against a physician and surgeon?
   a. 1374
   b. 1492
   c. 1957
   d. 1969

2. The implied attempt or threat to do harm to another is called
   a. assault
   b. battery
   c. negligence
   d. informed consent

3. The performance of a harmful act is called
   a. assault
   b. battery
   c. negligence
   d. informed consent

► **Table 2–1**

IMPORTANT INFORMATION CONTAINED IN A PATIENT'S CHART

Allergic history
Consent form
Physical examination
Prior surgical history
Patient's complaints
Diagnostic test results
Status of heparinization
History of hypertension
History of diabetes
Premedications

4. Behavior that does not conform to expected standards of care describes
   a. assault
   b. battery
   c. negligence
   d. informed consent

5. Any professional misconduct, unreasonable lack of skill in professional duties, or illegal or immoral conduct describes
   a. malpractice
   b. standard of care
   c. liability
   d. negligence

6. Every adult who has a sound mind has the right to determine what shall be done with his or her own body. This statement describes
   a. standard of care
   b. professional ethics
   c. informed consent
   d. professional negligence

7. A failure to perform adequate disclosure represents
   a. informed consent
   b. standard of care
   c. professional negligence
   d. patient acknowledgment

8. Informed consent is standardized at all hospitals.
   a. true
   b. false

9. The informed consent form should be signed in the presence of a third party.
   a. true
   b. false

10. Which contrast media are recommended for a high-risk patient?
    a. ionic contrast media
    b. negative agents
    c. nonionic contrast media
    d. oil-based agents

▶ STUDY QUESTIONS

1. Explain the basis for the lawsuit *Salgo vs Leland Stanford, Jr., University Board of Trustees*.

2. What is meant by the "law of contracts"?

3. Why is an informed consent form obtained from the patient?

4. Design an "informed consent" form and be prepared to defend your rationale for its contents.

5. What is meant by the "doctrine of liability for fault"?

6. Write a job description for your present position.

► CHAPTER THREE

► PHARMACEUTICALS AND CONTRAST AGENTS

► CHAPTER OUTLINE

Administration of Medication
Emergency Medications
Contrast Media
    Ionic Contrast Media
    Nonionic Contrast Media
    Ionic and Nonionic Comparisons
Arterial Injection: General Effects
Intravenous Injection: General Effects
Adverse Reactions to Contrast Media
    Vasomotor Effect
    Anaphylactic Reaction
        Treatment

    Vasovagal Reaction
        Treatment
    Contrast-Induced Renal Failure
Factors Predisposing to Contrast Media Reactions
    Injection of Impurities
    Quality Assurance
Anaphylactic Systemic Reactions
    Cardiac Responses
    Renal Responses
    Pulmonary Responses
    Central Nervous System Responses
Classification of Adverse Reactions

► CHAPTER OBJECTIVES

Upon completion of Chapter 3 the technologist will be able to:

1. Demonstrate how to look up a pharmaceutical in the *Physician's Desk Reference* (PDR)
2. List and describe the five routes of medication administration
3. Describe the four categories of adverse reaction to a contrast medium
4. List examples of the signs and symptoms for minor, moderate, and major adverse reactions
5. Explain the fundamental differences between ionic and nonionic contrast media
6. List the medications that should be available for emergency situations during angiography
7. List the general effects of intravascular injections
8. Explain the controversies that currently exist between ionic and nonionic contrast media
9. Describe the means by which potential impurities could be introduced into the vascular system
10. List at least four ways that contrast media would be considered spoiled and discarded
11. Define anaphylactic shock
12. Describe the current treatments for anaphylactic shock
13. Describe three signs of cardiac arrest

In the angiographic setting the technologist and a radiology nurse may be working together as part of the special procedure team. Currently an increasing number of radiology nurses are applying their skills in the radiology department. However, whether or not a radiology nurse is present, the technologist should have a basic knowledge and understanding of the pharmaceuticals and contrast agents that are used in conjunction with most interventional procedures.

▶ ADMINISTRATION OF MEDICATION

The technologist should be familiar with any and all pharmacologic preparations administered to the patient in conjunction with diagnostic and therapeutic interventional procedures. These "medications" would be drugs administered before, during, and after a procedure. Premedication is given to the patient prior to the procedure. During an invasive procedure, a contrast medium is often administered. Drugs have to be available in response to emergency reactions to the contrast medium. Following a procedure, a patient may receive medication for pain or for other adverse effects related to the invasive procedure. It is important for the technologist to be familiar with all the drugs that are frequently administered for invasive procedures. The technologist should be familiar with the written documentation that is included with a unit of medication or contrast medium. The contents of this packet include information regarding dosage, indications, contraindications, trade name, generic name, chemical composition, and side effects. This information is required by the United States Food and Drug Administration (FDA). In addition to package inserts, a good source of information for the technologist is the PDR.

Medications are administered by two primary routes: local and systemic. Local anesthetics are routinely injected into the tissues of the angiographic injection site. The loss of sensation to the injected and surrounding areas is almost immediate. The actions of medication administered systemically are much more complex than are those administered locally. Various results from these medications are possible, and it is essential that the medications are selected on the basis of the desired effect. Types of systemic administration are oral, sublingual, rectal, and parenteral.

Oral medications are available in many forms and are taken by mouth. Medications that are affected by gastric contents are not usually administered orally.

A *sublingual* medication dissolves immediately after being placed under the tongue. Sublingual medications are administered when immediate responses are desired, such as with nitroglycerin, a vasodilator used to treat the pain of angina.

Drugs that are administered *rectally* are usually given by this route because the patient is unable to take medication orally or because gastric secretions would destroy the drug.

Parenteral administration refers to the delivery of medication by way of an injection. Although the parenteral route is indicated when rapid drug action and a shorter duration are sought, it is also indicated when the oral route is not possible or advantageous. A parenteral injection is the route of choice when an oral medication is unpalatable or will cause mucosal irritation. In cases in which drugs cannot be absorbed by the gastric mucosa, the parenteral route presents a reasonable alternative.

There are five approaches for delivering medication parenterally.

A *subcutaneous* injection is an injection that takes place in the tissues beneath the skin. It is also referred to as a hypodermic injection. This injection is somewhat painful, and this discomfort can be minimized if the injection is made into the outer thigh or upper arm. A relatively small needle, 25-gauge, $\frac{5}{8}''$ to $\frac{3}{4}''$, is utilized to inject no more than 2 ml of medication.

An *intradermal* injection involves the administration of medication into the tissue substance. The intradermal injection can be administered in many locations, but the inner aspect of the forearm is the most common site. Like the subcutaneous method, the intradermal injection also uses a small, short needle.

An *intrathecal* (intraspinal) injection describes a group of injections that may also be specified as subarachnoid, subdural, or lumbar injections. Anesthesia administered intrathecally most often involves the insertion of a special needle that is $3\frac{1}{2}''$ long, containing a 16- to 25-gauge lumen. Spinal anesthesia is most often administered by an anesthesiologist. A contrast medium is frequently introduced into the subarachnoid space for cervical and lumbar myelography.

An *intramuscular* injection is given into the deep muscle when the substance must be absorbed at once. The gluteus maximus muscle of the buttock and the deltoid muscle at the shoulder are the two most common sites for intramuscular injections. The needle is usually $1\frac{1}{2}''$ in length and varies in gauge from 18 to 22. The thickness or viscosity of the medication determines the selection of an appropriate needle gauge.

The *intravenous* (IV) method of administration is preferred when rapid absorption is desired, when a fluid cannot be taken by mouth, or when the substance is too irritating to be injected into the skin or muscles. Blood transfusions, blood tests, and certain x-ray examinations are frequently conducted via the IV route. The IV approach is important during angiography for the purpose of maintaining hydration and providing a route for the administration of emergency, life-saving medications. Because medications are rapidly absorbed into hematopoietic tissues, the IV injection is a potentially hazardous route, and occasionally the patient's response to the injection may be instantaneous.

Medications can be administered intravenously in several ways. When a medication needs to be injected rapidly, it is referred to as a *bolus* injection. When medication is injected slowly, it is introduced by *infu-*

sion. Some IV injections may utilize an apparatus called a "butterfly" needle. This needle can be part of a "scalp vein" set that is used in infusions in infants or for infusing small veins in the hand or wrist (basilic or cephalic veins) or deep veins at the elbow. In the region of the elbow, the needle is usually inserted into the antecubital vein or accessory cephalic vein.

▶ EMERGENCY MEDICATIONS

In one or more locations of the radiology department one will find emergency medications. Depending on the radiologic services provided, one may find the medications housed in simple storage containers or in a modern mobile crash cart that consists of numerous drawers containing medications and other life-saving devices. The crash cart is usually mounted on a steel frame with stainless-steel casters. In the radiology department, it would be kept in an area that is easily accessible to all radiographic rooms. In the case of a special procedure suite, the crash cart would be stored in an adjoining room.

Although technologists are not expected to have the knowledge of a pharmacist, they have the responsibility of being familiar with the medications included in the crash cart, including their indications, average dosages, and routes of administration (Fig. 3–1).

Contained in the emergency crash cart are drugs and medications that can address any medical emergency. These medications are manufactured in many

ways. Medications can be found in small glass vials, unmixed (powdered concentrate), or premixed. They can also be found in ampules (in which the neck of the ampule is cut off with a razor blade) or in disposable syringes as a single-unit dose.

Although many of the drugs found in the crash cart have a life-saving ability, many also serve to counter allergic responses to contrast media. Epinephrine (Adrenalin) functions to stimulate the sympathetic nervous system and acts to constrict the blood vessels. This action in turn results in an increased cardiac output and produces a rise in the blood pressure. This action is useful in the treatment of allergic reactions. Dopamine hydrochloride (Intropin) is another drug that increases cardiac output. This is accomplished by a vasoconstrictive action on some of the vessels of the abdominal viscera. Patients experiencing hypotension could be given this medication. Isoproterenol hydrochloride (Isuprel) is an adrenergic that stimulates the central nervous system, resulting in vasoconstriction of blood vessels, increased cardiac output, rise in blood pressure, and relaxation of the smooth muscle lining of the respiratory tract. Isoproterenol hydrochloride is often used in cases of cardiogenic shock. Levarterenol bitartrate (Levophed) is used in maintaining blood pressure and in the treatment of hypotension. Procaine hydrochloride (Lidocaine), which is a local anesthetic, is used as a cardiac antiarrhythmic drug. *Digitalis* is a cardiac stimulant that is used to strengthen the heart beat and increase cardiac output. Hydrocortisone sodium succinate (Solu-Cortef) is an anti-inflammatory agent that is

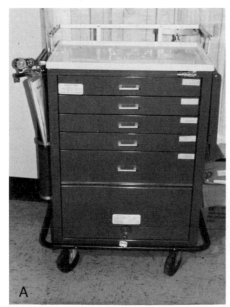
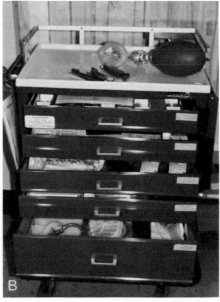
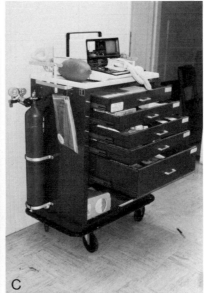

▶ **Figure 3–1**

A, Front view of a crash cart. Note the multiple drawers of varying depths, accessible countertop, and hard rubber casters, facilitating easy transport. **B,** Front view of a crash cart. Note how the drawer provides a comfortable capacity for miscellaneous items and how the countertop provides easy access to emergency equipment. **C,** Side view of a crash cart. Note that the crash cart can be placed at any location, occupying a minimum of space, while providing easy access to equipment. A canister of oxygen is mounted on the side of the cart.

used to counteract severe allergic reactions. Methylprednisolone (Medrol) is another anti-inflammatory medication that is used for allergic reactions. Diphenhydramine hydrochloride (Benadryl) is one of the more common antihistamines given to the patient who experiences a minor allergic reaction. This drug acts to overcome histamine liberation and sedates the central nervous system. Table 3–1 lists some of the emergency medications that could be utilized with an anaphylactic or idiosyncratic contrast media reaction.

▸ CONTRAST MEDIA

There are essentially two types of contrast agents used in radiography—positive and negative. A *positive* contrast agent absorbs x-rays and produces an opaque image on the finished radiograph. A *negative* contrast agent is a gas that absorbs lesser amounts of radiation and produces a radiolucent image. Further discussion of negative contrast agents is not appropriate for angiographic and other interventional procedures, thus the focus of discussion is limited to positive contrast agents.

The positive contrast agents used in angiography are in the form of *iodinated* compounds. These agents are categorized as *ionic* and *nonionic*. Many factors are involved when deciding which contrast agent should be used for an angiographic procedure. In order to produce adequate opacification of the radiographic image, the contrast medium must be injected at a high *molar* concentration. A contrast medium is injected into the vascular system at a rate that exceeds the rate of blood flow. At these high concentrations, the *density, viscosity,* and *osmolality* are much greater than are those of body fluids.[5] Plasma, for example, has a density of approximately 1.05 g/ml, a viscosity of 1.2 cP, and an osmolality of 0.3 osm/kg of water,[5] whereas angiographic contrast media at concentration of 380 mg I/ml would have a density of 1.51 g/ml, a viscosity of concentration of 12 cP, and an osmolality of 2.2 osm/kg of water.

Density represents the ratio of the mass of a substance to its volume. *Viscosity* represents the resistance to flow or the thickness of the agent and is strongly dependent on temperature and iodine content. *Osmolality* is defined as the concentration of a solution in terms of solutes (osmoles) per kilogram of solvent. It can also be described as the number of particles in a solution. Density and viscosity are both inversely related to temperature.

Ionic Contrast Media

The work of Wallingford and Hoppe and associates in the early 1950s led to the first tri-iodinated contrast agent. Derivatives of tri-iodobenzoic acid were developed and made soluble by salification with sodium, meglumine, or both, with added calcium or magnesium. Such ionic contrast media dissociate in solution to form an *anion* (negatively charged) and a *cation* (positively charged). Only the anion carries iodine atoms and is radiopaque. The cation has no function except to apply as a dissolving agent. Methylglucamine (Meglumine) salts of diatrizoate and iothalamate are frequently used in neuroangiography.

▸ **Table 3–1**
MEDICATIONS OFTEN AVAILABLE ON AN EMERGENCY CART

Drug	Action/Indication	Dosage
Epinephrine (Adrenalin)	Anaphylactic reaction	0.5—1.0 ml of 1:1000 solution IV*
Aminophylline	Acute bronchial spasms bronchodilator	6–10 mg/kg IV over 30 min
Atropine	Increase heart rate	1 mg IM/IV
Diphenhydramine (Benadryl)	Allergic reaction	25–50 mg IM/IV
Dopamine	Cardiac stimulant Bradycardia	800 mg in 500 ml of D5W
	Circulatory shock	D5W as drip, 2–5 μg/kg/min
Hydrocortisone sodium succinate (Solu-Cortef)	Allergic reaction bronchodilator	100–200 mg/vial
Isoproterenol hydrochloride (Isuprel)	Cardiac stimulant bronchodilator	IV infusion in D5W
Furosemide (Lasix)	Diuretic for pulmonary edema	40 mg/2 ml IV
Norepinephrine bitartrate (Levophed)	Increases blood pressure in profound hypertension	1–10 μg/min IV
Lidocaine (Xylocaine)	Ventricular fibrillation	50–100 mg IV
	Ventricular tachycardia	As a bolus
Morphine sulfate	Analgesic	2–20 mg IM,† SC‡
		5–10 mg IV
Nitroglycerin (Nitrostat)	Angina; chest pain; vasodilator	0.15–0.6 mg sublingually
Diazepam (Valium)	Convulsions	10 mg IV

* IV = intravenously.
† IM = intramuscularly.
‡ SC = subcutaneously.

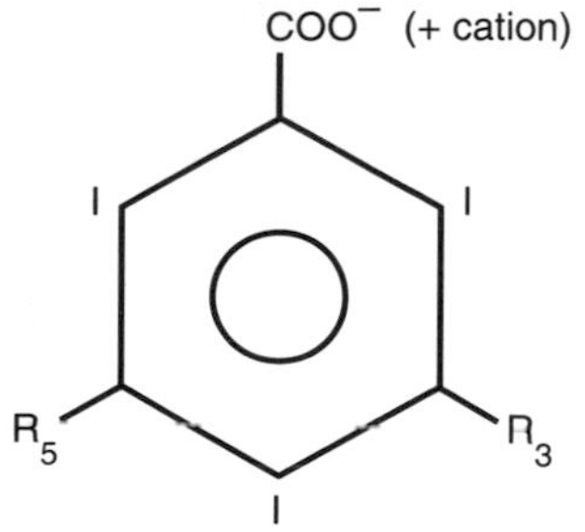

► Figure 3–2

Drawing of an ionic monomer, or ratio 1.5 molecule.

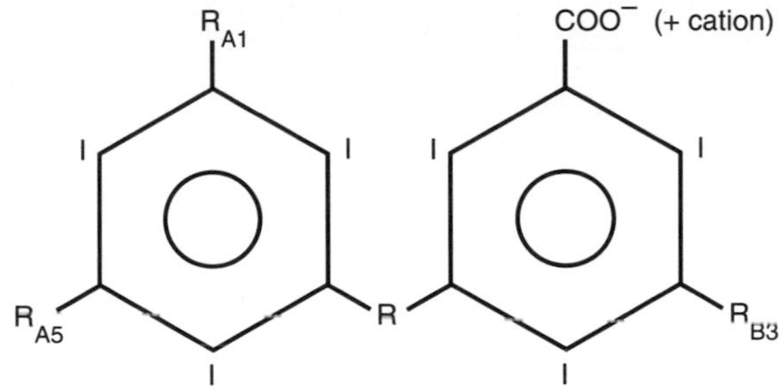

► Figure 3–3

Drawing of an ionic dimer, or ratio 3 molecule.

Conventional ionic contrast agents that are used in angiography exist in two generalized forms or structures.

A *monomer* is defined as a simple molecule that is capable of combining with a number of like or unlike molecules to form a polymer. A monomer, or ratio 1.5 molecule (Fig. 3–2), comes from the fact that a cation and an anion dissociate in solution, leaving three iodine molecules (attached to the benzene ring) for two particles in solution.[4] Table 3–2 lists the chemical and physical properties of ionic contrast media.

A *dimer* is defined as a condensation product that consists of two molecules. Only one ionic dimer, or ratio 3 molecule, is in use today and is called ioxaglate (Fig. 3–3). Ioxaglate consists of a solution of sodium and meglumine salts. This molecule is formed by joining two ionic monomer molecules at two R side groups. In addition, a carboxyl group (the monovalent radical, —COOH, found in organic acids called carboxylic acids) on one of the ionic monomers is replaced by an organic group (shown as R1 in Fig. 3–3). This leaves the dimer molecule with a valence of −1 and a ratio of 6 iodine atoms for two particles in solution or ratio 3.[4]

Nonionic Contrast Media

In 1969, a major advance in water-soluble contrast media was the synthesis of metrizamide (Amipaque) by Nyegaard of Oslo.[4] *Metrizamide* was the name given to the first nonionic contrast medium. The primary difference between ionic and nonionic contrast media is that nonionic media do not separate in solution as do their ionic counterparts. As a result, the solute concentration could be reduced without the loss of iodine content. Such nonionic contrast media do not require a salifying agent and, therefore, have a lower osmolality than do corresponding ionic contrast media.[5]

The nonionic monomer is a ratio 3 molecule (Fig. 3–4), whereas the nonionic dimer is a ratio 6 molecule (Fig. 3–5). These structures are quite comparable with ionic media except that the COO— portion of the ionic molecule is replaced by an organic R group. Because nonionic molecules do not dissociate (separate) in solution, such as ionic salts, the number of particles as well as the osmolality is reduced by one half. The current nonionic monomers include Amipaque, Isovue, Ultravist, iohexol (Omnipaque), and Op-

► Table 3–2

IONIC CONTRAST MEDIA: CHEMICAL AND PHYSICAL PROPERTIES*

Contrast Agent	Cation/Anion	Iodine (mg/ml)	Sodium (mg/ml)	Osmolality (mOsm/l)	Viscosity (cP) (25 to 37° C)	pH
Renografin-60	Meglumine diatrizoate (520 mg/ml), sodium diatrizoate (80 mg/ml)	292.5	3.76	1450	5.6/3.9	7.0–7.6
Hypaque, 60%	Meglumine diatrizoate	282	0.02	1415	6.17/4.12	6.5–7.7
Conray	Meglumine iothalamate (600 mg/ml)	282	0.03	1400	6.0/4.0	
Renografin-76	Meglumine diatrizoate (660 mg/ml), sodium diatrizoate (100 mg/ml)	370	4.48	1940	13.9/9.1	7.0–7.6
Hypaque-M, 75%	Meglumine diatrizoate (500 mg/ml), sodium diatrizoate (250 mg/ml)	385	9.0	2108	13.2/8.3	6.5–7.7
Hypaque-76	Meglumine diatrizoate (660 mg/ml), sodium diatrizoate (100 mg/ml)	370	3.68	2016	15.0/9.0	7.0/7.6
Vascoray	Meglumine iothalamate (520 mg/ml), sodium iothalamate (260 mg/ml)	400	9.4	2400	17.0/9.0	

* From Squibb Diagnostics; Winthrop Laboratories; Mallinckrodt, Inc., and from Kadir S: Diagnostic Angiography. Philadelphia, WB Saunders, 1986, p 30.

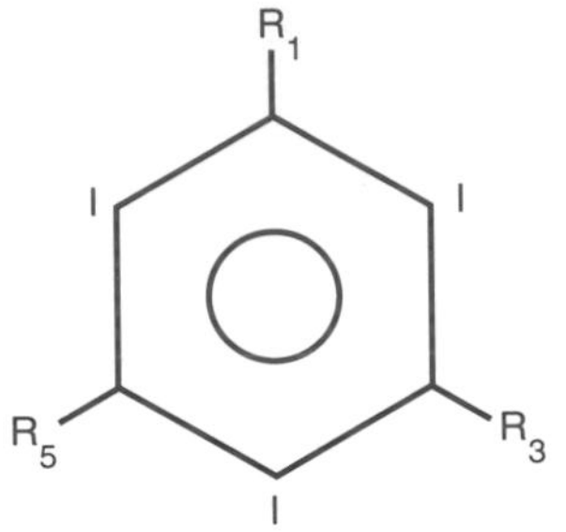

▶ **Figure 3–4**

Drawing of a nonionic monomer, or ratio 3 molecule.

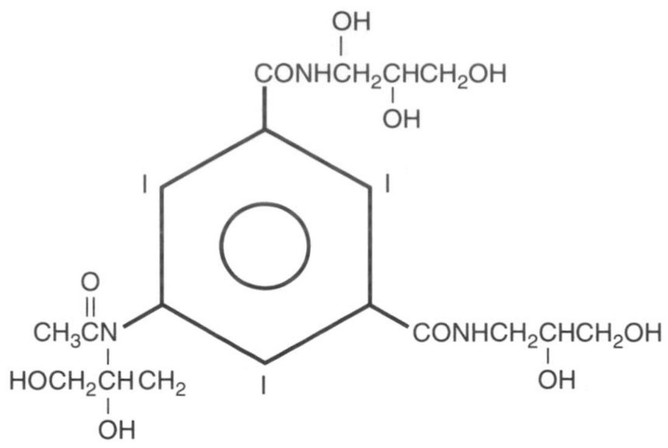

▶ **Figure 3–6**

Chemical symbol for a nonionic monomer—iohexol (Omnipaque).

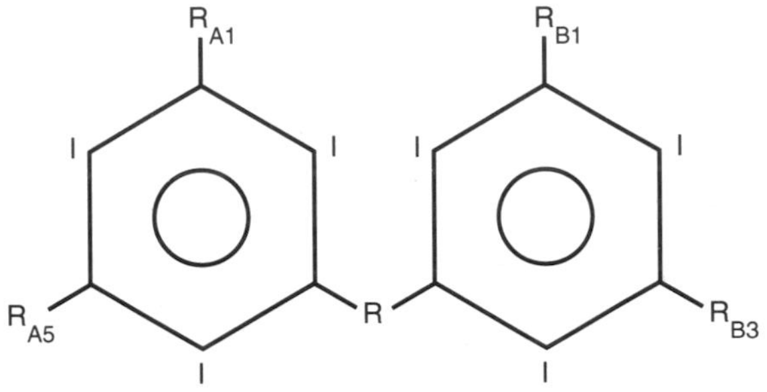

▶ **Figure 3–5**

Diagram of a nonionic dimer, or ratio 6 molecule.

tiray. Osmovist (Iotrol) is the only currently available nonionic dimer (Fig. 3–6). Table 3–3 lists the chemical and physical properties of low osmolality and nonionic contrast media.

Ionic and Nonionic Comparisons

Many viable studies comparing ionic and nonionic contrast media have been completed throughout the world, and the results are very similar. There is no longer any question as to the relative safety of nonionic contrast agents. The major dilemma is one of economics, not of quality medical care. Nonionic contrast media can cost up to or exceed 10 times the cost of ionic contrast media in the United States. Cost factors are greatly influenced by location. Most nonionic contrast media are manufactured in Europe. Improvements in imaging equipment, new molecules, and new manufacturing processes and locations within the United States will eventually reduce the cost of nonionic contrast media.

Osmolality appears to be the one factor that bears a relationship to contrast media reactions. Osmolality strongly depends on iodine concentration. That which has a lower iodine concentration also has a lower osmolality. There is also a difference in how these mediums interact with calcium. Ionic contrast agents have proved to be weak binders of ionic calcium, whereas nonionic contrast agents do not appear to bind ionic calcium and do not affect calcium activity. Calcium and magnesium ions are added to the contrast media because they reduce the disruption of the blood-brain barrier by minimizing an alteration of cerebral blood flow (Table 3–4).

▶ **Table 3–3**

LOW OSMOLALITY AND NONIONIC CONTRAST MEDIA: CHEMICAL AND PHYSICAL PROPERTIES*

Contrast Agent	Mol/Mol Wt	Iodine (mg/ml)	Osmolality (mOsm/l)	Viscosity (cP) (25° C/37° C)	pH
Amipaque	Nonionic monomer 789	482	484 at 300 mg I/ml at 37° C	12.7 at 300 mg I/ml at 20° C, 6.2 at 300 mg I/ml at 37° C	7.4
Hexabrix (ioxaglate meglumine 39.3%, ioxaglate sodium, 19.6%)	Ionic dimer 1269	320	600	15.7/7.5	
Iodecol	Nonionic dimer	300	260	7.2 at 37° C	
Iopamidol	Nonionic monomer 777	300	616	7.5/3.8	
Iohexol	Nonionic monomer 821	300	672	8.8 at 20° C/4.8	
Ioversol	Nonionic monomer 807.13	320	702	9.9/5.8	

* Modified from Winthrop Laboratories: Winthrop Laboratories Contrast Media Guide. New York, Winthrop Laboratories, 1982[6] and from Kadir S: Diagnostic Angiography. Philadelphia, WB Saunders, 1986, p. 30.[2]

▶ **Table 3–4**

COMPARISON BETWEEN IONIC AND NONIONIC
CONTRAST MEDIA

	Ionic	Nonionic
Osmolality	High	Low
Binder of calcium	Weak	No
Dissociates in solution	Yes	No
No. of particles in solution	More	−50%
Adverse reactions (all categories)	More	Less
Unit cost	Lower	Higher (+10 to +18)

▶ ARTERIAL INJECTION: GENERAL EFFECTS

Modern angiography encompasses the use of sophisticated equipment, such as catheters and injectors. One of the initial problems with hand injection was that the rate of injection was usually less than the flow rate within the vessel. Thus, when making an intra-arterial injection, one has to be cognizant of the injection rate as well as the flow rate of the vessel. In order to optimize the contrast on the finished radiograph, one has to ensure that the rate of injection, at a very minimum, is equal to the flow within the vessel. In addition to a loss of contrast, one also finds a loss in radiographic detail and a blurring of vessels. When we have inadequate images due to slow rates of injection, we have something called "streaming" of the media. The cross-sectional diameter of the vessel is misrepresented as a stenotic vessel and, therefore, presents the possibility of error in interpretation.

Fast arterial injection produces brief changes in vessel flow. The injection produces an initial increase in distal pressure and flow while producing a decrease in proximal flow. These effects last for only milliseconds. Fast arterial injection produces vasodilatation and may result in increased patient discomfort (heat or pain). Table 3–5 lists the acute effects of an arterial injection of contrast media.

▶ INTRAVENOUS INJECTION: GENERAL EFFECTS

Typically, IV injections involve much higher doses of a contrast medium compared with arterial injections. The major problem is that the contrast agent mixes with blood before it enters microcirculation. Because the average cardiac output is approximately 100 ml/sec, most contrast media are quite watered down before they reach the lungs. Bolus injections have been shown to demonstrate an initial increase in pulmonary artery pressure and cardiac output and a decrease in pulmonary and systemic resistances. In addition, the bolus injection produces hemodynamic changes in the vein. It has been suggested that a bolus injection of contrast media can produce some minor patient discomforts, such as burning, the feeling of warmth or flushing, or a metallic taste in the mouth. These common occurrences associated with bolus injections of contrast media are referred to as the *vasomotor effect*. Currently, most contrast media are eliminated through the kidneys. With kidney dysfunction, glomerular clearance takes place slowly through the liver and gastrointestinal system for both arterial and IV injections. Table 3–6 lists the acute effects of an IV injection of contrast media.

▶ ADVERSE REACTIONS TO CONTRAST MEDIA

Four major categories of adverse reactions have been identified with regard to the administration of ionic contrast media: (1) the vasomotor effect, (2) the anaphylactoid (idiosyncratic) reaction, (3) the vagal reaction, and (4) acute renal failure (Table 3–7).

Vasomotor Effect

The vasomotor effect is frequently confused with the vagal effect or the more severe anaphylactic reac-

▶ **Table 3–5**

ACUTE EFFECTS OF ARTERIAL INJECTIONS

- Force of injection results in increased distal pressure and flow and decreased proximal flow.
- Higher viscosity results in increased resistance and decreased flow.
- Higher osmolality causes water flux from erythrocytes and tissue to the plasma, and contrast media molecules enter the interstitial fluid.
- Vasodilatation decreases resistance and may cause a feeling of warmth or pain.
- Water and contrast media fluxes are reversed.
- Contrast agent is washed out of the local vascular bed by isotonic blood.
- Physiologic status reverts to preinjection levels.

▶ **Table 3–6**

ACUTE EFFECTS OF INTRAVENOUS INJECTION OF CONTRAST MEDIA

- Higher osmolality causes water flux from erythrocytes and endothelial cells to the plasma.
- Hypertonic, hyperviscous mixture reaches the lungs, where further fluid shifts occur and where the lung parenchyma receives contrast media. An increase in plasma protein to the lung may occur.
- Increase in pulmonary artery pressure and cardiac output.
- Decrease in pulmonary resistance, systemic pressure, and hematocrit occurs.
- The fluid mixture enters the systemic vascular beds, where additional water shifts occur and media molecules enter the interstitial space.
- Water contained within isotonic blood moves from the lung capillaries back into the hypertonic tissues; the process is repeated in systemic tissues.
- Physiologic status reverts back to preinjection levels.

tion. Ionic contrast media are *hypertonic* (pertaining to or characterized by an increased tonicity or tension) and result in *hemodynamic* (alteration of blood flow) changes initially, during, and after the injection. Sensations of warmth and heat are not uncommon. In addition, the patient could complain of a metallic taste in the mouth as well as a tingling sensation. The patient may exhibit signs of nausea; however, if the patient takes some deep breaths through his or her mouth, this problem should be alleviated.

Some degree of pain often accompanies the intra-arterial injection. Most patients who have computed tomography (CT) scans are injected or infused, and about half experience vasomotor symptoms. Vasomotor reactions for the most part are not complex and thus are not life threatening. Vasomotor responses can be minimized by a slower rate of injection, heating of the contrast media, and use of nonionic contrast media.

Anaphylactic Reaction

Minor adverse reactions with perhaps mild flushing, erythema, and scattered urticaria are common patient responses with current ionic contrast agents. Studies indicate that 5 to 6% of patients have a mild adverse reaction. Some of these symptoms are the result of the vasomotor effect. *Anaphylactic* (idiosyncratic) reactions are not common and occur (moderate reactions) in fewer than 2% of examinations. Severe life-threatening reactions occur at a rate of 1 to 2/1000 examinations. The mortality rate of ionic intravascular injections ranges from one in 10,000 to one in 75,000 examinations.[4]

▶ **Table 3–7**

FOUR CATEGORIES OF ADVERSE REACTIONS TO CONTRAST MEDIA

1. Vasomotor effect
2. Anaphylactic/idiosyncratic reaction
3. Vagal reaction
4. Acute renal failure

Although investigators have attempted to link hypersensitivity or allergic reactions with an anaphylactic response, most investigators have not been able to link the two conclusively. The exact cause of an anaphylactic reaction is still being debated. Theories involve the liberation of histamine, the central nervous system, a history of atopy (clinical sensitivity with hereditary predisposition), and emotional responses (e.g., fear or stress). Although certain patients historically have a higher rate of reaction than do others, inconsistencies still remain. For example, one survey indicated that patients who are allergic to shellfish may not be allergic to other foods that contain iodine. One of the latest theories is that in systemic anaphylactic reactions the carrier protein is more likely to be the culprit than is the iodine itself. This finding may correlate with the appearance of a charged molecule in ionic contrast media.

Studies have revealed that anaphylactic reactions involving ionic contrast agents are more common in the 20- to 29-year-old age group. However, in the fatalities that have been documented, patients appear to be older than 50 years of age. There does not seem to be a gender dominance of fatal reactions: they occur equally. Generally, anaphylactic reactions are less common in the very young and in the elderly. There is a higher rate of reaction involving IV injections than intra-arterial injections.

Patients who have a history of prior reactions seem to be at the highest risk for an anaphylactic reaction. The severity of the second reaction may or may not be worse than the initial reaction. This finding is at best inconclusive.

Treatment

Patients with minor reactions to ionic media often do not require any treatment other than observation. Urticaria and pruritus represent the most common types of allergic reactions. Usually, 50 mg of diphenhydramine (Benadryl) administered orally, intramuscularly, or intravenously will provide symptomatic relief; however, there is no evidence that diphenhydramine will reduce the severity of a cutaneous reaction. Drowsiness is often a complication of diphenhydramine, and this fact must be taken into account in the case of outpatients. Patients with respiratory problems should receive oxygen via a nasal cannula (initially 2 l/min). It is possible that a patient's initial reaction may be moderate to severe. In these events, the reactions are often referred to as "accelerating." Symptoms and signs such as laryngospasm, bronchospasm, angioedema, and hypotension require quick treatment. In addition to maintaining an open airway, administration of oxygen and establishment of an IV catheter pathway for further treatment are the initial steps in this type of reaction. *Adrenergic* drugs are used to address physiologic changes in cardiac behavior. *Epinephrine* is the primary drug for treating a moderate *anaphylactic* reaction. An initial dose of up to 0.3 ml of a 1 : 1000 concentration is injected subcutaneously in all except extremely hypotensive patients and can be repeated twice at 15- to 20-minute intervals.[1] If epinephrine does not relieve the bronchospasms, *aminophylline* (a bronchodilator) can be administered. An initial IV dose of 250 mg in 5% dextrose in water administered for 10 to 20 minutes and followed by a maintenance dose of 0.4 to 1 mg/kg/hr can be given.[1] However, care must be taken, because aminophylline can cause an abrupt hypotensive condition.

Vasovagal Reaction

The cause of the *vasovagal* reaction is not yet known. Vasovagal reactions are also observed following contrast media injections, but the symptoms differ greatly from anaphylactoid reactions. Interestingly, vasovagal reactions are seen with other procedures such as cholangiography and barium enemas. Vasovagal responses are directly related to cardiac changes. There is depressed sinoatrial (SA) node activity and interference of the atrioventricular (AV) conduction system. There is peripheral vasodilatation. The patient appears to be bewildered, anxious, and diaphoretic. Hypotension (<80 systolic) and a sinus bradycardia pulse rate of less than 50 are also noted. If the decrease in blood pressure is not treated immediately, then the patient may become unresponsive and may even go into cardiac arrest.

Treatment

It is essential that the diagnosis of a vagal reaction not be confused with an anaphylactic reaction. The patient's legs should be elevated (Trendelenburg position) and IV (isotonic) fluid should be administered. Atropine (an anticholinergic) may be given to overcome the bradycardia (0.5 to 2 mg). Initially, a 1-mg dose of atropine is administered intravenously, followed in 1 to 2 minutes with another 1-mg dose if bradycardia persists. The pulse rate is monitored to determine whether or not additional therapy is necessary. Atropine serves to block the vagal cardiac slowing but does nothing to alter the peripheral dilatation.

Ephedrine is another drug that is used to treat the vasovagal reaction. Even though atropine acts to block the vasovagal cardiac slowing, it does not correct peripheral vasodilatation. Ephedrine is a vasoconstrictor that directly stimulates the heart and provides peripheral vasoconstriction. A dose of 10 mg of ephedrine is usually administered intravenously.

Contrast-Induced Renal Failure

The problem of renal failure is a direct complication of performing a contrast procedure on a patient who has renal dysfunction. The examination risk is proportional to the level of renal dysfunction. Renal shutdown as the result of a contrast medium infusion is often the result observed in patients with small vessel renal disease, diabetic renal disease, multiple myeloma, low cardiac output, or advanced age. Table 3–8 shows the adverse effects of contrast media, major symptoms, and the primary modes of treatment.

► FACTORS PREDISPOSING TO CONTRAST MEDIA REACTIONS

Palmer[3] reported an incidence of severe reactions of approximately 1 : 1000 and a mortality rate of 1 : 14,000 to 1 : 90,000, with 1 : 40,000 being a commonly accepted figure for ionic contrast media. Overall, 6% to 8% of all contrast injections—more than 10 million are done in the U.S. each year—cause a reaction. Three out of every 1000 cause severe reactions requiring hospitalization.[3]

Patients who have a history of allergic reaction to ionic contrast media have an increased probability of allergic reaction if that contrast medium is received again (up to 11 times). Patients with an asthmatic and cardiac history also have an increased probability of having an adverse reaction to ionic contrast media (twice up to 4.5 times, respectively). Other patients

► **Table 3–8**

SYMPTOMS AND TREATMENTS FOR ADVERSE EFFECTS OF CONTRAST MEDIA

Effect	Major Symptoms	Primary Treatment
Vasomotor effect	Warmth Nausea Vomiting	Reassurance
Anaphylactic reaction	Urticaria Bronchospasm	Adrenergics
	Hypotension Tachycardia	Inhaled β-adrenergics
Vagal reaction	Hypotension Bradycardia	Fluids (IV*) Atropine (IV)
Nephrotoxicity	Acute renal failure	Avoidance (other tests) Hydration Diuretics

* IV = intravenously.

who are at high risk of having adverse reactions are those who are dehydrated or have a history of diabetes mellitus, sickle cell anemia, chronic obstructive pulmonary disease, renal insufficiency, central nervous system lesions, or multiple myeloma or patients who are apprehensive or emotionally upset.

Since the cost factor of nonionic contrast agents is so much greater than that of ionic contrast media, studies are being initiated to determine whether the widespread use of nonionic agents and increased safety can justify the greater expense. Overall, the risk of a severe reaction is 5.75 times greater with ionic than nonionic media. Rapid injections are more likely to produce a reaction than a slow injection.[3]

According to Palmer,[3] the procedure that has the highest incidence of reactions to ionic contrast media is CT scanning. CT scanning yielded an incidence reaction percentage of 6.8%, followed by urography, 5.7%; vascular procedures averaged slightly less than 2.5%. A study that was conducted in 1987 by the Royal Australian College of Radiologists indicated the incidence of severe reaction to contrast media (61,000 studies) in high-risk patients. For ionic contrast media the risk recorded was 0.31%, and for nonionic media the risk recorded was 0.03%.

Latshaw reported in the August 1991 issue of *Administrative Radiology* the average cost for adverse reactions. The treatment costs, respectively, for mild reactions is $148; for moderate reactions is $1040; and for severe reactions is $6425. Based on a 300-bed hospital, 20 procedures/day, 6 days/wk for 52 weeks, the number of reactions utilizing ionic contrast media (312) cost a total of $109,000. The number of reactions utilizing nonionic contrast media (75) cost a total of $26,000.

Selected results from a 1988 nationwide survey of 244 responses by radiologists indicated the following: 75% indicated that nonionic contrast agents were diagnostically equivalent or superior to ionic agents; 68% reported a lesser risk of serious reaction; and 86% reported less patient discomfort upon injection, when using nonionic contrast agents. In answer to the question—if low osmolar media were not so expensive, they would completely replace the use of conventional media in most (if not all) procedures—92% responded to this question in the affirmative.

Table 3–9 identifies patients who present an increased risk for contrast media reaction.

Injection of Impurities

Some disposable plastic syringes used for contrast media injections have been found to contain foreign substances. These substances include a *lubricant* coated on the plunger and particles of *rubber,* also from the plunger. The lubricant is supposed to prevent the plunger from sticking in the barrel and to facilitate easier syringe loading (by hand or with power injector). Contrast media in the filled syringe may be in contact with the rubber portion of the plunger. Prolonged contact may cause changes in the integrity of the rubber. Rubber particles could enter the blood stream upon injection.

It has been suggested that, upon opening a sterile disposable syringe, one should carefully separate the plunger from the barrel and rinse both pieces with several milliliters of saline. It is also advisable to store bottles of contrast media in an *upright* position in order to minimize contact of the rubber stopper with the contrast media.

Heating of contrast media may increase the likelihood of contamination from impurities. Syringes are now being manufactured with a unit dose injection. During the manufacturing process, the contrast media–filled syringe is not touched by human hands

▸ **Table 3–9**

PATIENTS AT INCREASED RISK FOR CONTRAST MEDIA REACTION

Idiosyncratic or Anaphylactic Reaction
1. Previous reaction to contrast media
2. Multiple food or medication allergies
3. Asthma/hay fever

Nonidiosyncratic Reaction
1. Contrast-induced renal failure (nephrotoxicity)
   • Azotemia
   • Diabetes mellitus
   • Congestive heart failure
   • Dehydration
   • Multiple myeloma
2. Aggravation of pre-existing disease
   • Cardiac arrhythmias
   • Congestive heart failure
   • Sickle cell anemia
   • Pheochromocytoma
   • Severe hyperthyroidism
3. Other (proposed, but unconfirmed mechanisms)
   • Anxiety and emotions
   • Age: infants and the elderly (more susceptible to radical fluid shifts)

and is wrapped in a sterile package or container. Despite the manufacturer's assurance of sterility, one must be sure to check the syringe for any defects.

Quality Assurance

All medications and contrast agents must be checked for spoilage. Contrast media and emergency medications can be spoiled in many ways. They are usually contained within clear glass containers (e.g., vials, bottles, ampules). These glass containers should be stored upright at room temperature in a location that is out of direct contact with white light, fluorescent light, or sunlight. Exposure to light could chemically alter the substance and spoil it. Storage of the substance near water pipes or heating elements could also compromise the integrity of the material. The easiest way to determine the quality of the solution is by observation. Clear glass makes it possible to see particulate matter or precipitate floating in the solution. It also allows the technologist to look for any discoloration or separation of the contents. Some medications must be refrigerated. Check the manufacturer's indication for proper storage instructions. If the date of expiration has been exceeded, the material should be discarded.

If a bottle, vial, or ampule is opened, it is spoiled and must be discarded. If the expiration date has been exceeded, it is spoiled. It must also be discarded if the media/medication is *discolored* or *separated* or presents a suspended *precipitate* or *particulate* matter in the solution. A protocol should be established to ensure that all medications and contrast media are checked for spoilage and are replaced after use. Table 3–10 lists the ways in which spoilage of contrast media can occur.

► ANAPHYLACTIC SYSTEMIC REACTIONS

Anaphylactic reactions to contrast media may be the result of complex interactions among several mediator systems, as yet unknown.[5] Adverse reactions are classed as minor (mild), moderate (intermediate), and major (severe). Anaphylactic reactions do not necessarily follow a uniform pattern. Most reactions are minor and require little or no treatment. Some reactions linger and progress to the next level of severity.

On rare occasions, a patient may initially suffer a major response and require life-saving measures. Table 3–11 presents a summary of the signs and symptoms of anaphylactic reactions.

Contrast media reactions result in certain physiologic responses (as follows).

Cardiac Responses

Many serious reactions are believed to have a cardiovascular cause.[5] The circulation of older adults is often compromised by arteriosclerosis. The very young are influenced by profound fluid shifts and changes in blood volume. The high osmolar concentration of ionic contrast media is primarily responsible for the hemodynamic changes caused by the fluid shifts. The high osmolar media draw fluid from the extravascular space, from the red blood cells, and from endothelium, initiating reflexes that cause others. In contrast, low osmolar media produce lesser alterations in the hemodynamic status because of less pronounced fluid shifts.[4]

Intra-arterial injections of radiopaque contrast media in the coronary artery cause myocardial depression, bradycardia, electrocardiographic changes, arrhythmias, and occasionally ventricular fibrillation.

Cardiac arrest is an unexpected and sudden halt of heart action. The electrical impulses that trigger heart muscle action cease, or ventricular fibrillation occurs. Many patients have a history of cardiac disease, and thus their only chance of survival is immediate implementation of emergency cardiac care.

Renal Responses

The kidneys are responsible for clearing (removing) more than 99% of conventional contrast media from the body. The remaining material is removed by the intestine. Regardless of where the injection takes place, the contrast media reach high concentrations in the renal collecting system and renal tubules. Intra-arterial and IV injections have an effect on renal hemodynamics and function. Changes in blood flow are accompanied by changes in glomerular filtration. In normal kidneys, the effects of contrast media are usually of little concern. In a diseased kidney, changes in blood flow can lead to ischemia. The greatest potential for acute renal failure is when contrast media is delivered directly into the renal artery by way of se-

► **Table 3–10**
SPOILAGE OF CONTRAST MEDIA

Check all contrast agents and medications for:
  Date of expiration
  Discoloration of media
  Separation of media
  Precipitate suspended in media
  Broken seal

► **Table 3–11**
FOUR MAIN SYSTEMIC RESPONSES TO AN ANAPHYLACTIC REACTION

1. Cardiac responses
2. Renal responses
3. Pulmonary responses
4. Central nervous system responses

lective catheterization (renal arteriography). Patients who have renal dysfunction, who are elderly, who have diabetes, and who are dehydrated present the greatest risk for nephrotoxicity.

Pulmonary Responses

IV injections of contrast media and injections into the right ventricle or pulmonary artery produce relatively high concentrations of contrast media in the lungs. The effects of these injections include elevations in pulmonary artery and vein pressures, increases in cardiac output, and increases in lung water and pulmonary edema.[4]

Pulmonary responses that are the most common include cough, dyspnea, tachypnea, bronchospasm, and respiratory arrest.

Central Nervous System Responses

Hemodynamic responses take place within the central nervous system during an intra-arterial injection. The change in blood flow is determined by the site of injection: intracarotid, brachial, or transfemoral.

Some of the responses include vasodilatation (vasospasm); hypotension; bradycardia or tachycardia; increased blood viscosity; red blood cell crenation and aggregation; and alterations in blood coagulation, fibrinolysis, and platelet aggregation. All of these factors could lead to some modification of cerebral blood flow.

Changes in cerebral arterial circulation and *blood-brain barrier* permeability are significantly affected by high osmolar contrast agents. Central nervous deficits to the blood-brain barrier following cerebral angiography may be caused as a result of damage to the blood-brain barrier.

▸ CLASSIFICATION OF ADVERSE REACTIONS

Systemic contrast media reactions are usually ranked in order of severity: *minor* (mild), *moderate* (intermediate), and *major* (severe). The signs and symptoms for these reactions are listed in Table 3–12.

▸ REFERENCES

1. Kadir S: Current Practice of Interventional Radiology. Philadelphia, BC Decker, 1991.
2. Kadir S: Diagnostic Angiography. Philadelphia, WB Saunders, 1986.
3. Palmer F: Contrast media reactions. Br J Radiol 56:653, 1983.
4. Parvez Z, Moncada R, and Sovak M: Contrast Media: Biologic Effects and Clinical Application, Vol II. Boca Raton, FL, CRC Press, 1987.
5. Skucas J: Radiographic Contrast Agents, 2nd ed. Rockville, MD, Aspen Publishing Co., 1989.
6. Winthrop Laboratories: Winthrop Laboratories Contrast Media Guide. New York, Winthrop Laboratories, 1982.

▸ BIBLIOGRAPHY

Abrams HL: Abrams Angiography: Vascular and Interventional Radiology, 3rd ed. Boston, Little, Brown, 1982.
Brasch RC: Contrast Media Choices: What Are The Differences? What Are the Advantages (Published Paper)? San Francisco, University of California, 1991.
Erlich RA and McCloskey ED: Patient Care in Radiography, 3rd ed. St Louis, CV Mosby, 1989.
Hitner H and Nagle BT: Basic Pharmacology for Health Occupations, 2nd ed. Encino, CA, Glencoe Publishing Co., 1987.
Hoppe JO, Larsen HA, and Coulston FJ: Observations in the toxicity of a new urographic contrast medium, sodium 3, 5-diacetamido-2, 4, 6, tri-iodobenzoate (Hypaque so-

▸ **Table 3–12**
THREE MAJOR TYPES OF ADVERSE REACTIONS

Reaction	Signs and Symptoms
1. Minor (mild) reaction	Warmth Itching Urticaria (mild) Angioedema Flushing Coughing Sneezing Metallic taste in mouth Pallor Sweating Tachycardia Bradycardia Nausea Vomiting
2. Moderate (intermediate) reaction	Hives that don't respond to initial treatment Mild bronchospasms Rapid weak pulse Mild hypotension Pulmonary edema Anxiety Severe vomiting Dyspnea
3. Major (severe) reaction	Severe bronchospasms Laryngospasms Epiglottal edema Severe hypotension Cardiac arrhythmia Ventricular fibrillation Dyspnea-cyanosis Pulmonary edema Cramps Paralysis Seizures Coma Pulmonary or cardiac arrest

dium) and related compounds. J Pharmacol Exp Ther 116:394, 1956.

Johnsrude I and Jackson D: A Practical Approach to Angiography, Boston, Little, Brown, 1979.

Larson E: Innovations in health care: Antisepsis as a case study. Am J Public Health 79:92, 1991.

Lasser EC: Basic mechanisms of contrast media reactions—theoretical and experimental considerations. Radiology 91:63, 1968.

Lasser EC, Farr RS, Fujimagari T, and Tripp WN: The significance of protein binding of contrast media in roentgen diagnosis. Am J Roentgenol, Radiotherapy Nuclear Medicine 87:338, 1962.

Lasser EC, Reuter WA, and Lang J: Histamine release by contrast media. Radiology 100:683, 1971.

Lipton MJ: Contrast Media: The Worldwide Experience (Published paper). Chicago, University of Chicago, 1991.

Reuter S, Redman H, and Cho K: Gastrointestinal Angiography, 3rd ed. Philadelphia, WB Saunders, 1986.

Schechter M, et al: Putting New Low Osmolality Agents Into Perspective: An Interview, Booklet, Clinical Perspectives and Practical Insights. St Louis, Mallinckrodt, Inc., 1987.

Snopek AM: Fundamentals of Special Radiographic Procedures, 2nd ed. Philadelphia, WB Saunders, 1984.

Stark DD: Contrast Media Choices: What are the Differences? What are the Advantages (Published paper)? Boston, Massachusetts General Hospital, 1989.

Swamy S, Segal L, and Mouli S: Percutaneous Angiography. Springfield, Charles C Thomas, 1977.

Torres LS: Basic Medical Techniques and Patient Care for Radiologic Technologists, 3rd ed. Philadelphia, JB Lippincott, 1989.

Tortorici MR: Fundamentals of Angiography. St Louis, CV Mosby, 1982.

Watson JC: Patient Care and Special Procedures in Radiologic Technology, 4th ed. St Louis, CV Mosby, 1974.

White RI: Fundamentals of Vascular Radiology. Philadelphia, Lea & Febiger, 1976.

Winfield AC: Contrast Media Choices: What Are The Differences? What Are The Advantages (Published paper) Nashville, Vanderbilt University Medical Center, 1991.

Zelch JV: Can we afford not to use nonionic contrast media? In Practical Considerations for Reimbursement of Nonionic Contrast Media: Diagnostic Imaging 2:251, 1989.

► SELF-ASSESSMENT QUIZ

1. Medications are administered by two primary routes:
   a. internal and external
   b. oral and parenteral
   c. local and systemic
   d. topical and internal

2. Which of the following are examples of systemic administration?
   1. oral
   2. sublingual
   3. rectal
   4. parenteral
      a. 1 only
      b. 1 and 2
      c. 1, 2, and 3
      d. 1, 2, 3, and 4

3. Medications that are affected by gastric contents are not usually administered orally.
   a. true
   b. false

4. Parenteral administration refers to the delivery of medication
   a. by mouth
   b. by injection
   c. placed under the tongue
   d. by rectal insertion

5. Which of the following are examples of iodinated contrast media?
   1. barium
   2. ionic
   3. negative
   4. nonionic
      a. 1 and 2
      b. 2 and 4
      c. 1, 3, and 4
      d. 1, 2, 3, and 4

6. Which represents the ratio of the mass of a substance to its volume?
   a. density
   b. viscosity
   c. osmolality
   d. molar concentration

7. Viscosity represents the
   a. resistance to flow or thickness of the agent
   b. iodine concentration
   c. osmolality of the agent
   d. density of the agent

8. Isuprel is an example of what class of medication?
   a. analgesic
   b. adrenergic
   c. antiemetic
   d. antihistamine

9. Benadryl is an example of what class of medication?
   a. analgesic
   b. adrenergic
   c. antiemetic
   d. antihistamine

10. Which medication is administered intravenously in response to metabolic acidosis?
    a. diphenhydramine hydrochloride (Benadryl)
    b. digitalis
    c. sodium bicarbonate
    d. isoproterenol hydrochloride (Isuprel)

11. Epinephrine
    1. stimulates the sympathetic nervous system
    2. is a vasoconstrictor
    3. raises blood pressure
    4. is useful in treatment of allergic reactions
       a. 1 only
       b. 1 and 2
       c. 1, 2, and 3
       d. 1, 2, 3, and 4

12. Compared with the sodium ion, meglumine ion is
    a. heavier
    b. equivalent
    c. lighter

13. When discussing the factor of ''opacification,'' which would usually produce an image of higher contrast?
    a. sodium
    b. meglumine

14. When discussing the factor of ''safety,'' which could be the contrast medium of choice?
    a. sodium
    b. meglumine

15. Torsten Almen is best known for the development of
    a. opaque contrast media
    b. water-soluble contrast media
    c. ionic contrast media
    d. nonionic contrast media

16. Metrizamide was the name given to the first
    a. opaque contrast media
    b. ionic contrast media
    c. water-soluble contrast media
    d. nonionic contrast media

17. Low osmolar contrast agents are typically
    1. nonionic
    2. ionic
    3. more expensive
    4. less expensive
    5. safer to use
       a. 1, 3, and 5
       b. 2, 3, and 5
       c. 1, 4, and 5
       d. 2, 4, and 5

18. Osmolality is strongly dependent on iodine concentration.
    a. true
    b. false

19. In terms of unit cost, ionic contrast agents are
    a. more expensive
    b. of equal cost
    c. less expensive

20. If the rate of injection is slow compared with the flow rate in the vessel, the contrast medium will not mix with the blood uniformly and the images will be inadequate. This statement describes
    a. delay flow
    b. streaming
    c. concentric flow
    d. transient flow

21. What organ(s) is or are responsible for the removal of contrast media from the body?
    a. liver
    b. intestine
    c. kidneys
    d. adrenal glands

22. Which of the following is or are related to contrast medium reactions?
    1. vasomotor effect
    2. anaphylactoid reaction
    3. vagal reaction
    4. acute renal failure
       a. 1 only
       b. 1 and 2
       c. 1, 2, and 3
       d. 1, 2, 3, and 4

23. Atropine may be administered
    a. to overcome bradycardia
    b. to treat urticaria
    c. to overcome tachycardia
    d. to treat hypertension

24. All of the following are examples of contraindications to administration of contrast media, except
    a. multiple myeloma
    b. diabetic renal disease
    c. low cardiac output
    d. advanced age
    e. history of allergy

25. Medications are considered to be spoiled when
    1. contents separate
    2. precipitate is present
    3. contents are discolored
    4. expiration date is exceeded
    5. original seal is broken
       a. 1 only
       b. 1 and 2
       c. 1, 2, and 3
       d. 1, 2, 3, and 4
       e. 1, 2, 3, 4, and 5

26. Pulmonary arrest is defined as an unexpected and sudden stoppage of heart action.
    a. true
    b. false

27. Flushing, nausea, vomiting, and pallor are found with which type of adverse reaction?
    a. minor
    b. moderate
    c. major

28. When hives do not respond to initial treatment, the reaction is considered to be
    a. minor
    b. moderate
    c. major

29. When bronchospasms are not relieved by initial treatment, the reaction is considered to be
    a. minor
    b. moderate
    c. major

30. Following an intravascular injection of an iodinated contrast medium, when is it considered safe to leave the patient completely unattended?
    a. while the films are being checked
    b. after about 5 minutes have elapsed
    c. after about 15 minutes have elapsed
    d. never

▶ STUDY QUESTIONS

1. What medications should be included in an emergency crash cart?

2. List several advantages and disadvantages for nonionic/low osmolar contrast media.

3. Describe the acute effects of arterial injections on the heart, kidneys, and central nervous system.

4. Describe the term ''osmolality.''

5. How is the blood-brain barrier affected by intravascular contrast media injections?

6. Explain what is meant by an ''idiosyncratic'' reaction.

7. Describe the factors that, when present, would put the patient at risk for an injection of contrast media.

8. List and describe several symptoms and signs of a major anaphylactoid reaction.

9. What is the primary difference between an anion and cation?

10. List and describe the four major categories of adverse reactions to contrast media.

► CHAPTER FOUR

► **PATIENT CARE PROCEDURES**

► CHAPTER OUTLINE

Preprocedural Assessment
Procedural Indications
Preprocedural Protocol
    Premedication Guidelines
    Types of Premedication
Technologist-Patient Communication
Medical/Surgical Asepsis
Transmission of Infection
Isolation Techniques
Surgical Asepsis
    Rules for Surgical Asepsis
Proper Handling of Sterilized Equipment

Invasive/Interventional Procedures: Personnel
Procedural Supplies
    Standard Essentials: Angiographic Procedural
      Tray
    Dedicated Procedural Tray-Sets
    Regional Site Preparation
    Specific Site Preparation
Postprocedural Orders
Radiation Protection and Safety Procedures
    Sources of Scatter and Primary
      Radiation
    Methods to Reduce Radiation Exposure

► CHAPTER OBJECTIVES

Upon completion of Chapter 4 the technologist will be able to:

1. List three primary indications for invasive/interventional procedures
2. Explain what is meant by preprocedural protocol
3. List the primary laboratory tests that may be ordered for patients who have cardiovascular/interventional procedures
4. Explain the purposes of the following tests: hematocrit, prothrombin time (PT), partial thromboplastin time (PTT), and activated partial thromboplastin time (APTT)
5. List the drugs used in premedication and their primary actions
6. List and describe the five primary routes of disease transmission
7. Explain what is meant by "body substance precautions"
8. List and explain the four primary types of isolation
9. Describe the procedure for disposing of contaminated articles
10. Explain the role of the special procedures technologist with regard to patient care and communication
11. List five to seven items that are included in a standardized angiographic tray
12. List and describe the steps for regional site preparation
13. Explain what patient considerations must be addressed for an invasive procedure
14. Describe the role and specific functions of the technologist as a team member in cardiovascular/interventional technology
15. List the primary precautions regarding safety that have an impact on the technologists and physicians working in cardiovascular/interventional procedures
16. List the required lead equivalents for protective safety equipment used in the work environment
17. List and describe the important pieces of radiation protection used in the work environment

A technologist working in the cardiovascular/interventional department interacts with the patient very closely and may be the one person who is solely responsible for independent direct patient care during the procedure. The relationship between the technologist and the patient and the communication skills of the technologist can play a major role in determining the success of a cardiovascular/interventional procedure.

▶ PREPROCEDURAL ASSESSMENT

The decision to perform an arteriogram or interventional procedure is made in conjunction with the vascular radiologist and the patient's referring physician. This consultation generally takes into consideration the patient's history, the previous diagnostic evaluations, and the expected therapeutic or diagnostic result. Vascular radiology is associated with low morbidity and mortality, yet it is still an invasive procedure. Bearing this in mind, the referring physician and the radiologist must consider the diagnostic results to be obtained and weigh the potential risks of the procedure.

▶ PROCEDURAL INDICATIONS

There are several primary indications for ordering an invasive or interventional procedure:

1. Other conventional, less risky examinations and study regimens have produced negative or inconclusive results for diagnosis.
2. Conventional medical investigation demonstrates a disease process, but more information is needed concerning its nature, its extent, and the feasibility of other medical or surgical interventions.
3. Emergency situations in which an invasive diagnostic procedure may be the initial diagnostic or treatment regimen required.
4. Interventional and therapeutic procedures aimed at alleviating or treating a disease process, often resulting in less mortality and morbidity than does conventional surgical management.

▶ PREPROCEDURAL PROTOCOL

On the day before the procedure, an initial consultation takes place between the physician performing the procedure and the patient who will be the recipient of this procedure. This initial consultation serves to establish a bridge in the physician-patient relationship. This relationship enhances the performance of the procedure and a well-informed patient who possesses a positive attitude toward the procedure helps to make everyone's job easier. Second, if any complications occur, this relationship may lessen the likelihood of a lawsuit. All pertinent information must be explained in terms that the patient can understand. These terms should be in written form and constitute an "informed consent" form. This form contains an explanation of the intended procedure, what is expected of the patient during the examination, and any complications that can occur during the procedure or during recovery. The patient should be advised of the anticipated length of bed rest that will follow the procedure. The informed consent must be written, witnessed, and signed.

The preangiographic visit enables the radiologist to assess the patient's relative condition and medical history and permits a chart inspection focusing on the patient's cardiac, hepatic, pulmonary, and renal functions. This medical history is important, because the patient is being subjected to a procedure that places an increased workload on the heart, lungs, kidneys, and other vital organs. Contrast agents, injected directly into the vascular system, will greatly influence organ and organ/system function. For example, patients with chronic obstructive pulmonary disease (COPD) may be respiratorily depressed by barbiturate administration; the patient may be on oral or intravenous (IV) anticoagulants; the patient may have an allergic history to iodine; or the patient may not have good cardiac or renal output. Thus, the preangiographic assessment requires an informed consent, an explanation of the procedure, preangiographic orders, and a physician's (radiologist) evaluation of the patient's physical and vascular condition.

In addition to the patient's past and current medical history, laboratory data are reviewed and specific questions are asked with regard to past studies in which a contrast agent was used. Information concerning prior reactions and specific allergies to medications, foods, and so forth are added to the patient's chart.

A review of renal function tests, such as creatinine and blood urea nitrogen (BUN), must be included as should the hematocrit and bleeding parameters. Many patients with peripheral vascular-associated diseases receive anticoagulant therapy. Hemorrhage is always the major toxicity associated with the use of an anticoagulant. The bleeding parameters are strongly influenced by the quantity of anticoagulant as well as by when the patient was last medicated. Hematocrit, PT, PTT, APTT, and platelet count (thrombocytes) are all tests used to determine bleeding parameters.

Hematocrit is a measure of the concentration of red blood cells in the total blood volume. Hematocrit can also be an indicator of the hydration status of the patient. Low hematocrit levels are usually found in patients who are anemic or who have leukemia.

PT (prothrombin time or Pro-time) is one of the tests that is usually performed to test clot formation and monitor oral anticoagulant therapy. The PT measures the clotting ability of factors I (fibrinogen), II (prothrombin), V, VII, and X. Alterations of factors V and VII will prolong the PT for approximately 2 seconds, or 10% of normal. In liver disease, the PT is usually prolonged, since the liver cells cannot synthe-

▶ **Table 4-1**

LABORATORY TESTS FOR KIDNEY FUNCTION
AND BLOOD CLOTTING

Kidney function	• Blood urea nitrogen
	• Creatinine
Red blood cell volume	• Hematocrit
Blood coagulation	• Prothrombin time
	• Partial thromboplastin time
	• Activated partial thromboplastin time

size prothrombin. The normal value for the PT of an adult or a pediatric patient is 10 to 13 seconds, depending on the method and reagents used, or 70 to 100%. Anticoagulant therapy is 2 to 2.5 times the control in seconds, or 20 to 30%.

The PTT (partial thromboplastin time) is a screening test used to detect deficiencies in all clotting factors except factors VII and XIII and to detect platelet variations. The PTT is more sensitive than is the PT in the detection of minor deficiencies but is not as sensitive as the APTT. The normal range of a PTT is 22 to 35 seconds.

The APTT (activated partial thromboplastin time) is similar but is more sensitive than the PTT because of a special additive (kaolin, celite, or ellagic acid) that shortens the clotting time, thus permitting detection of minor clotting deficiencies. The normal range for an APTT is 30 to 45 seconds (>50 seconds is abnormal). Table 4-1 summarizes the screening tests for kidney function and blood clotting disorders.

Orders written by the attending physician will indicate specific instructions to nursing personnel regarding the patient and the special procedure that will be performed on the following day. The patient is usually not allowed to eat any solid food for at least 5 to 6 hours before the procedure. Food is withheld to avoid any sickness that may occur after the administration of any scheduled premedication. Special attention must be paid to the scheduled time of the procedure and whether there may be special instructions (e.g., for the diabetic patient). Most vascular studies (arteriograms or angiograms) will take an average 2 to 3 hours from start to finish. Thus, an IV line is established in an elbow or forearm vein. The IV line should be placed on the arm side opposite the anticipated vascular puncture site. High-risk patients (e.g., diabetics) should be hydrated overnight. Table 4-2 presents an example of preprocedural orders.

Premedication Guidelines

Both the nursing and angiographic personnel must pay close attention to premedication guidelines. The patient should empty his or her bladder before these medications are administered. Patients are usually catheterized prior to a cardiovascular or interventional procedure. Premedication should be administered about 1 hour before the scheduled procedure. Although the specific type of patient preparation may vary according to the type of procedure ordered, the patient's intestines should be as empty as possible to alleviate any physical discomfort and avoid the patient's having to move his or her bowels during the examination.

On certain occasions a patient should *NOT* be premedicated. These contraindications include increased intracranial pressure, COPD, and patients who have a significant deficiency in the amount of circulating plasma in the body. There are also situations in which a great deal of care should be taken when premedication is to be administered. Elderly patients are always at risk for almost any invasive procedure because of many chronic illnesses and conditions of aging. Any patient with hepatic, renal, respiratory, or cardiovascular disease must be watched carefully. There is also increased risk in patients with primary and metastatic cancer, especially intracranial lesions. Pediatric patients usually do not have fluids withheld. Children are subject to dramatic shifts in fluid electrolytes and are often sedated so that their cooperation can be achieved during the procedure.

▶ **Table 4-2**

PREPROCEDURAL ORDERS ISSUED BY THE ATTENDING PHYSICIAN

1. The patient must sign a consent for an angiogram procedure before premedications are given.
2. A *clear liquid diet* is given after 8 PM on the night before an angiogram is done.
3. The patient may have a clear liquid diet for breakfast in the morning just before the angiogram is done (at least 15 minutes before transport to Diagnostic Radiology).
4. *Encourage administration of clear oral fluids on the night before and on the morning when the angiogram is done. The patient must be well hydrated.*
5. Prothrombin time, patient count, APTT,* BUN,† and creatine are checked.
6. Stop heparin therapy 4 hours before the angiogram is done.
7. Pentobarbital, 50 mg and promethazine hydrochloride (Phenergan), 25 mg are given IM at ___ AM (or on call) and valium, 10 mg.
8. The patient must be in Diagnostic Radiology on a cart by ___ AM with the chart.
9. Start intravenous line using left arm, using dextrose 5% ½ normal saline at 150 ml/hr.
10. If there are any questions, telephone the Radiology Supervisor at extension ■■■■.

* APTT = activated partial thromboplastin time.
† BUN = blood urea nitrogen.

The purpose of premedication is to relax and calm the patient so that he or she can be cooperative during the procedure.

Each patient's premedication is individually tailored according to age, weight, physical condition, allergic history and information relative to past drug reactions, and history of drug or alcohol abuse. Finally, the emotional state of the patient should be noted; adverse incidents are more common when the patient is in a state of emotional unrest.

Types of Premedication

Tranquilizers are mild sedatives that act to control anxiety by depressing the central nervous system and by reducing mental activity. Some of the more mild sedatives include hydroxyzine pamoate (Vistaril), diazepam (Valium), chlordiazepoxide hydrochloride (Librium), and meprobamate (Miltown).

When the radiologist discusses the examination with the patient on the day before the special procedure, he or she also indicates what medications will be ordered for the patient if the patient has pain during or after the procedure.

Meperidine hydrochloride (Demerol) and morphine are used to eliminate pain. Meperidine hydrochloride is a synthetic analgesic and may be used in place of morphine, because it is less potent and it has a slight sedative effect. Both meperidine hydrochloride and morphine frequently cause nausea and vomiting and result occasionally in respiratory depression and hypotension. Atropine is frequently used to help minimize the build-up of secretions in the respiratory passages.

Before coming to the radiology department, the patient is often catheterized, and all interfering objects are removed (including dentures, hearing-aids, all metallic objects, and jewelry). All private property should be itemized, indexed, and recorded before he or she leaves the hospital room. This task should also be signed and witnessed. If ancillary equipment is to accompany the patient to the radiology department (e.g., a cardiac monitor, oxygen), radiology personnel should be notified in advance. Once in the radiology department, a technologist team member should acknowledge the arrival of the patient. The patient at this point may be quite apprehensive, and the technologist should assist by discussing the procedure with the patient. It is important for the patient to realize that there may be some discomfort, and it is essential that he or she remain as still as possible during the procedure. The designated team member should thoroughly review the patient's chart and should double-check all pertinent data (Fig. 4–1). The technologists as a "team" may want to review the patient's chart with the radiologist before the procedure in order to discuss any important facts regarding the patient's status. The patient's film folder should be kept at hand in case prior radiographs need to be reexamined.

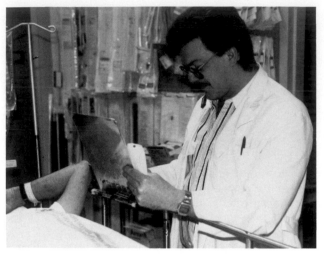

▸ **Figure 4–1**

A technologist is reviewing the patient's chart and discussing the expectations of the examination with the patient.

▸ TECHNOLOGIST-PATIENT COMMUNICATION

During the pre-examination phase the personal relationship between the technologist and the patient is established. Patients arrive in the radiology department in a wide variety of physical, mental, and emotional states. Many of the patients' attitudes may be immediately apparent. It is very important that everyone is prepared and that everything is organized when the patient arrives. Every patient will arrive in a specific anxiety state and will often be very fearful of the scheduled procedure. As an individual with a distinct personality, each patient has needs that vary and are often dictated by the patient's illness. The illness may be chronic, recent, or perhaps an "acute emergency" that requires immediate attention. Many messages conveyed by the patient are nonverbal, and it is essential that the technologist establish a rapport with the patient at an early stage and be aware of any nonverbal cues that the patient may convey.

During this period, the technologist should communicate openly with the patient and should give an explanation of the procedure, what will take place, and, most important, what will be expected of the patient. If the patient is informed, he or she will be more likely to cooperate. At this point the technologist should answer any questions that the patient may have. It is important to gain the patient's confidence, despite his or her ever-present anxiety. The patient should be made to feel secure. We believe that successful completion of the examination is strongly influenced by direct patient care and by good communication between the patient and the technologist. The patient should be made to feel that he or she is "sharing" in his or her medical care. Thus, the patient should be a part of the "team" during his or her brief stay in the angiographic/interventional suite.

The parameters of the procedure are complex for the technologist and include patient care and communication; patient monitoring; management of the numerous imaging modalities (e.g., radiography, fluoroscopy, digital); and direct assistance to the radiologist.

Thus, in order to achieve a successful outcome, the technologist must develop good communication skills and subjective problem-solving techniques. These must include affective skills, such as listening; empathy; understanding the patient's denial, anger, and needs; and the ability to use the spoken word therapeutically to motivate and calm the patient in order to achieve established goals for a successful outcome.

► MEDICAL/SURGICAL ASEPSIS

The hospital environment began to change from being a site of disease and death from sepsis to a place of potential healing due to the work and influence of people such as Semmelweis (in obstetrics in Vienna), Joseph Lister (in surgery in Scotland), and Florence Nightingale (in nursing in London). The decrease in morbidity and mortality was dramatic and was a direct result of hand washing technique and the use of antiseptics before and after contact with patients.

► TRANSMISSION OF INFECTION

There are two methods of controlling contagious diseases: disinfection and isolation. The primary types of disease transmission are contact, droplet, vehicle, and air-borne. The terms aseptic and surgical asepsis are familiar to personnel who are associated with operating room procedures and with the percutaneous invasive procedures that are commonly seen in the special procedures/angiographic suite. They refer to the vital function of controlling and stopping the transmission of infectious microorganisms. Table 4–3 lists and describes the types of disease transmission.

Infections are prevented by eliminating the infective agent by disinfection, sterilization, or elimination of the method of transmission through the use of sterile gloves, gowns, and barriers.

In the vascular suite, the primary source of infections are by way of the angiographic personnel, selected instruments, catheters, guidewires, and specialized imaging equipment.

Angiography and interventional procedures require the catheterization of an artery or vein or by the introduction of a needle or catheter system that leads directly into an organ. It is essential that the technologist is skilled in surgical asepsis. It is the responsibility of all participating personnel to maintain strict surgical aseptic technique at all times, because the patient's well-being is at stake. All primary patient-contact surfaces are cleaned with viricidal agents. Lead aprons are frequently contaminated by a patient's body fluids and should also be cleaned and

► **Table 4–3**
TRANSMISSION OF INFECTION IN THE HOSPITAL

Contact:	Direct transmission from one infected person to another
Indirect contact:	Transmission from infected equipment or objects to a host
Droplet:	Transmission by way of the nose or mouth
Vehicle:	Transmission by way of contaminated equipment (e.g., catheters, drugs, and blood)
Airborne:	Infected agents are suspended in air or dust

disinfected with bactericidal and viricidal agents. The Centers for Disease Control (CDC) publish guidelines for the handling, cleaning, and disposal of contaminated articles. The CDC's guidelines related to ''Body Substance Precautions'' should be displayed visibly within the work area. All personnel, (e.g., technologists, physicians, and nurses) who work in the cardiovascular/interventional suite should be proficient in the handling of contaminated articles.

► ISOLATION TECHNIQUES

There are four primary types of isolation: (1) respiratory; (2) enteric; (3) strict; and (4) protective. The importance of the control of infection in the invasive procedures' environment cannot be emphasized enough. Each of the four specific types of isolation may be encountered by the technologist in the radiology department. Although each method is important, the occurrence of human immunodeficiency virus (HIV), hepatitis A and B, and other opportunistic diseases requires serious consideration for those providing direct patient care during any percutaneous procedure.

The process of determining the proper isolation technique begins with an examination of the patient's clinical history, which is recorded on his or her chart. The technologist should note any significant history of the following types of infection: (1) blood-borne; (2) respiratory; (3) resistant to antibiotics; and (4) any specific indication such as transplant surgery. Patients with transplants are often immunosuppressed, and extreme care with regard to cross-infection must be observed in these situations.

Many institutions have begun an infection-control process called ''Body Substance Precautions.'' This process assumes that all body fluids are contaminated and that any possible contact with a particular patient (via fluid) dictates the degree of protection needed. It is essential that the technologist should wear protective gloves whenever body substances are present. For example:

1. Does the patient have an IV line?

Technologists should know how to properly handle and dispose of an IV needle that has been removed from a vein. IV needles can slip out of a vein. Exposure to contaminated blood at the injection site must be considered. Accidental skin punctures by a contaminated needle pose potential hazards to anyone handling an IV line.

2. Are there draining wounds with wet dressings?

Dressings are frequently soiled with body fluids from draining wounds. Any dressing that is moist or wet is considered to be contaminated and should not come in contact with unprotected skin. Some types of drainage are sanguineous (bloody) or purulent (containing pus) and often have a noxious odor.

3. Does the patient have a tracheostomy that needs suctioning?

Patients with tracheostomies often require frequent suctioning due to the build-up of secretions. The secretions are also forcibly expelled when the patient coughs. Nursing personnel often provide assistance to the technologist by keeping the patient's airway open and unobstructed of thick secretions. All personnel should take precautions from potential interaction with mucoid secretions when performing procedures on patients with tracheostomies.

4. Does the patient's social history indicate any exposure to HIV?

The patient's social status is not always known, but it is necessary to be careful and to follow "universal precautions" when in contact with a patient's body fluids (especially blood).

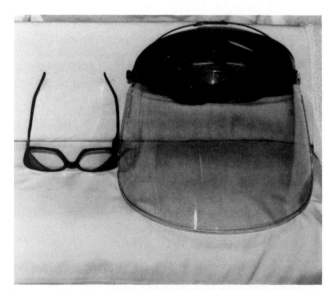

▶ **Figure 4–2**

Examples of protective shielding worn by the radiologist during the procedure.

Radiology departments today are mandated to protect their technical staff and patients during a given invasive procedure. Our department provides protection by supplying sterile gloves, visors, gowns, masks, hats, and shoe covers in each room. Each room is equipped with an approved disinfectant/virucidal solution for decontamination of the radiographic environment, including all equipment that might come in contact with the patient (Fig. 4–2).

Fluid-contaminated disposable items and bedding should be disposed of according to the written policies of the institution. Linen bags and plastic trash bags should be labeled as "contaminated" in order to dictate special handling by laundry and sanitation disposal crews. Policies should be established that indicate the proper disposal of single-use products such as needles and syringes (Fig. 4–3).

▶ SURGICAL ASEPSIS

Before the patient arrives in the radiology department, the special procedure technologists must prepare sterile examination trays and check out all equipment to ensure that it is in operating order. Once the patient arrives, the injection site is cleansed and prepared. Surgical asepsis is defined as the complete removal of all organisms and their spores from equipment used to perform patient care or procedures.[2]

Rules for Surgical Asepsis

1. If the sterility of an object is in doubt, it is not considered to be sterile.

2. Sterile objects and persons should avoid unsterile areas.

3. When any sterile item becomes contaminated, it must be replaced immediately.

4. Personnel must be clothed in sterile gowns and gloves if they are considered to be sterile.

5. If a sterile person's gown or gloves become contaminated, the item(s) must be discarded.

6. If a person working in a sterile area thinks that he or she might be contaminated, the articles in question should be treated as if contaminated and should be discarded.

7. Any sterile area or instrument touched by an unsterile object or person is considered to be contaminated.

8. A sterile area should be created prior to its use.

9. Once a sterile area is created, it should not be left unattended.

10. All articles within the sterile area should be no lower than the table-top level. The only parts on a sterile gown that are considered to be sterile are from the waist to the shoulders, the front (anterior body surface), and the sleeves.

11. If a solution soaks through a sterile area, that area must be covered by a sterile towel of double thickness.

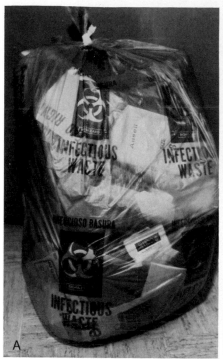
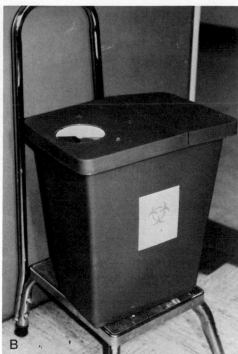

▶ Figure 4–3

A, Plastic bag designed specifically for infectious waste material. B, A receptacle designed for collection of hazardous materials such as syringes, needles, and scalpel blades.

12. Unsterile persons should not reach above or over a sterile area. The chance of contamination can be reduced if unsterile individuals are kept away from the sterile area.

13. Sterile-wrapped angiographic supplies should be preinspected for moisture and wrapping integrity before being introduced into a sterile area. Any material or pack that becomes damp or wet is contaminated.

14. The technologist should keep his or her sterile gloved hands above the waist at all times and in front (*not in contact with*) of the chest.

15. When pouring a sterile solution, the technologist should not touch the inside of the lid, and care should be taken not to splash contents on a sterile area.

16. Containers of sterile solution should be placed strategically in a corner edge of the sterile field.

17. All equipment and work areas (including floors) should be cleaned with a disinfectant after every procedure.

18. Air conditioning and laminar flow ducts must be cleaned, dusted, and disinfected periodically.

▶ PROPER HANDLING OF STERILIZED EQUIPMENT

Other than the commercially prepared tray sets, both the "sterile" special procedures technologist and an assistant will be handling cloth-wrapped packs. Sterilization is a process that kills microorganisms and their spores. Although there are several methods of sterilization, cloth-wrapped packs are best prepared using steam under pressure. Under ordinary means (without pressure), steam cannot kill microorganisms. However, when steam is pressurized, temperatures can be reached that result in the killing of microorganisms. The chamber responsible for this sterilization process is the *autoclave*. The autoclave sterilizes surgical supplies by pressurized steam. Procedural trays containing surgical instruments (reusable) and supplies (e.g., sheets, drapes, 4 × 4s) may be sterilized for use in a particular cardiovascular/interventional procedure. Once removed from the autoclave, the tray must not be used until it is completely dry. After the outer wrapping is placed around the procedure tray, a special tape is used to secure the tray. This special tape has diagonal lines on its surface that darken or change color when sterilization and drying is complete. Also, an indicator is often placed inside the pack. However, care must be taken, because when the packs are removed from the autoclave, they are still damp. When damp, the indicator tape will not fully reveal darkening of the diagonal lines. The pack is only considered to be sterile for use when the diagonal lines are darkened.

Cloth-wrapped packs can be opened by the unsterile technologist and carefully "dropped" onto the sterile field, or the packs can be carefully unwrapped by the unsterile technologist and the uncontaminated (inner) portion can be handed to the sterile technologist (Fig. 4–4). When one opens a cloth-wrapped pack, the pack should be placed with the triangular flap facing the technologist. This flap is carefully lifted

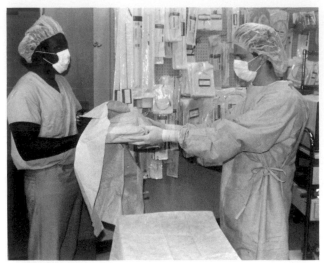

▶ **Figure 4–4**

An unsterile technologist handing a sterile tray to a sterile technologist.

up and away from the technologist (Fig. 4–5A). The next two visible flaps are opened to the side (laterally) (Fig. 4–5B and C), and the last flap opens toward the body (Fig. 4–5D). As with the prepared pack, it can be picked up for placement on the field or handed to the sterile technologist for placement.

▶ INVASIVE/INTERVENTIONAL PROCEDURES: PERSONNEL

In modern-day hospital radiology departments, invasive/interventional procedures are conducted in a dedicated area. Depending on the size of this section or department, two or more technologists may be assigned on a full-time basis to this area. In some hospitals, technologists may be assisted by a radiology nurse. All personnel working in this section or department are specially trained and do not usually rotate through other radiology work stations. Tech-

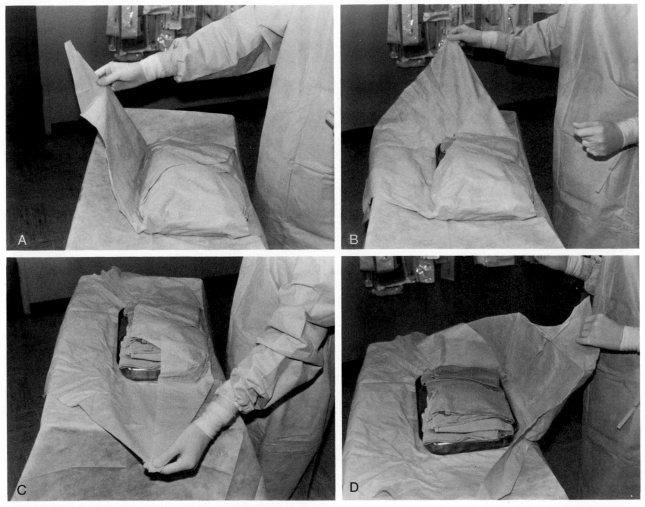

▶ **Figure 4–5**

A, Technique for opening up a sterile pack by a sterile technologist. The top flap is carefully brought back away from the technologist and is allowed to rest on the sterile sheet/examination cart. B, The second flap is opened to the right. C, The third flap is opened to the left. The contents of the examination tray are now partially exposed. D, The final flap is brought back toward the sterile technologist. The entire inner surface of the cloth/paper tray cover is now exposed and is completely sterile.

nologists functioning in this environment frequently work closely with diagnostic radiologists who have additional education and training in special procedures. Within this highly specialized environment, the professional staff members concentrate on providing the patient with the best possible care. A basic ingredient of this total care concept is the working relationships among the physicians, technologists, radiology nurses, and other support personnel. We realize that their perceptions and criteria may differ from other similar working environments; however, despite those differences, the primary goal is to provide total patient care. Communication and cooperation are essential ingredients for total patient care, regardless of the differences that may exist in a clinical environment.

► PROCEDURAL SUPPLIES

Standard Essentials: Angiographic Procedural Tray

The angiographic tray should be placed on a stainless-steel table that is at least $2\frac{1}{2} \times 3\frac{1}{2}'$. The table should contain sturdy metal casters that provide easy maneuverability and that are easy to keep clean.

The angiographic tray should contain instruments and accessories that are dictated by the type of procedure being performed. However, for the purposes of continuity and convenience, we suggest a "standardized" tray assembly for all interventional procedures. Other items that are not used routinely can be kept accessible for immediate use (Fig. 4–6).

For guidewire or catheter placement, one will want to include a large basin that contains a sterile solution used to flush the catheter in use. A quantity of 1000 ml

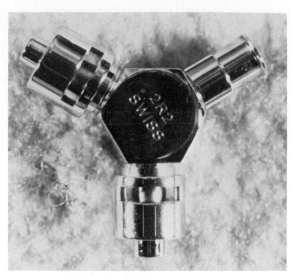

► Figure 4–7

A stainless-steel three-way stopcock.

of normal saline with 3000 units of heparin is standard in most angiographic set-ups, as is an IV flush administration set with a three-way stopcock (Fig. 4–7). Two large stainless-steel bowls are included for disposal of aspirates. One small cup should be available for a contrast medium. A generous supply of 4 × 4″ gauze sponges (20) and at least six sterile cloth towels should be included. It might be important to note that the quality of gauze sponges may vary. Some sponges consist of fabrics that "shed" fibers with routine angiographic use. These sponges should be used only for preprocedural cleansing of the proposed injection site. For the angiographic tray, the technologist should include only gauze sponges that do not leave remnants over or in the sterile field (Fig. 4–8).

► Figure 4–6

The contents of the sterile examination tray are carefully removed and are placed strategically on the sterile surface of the examination cart. Note that the angiographic needle, guidewire, and other items are placed in the large sterile basin that will be immersed in a heparinized solution. When arrangements are complete, the examination cart and instruments are covered with a sterile sheet while awaiting the arrival of the patient.

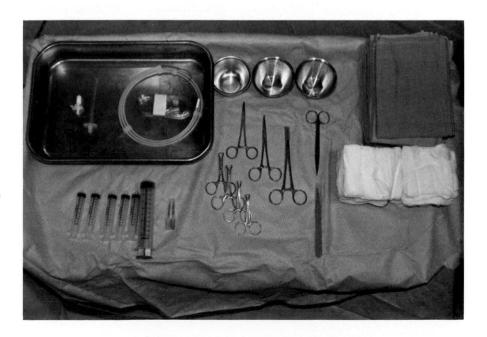

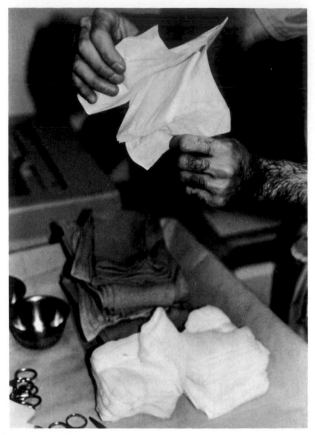

The unsterile technologist is demonstrating how sterile 4 × 4's are removed from their packaging and placed onto the sterile examination tray.

Sterile table covers, drapes, and gowns could be included as part of the sterilized angiographic tray or should be prepared individually in sterile packs. In either case, extra sterilized packs of linen goods should be available for immediate use.

It is assumed that in modern-day angiography most trays contain disposable products. Disposable products are intended for one-time use only and are designed to eliminate the possibility of cross-contamination. However, the specifics of tray contents are usually indicated by the preference of the physician or radiologist performing the interventional procedure.

Disposable products such as needles are usually added to the sterile tray by the "sterile" technologist who is gowned and gloved. In order for disposable sterile items to be removed from their packages without contamination, the sterile technologist is assisted by another member of the angiographic team. Needles of various sizes are included for the radiologist to select from. The needles can then be affixed to the syringes that carry out the various functions. A 25-gauge × $\frac{5}{8}$″ needle and a 22-gauge × $1\frac{1}{2}$″ needle should be used for injecting the local anesthetic. One 18-gauge × $1\frac{1}{2}$″ needle is used to aspirate local anesthetic

from the vial. One 18-gauge × $2\frac{3}{4}$″ needle is included for percutaneous access. A fingertip control Luer-Lok 10-ml syringe is used to inject local anesthesia. To make an incision in the skin, a No. 11 blade should be provided. Once a skin incision is made, a 5″ curved mosquito hemostat is used to divide the superficial soft tissues. A three-way plastic stopcock should be included for attachment to the proximal end of the catheter. Procedural trays are often prepared for use according to an "equipment list" provided in advance by the radiologist. This list identifies the radiologist's personal preferences. Specific catheters and guide-wires, needles, forceps, and scalpel blades are examples of items selected by the radiologist. In other cases, radiologists are satisfied with commercially prepared trays designed for one-time use (disposable).

Dedicated Procedural Tray-Sets

It is economically practical to purchase commercially prepared, disposable tray-sets for specialty procedures that necessitate the use of special instruments and needles. Many nonvascular interventional percutaneous procedures such as nephrostomy, biliary decompression, biopsy, and drainage employ these specially dedicated procedural tray-sets. These prepared tray-sets are usually sealed in plastic to ensure outside barrier and long-term sterility. Before opening any sterile package, it should be inspected to ensure that the package is intact and definitely sterile. The tray-set can be opened completely so that the "sterile" technologist can pick it up or the contents can be dropped carefully onto the sterile field.

Regional Site Preparation

Percutaneous invasive procedures require the complete removal of regional hair and a thorough cleaning or cleansing of the region. Regional hair removal requires a physician's order. Hair removal may take place in the patient's hospital room or in the radiology department. If hair removal is to be completed in the radiology department, it is preferred that the patient be prepared while on the "cart," before being placed on the angiographic table. This decreases the chance of particulate contamination caused by hair and other particulate matter possibly settling on the regional site or other clean areas when the patient is being transferred.

Patient transfer should be performed by an unsterile technologist. The patient should be told what is going to take place during every step. Angiography requires that a percutaneous needlestick be applied to various areas of the body. These areas must be prepared so that the injection site is as clean as possible. Regardless of where this initial preparation takes place, it is essential that the patient be informed about what you are about to do and why you are doing it.

Every attempt should be made to recognize the patient who is self-conscious. This is inclusive of both males and females and especially pediatric patients. The patient often communicates his or her uneasiness nonverbally by facial expression and by other body mechanics. Patients are often too embarrassed to voice an objection. The technologist must be observant and should always be sensitive to the patient's feelings or to situations that may require extra consideration. Patients who are frightened, embarrassed (due to being undraped during the removal of body hair), or in pain often require extra assurance. Patients may have had a bad experience with a procedure that was performed previously. It is good practice for the technologist to assess the patient at the outset of patient preparation.

The first step in regional site preparation is hand washing. Throughout the medical profession, the process of hand washing should be second nature to all health care professionals. The technologist washes his or her hands before gowning and gloving. Percutaneous invasive procedures require the complete removal of regional hair and a thorough cleaning or cleansing of the region. A hospital orderly may prepare the patient in his or her room, or a technologist may prepare the patient while he or she is lying on the cart in the radiology department. Before shaving, the region is saturated with a solution of surgical soap and tepid tap water. The air temperature in the angiographic suite is often noticeably cooler than that of the holding or recovery area. Cold solutions that come into contact with the skin merely add to patient discomfort and anxiety. One might consider warming the solutions in a 37 to 40° C water bath. Parker Laboratories manufactures an apparatus that is a gel warmer for ultrasonic gels. This instrument can also be used to warm the preparation solutions.

Surgical soaps such as chlorhexidine gluconate (Hibiclens) and pHisoHex (a trademark for an emulsion containing hexachlorophene that is used as a skin cleanser) serve many purposes. The soap tends to "lubricate" the regional hair and facilitate a smoother, less resistive stroke with the razor blade; the soaps are hypoallergenic, thus reducing skin irritation, and they are germicidal in their action. Hair from the proposed injection site and the surrounding area (6 to 10″ surrounding the injection site) is shaved with short, firm strokes. For an inguinal or axillary preparation, the technologist must be sure to hold the skin taut and shave in the direction of hair growth (Fig. 4–9).

Once the hair has been removed from the surrounding region, the surfaces are rinsed and excess soap is removed. The region is patted dry and covered with a sterile towel. The technologist must discard all contaminated articles, including the gown and gloves. Once this is done, the technologist can now move the patient onto the angiographic table. Scout films (usually taken in two planes, such as anteroposterior and lateral) are taken. In addition to establishing positioning and technique protocols, the technologist should again verify patient information and ensure that the images reverify patient identification and that directional leaded markers are visible within the film emulsion.

Once the scout films have been taken, the technologist starts to complete the next step in preparation of the injection site. The work station is re-established; an antiseptic scrub set is prepared; and sterile gloves and a new gown are now worn. With the regional site,

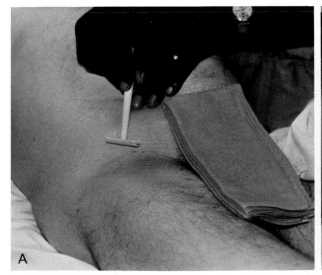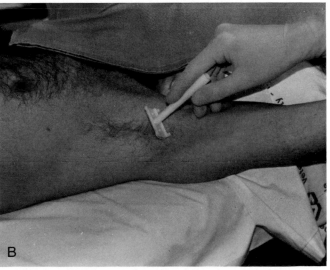

▶ **Figure 4–9**

A, The technologist is performing an inguinal preparation of the injection site. After being washed and lubricated with a soap solution, the skin is shaved with a disposable safety razor. Note that the technologist is facilitating a smooth, clean stroke by carefully applying some skin traction. *B,* The technologist is shaving the axilla in preparation for an percutaneous axillary approach. Note that the arm is raised over the head, resulting in tautness of the skin surface, facilitating a smooth, clean stroke of the safety razor.

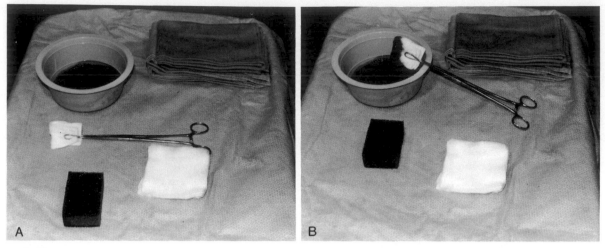

▶ **Figure 4–10**

A, Typical preparation tray set-up: sterile towels, several sterile 4 × 4's, a sterile plastic basin containing povidone-iodine (Betadine) solution, a povidone-iodine–impregnated sponge, and a long forceps. Note that the 4 × 4 is folded into quarters and secured by the teeth of the forceps. *B*, The forceps with a sterile gauze has been immersed into povidone-iodine solution in preparation for the application to the skin.

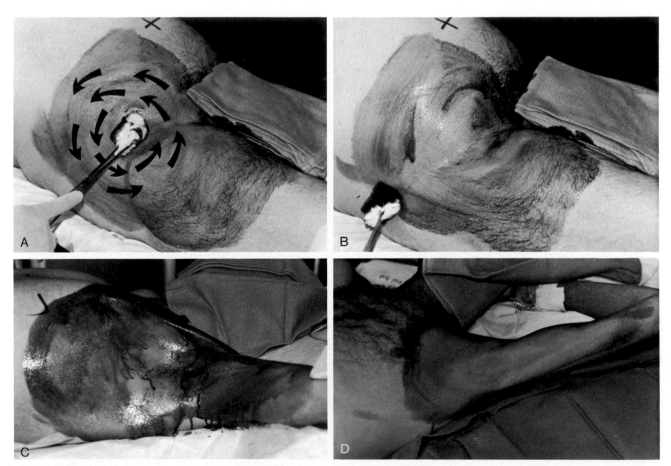

▶ **Figure 4–11**

A, With the genitals covered wtih a sterile cloth, the technologist begins a surgical scrub of the inguinal region at the approximate site of injection, working in a clockwise or counterclockwise motion. *B*, The circular motion enlarges until a significant surface has been covered. Note the "x" that marks the site for entrance of the x-ray beam. This mark was made during scouting. *C*, An example of an axillary surgical scrub. *D*, A completed axillary scrub. The surface will then be draped.

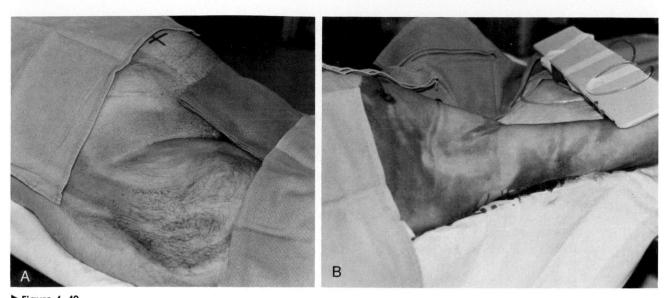

► **Figure 4–12**

A, The inguinal region is now prepared. The surrounding surfaces are covered with cloth drapes, creating a rectangular field. *B,* A rectangular field is now created for an axillary approach.

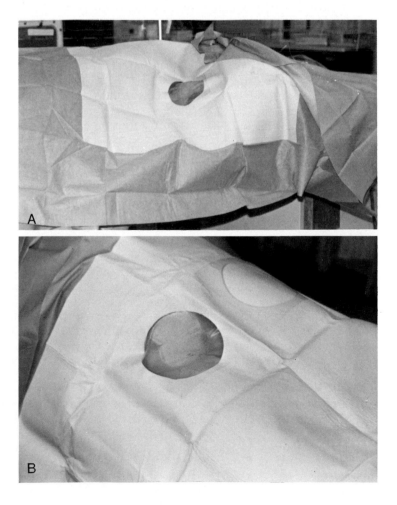

► **Figure 4–13**

A, Single-hole barrier drape. *B,* Bilateral femoral barrier drape.

which is free of external hair, the exposed surface area is now cleansed with antiseptic solutions. Povidone-iodine (Betadine) and alcohol are two frequently used antiseptics. Povidone-iodine is a widely used antiseptic whose action typically lasts longer than do iodine solutions. With regard to patient discomfort, nothing could be worse than applying alcohol to a freshly shaved region. Occasionally, one encounters a patient who is allergic to iodine or has very sensitive skin, and an alternative antiseptic will have to be sought (e.g., hypoallergenic Hibiclens or pHisoHex (Fig. 4–10).

The scrub begins at the site of injection, and a firm clockwise or counterclockwise stroke is applied, moving outward and expanding the border (Fig. 4–11). A long-handled applicator helps to facilitate the cleansing motion. Each time that the sponge completes its circular path, it is discarded. Friction by way of good skin contact is a good way of mechanically removing microorganisms from the exposed area. This scrub is repeated several times. Once the scrub is complete, the area is allowed to air-dry. Once the skin surface is dry, the technologist proceeds to apply sterile drapes to a confined region that surrounds the injection site. The large surface area of skin that was just prepared is now covered with sterile drapes. Cloth or paper drapes will mask the surrounding region, and a smaller area surrounding the site of injection is isolated within a rectangular field. One side of the paper drape contains a sheet of thin plastic that helps to secure the drape to the surrounding region while keeping the skin clean and dry. With cloth drapes, towel clips can be utilized to prevent unnecessary movement or slippage of the drape. Once the region is bordered, the sponge is discarded (Fig. 4–12).

The region should be scrubbed for no less than 3 minutes. We recommend a 10-minute scrub. Upon completion, the region is rinsed with sterile water and patted dry with a sterile towel. A circular drape is placed over the prepared area in final preparation for entrance of the needle (Fig. 4–13).

Almost all foreign objects that enter the vascular system are thrombogenic or clot-forming. Clot formation within the vascular system is the most significant complication that can occur during angiography. These clots form on the surface of guidewires and catheters; they have the potential to travel within the vascular system and can result in fatal occlusions of the brain and heart. Many patients who require angiography are older than 50 years of age and suffer from the effects of advanced peripheral vascular disease. Heparinization, therefore, is required for most of these patients. At our facility, the radiologists prefer to employ "systemic" heparinization. The longer time that a procedure takes to complete, the greater is the chance of thrombi forming on the needle, guidewire, or catheter. For procedures that do not extend beyond 45 minutes to 1 hour, one may choose to employ "intermittent" heparinization by which hand injections are made every 2 minutes without interrup-

tion. At our facility, the radiologists have chosen to use 1 to 2000 units of heparin/500 ml of a 5% dextrose and water or normal saline solution. This method provides constant irrigation and is the best method for minimizing thrombi formation.

The individual components of systemic heparinization are shown in Figure 4–14A. The designated amount of heparin is drawn into a 3-ml syringe (Fig. 4–14B). The heparin is then injected into the tubing of the heparin bag (Fig. 4–14C). Plastic tubing is then inserted into the heparin bag (Fig. 4–14D). A pressure gauge is attached to the bag as it is suspended on a standard IV stand, and the bag is then inflated to the desired pressure, which is usually slightly above the patient's systolic pressure (Fig. 4–14E). The heparinized solution flows through the tubing into the patient's vascular system by overcoming the resistance of the arterial pressure.

Once the patient preparation is complete, all pieces of equipment are made ready. The film changers are loaded; all systems are double checked; and the team awaits the arrival of the radiologist. When the radiologist arrives, he or she will review the patient's chart and scout films with one of the technologists. The filming sequences are selected and programmed into the appropriate devices: rapid film changer, x-ray control panel, and automatic injector. Before donning the gloves and gown, the radiologist scrubs his or her hands for 5 to 10 minutes using a disposable stiff brush that contains an antimicrobial agent. The time taken for hand scrubbing varies from one hospital to another. Upon completion of the surgical scrub, the technologist assists the radiologist with the gowning and gloving procedures. The radiologist first opens the sterile gown pack (Fig. 4–15A), then picks the inner portion of the top flap of the sterile gown (Fig. 4–15B), unfolds the gown to its full length (Fig. 4–15C), and inserts his or her arms into the gown with the assistance of the technologist, who pulls the excess material back and secures the gown at the neck (Fig. 4–15D). The unsterile technologist receives a sterile paper waist belt (while in sterile wrapper) (Fig. 4–15E). The radiologist turns in a circular manner (while the belt wraps around the waist), grasps both ends of the belt, and secures it (Fig. 4–15F).

After gowning and gloving, the radiologist greets the patient, reaffirms what is to take place, and prepares to initiate the procedure. A local anesthetic is drawn into a 5-ml syringe (Fig. 4–16). The local anesthetic is injected subcutaneously into loose connective tissue layers under the skin surrounding the injection site. The local anesthesia is rapidly absorbed and quickly desensitizes the area to pain.

Once the site has been anesthetized, the radiologist percutaneously passes an angiographic needle into the target vessel (frequently the femoral artery) and subsequently performs the Seldinger technique (needle-guidewire-catheter). Some radiologists perform a cut-down (incision) to expose the target artery.

The unsterile technologist opens a bottle of contrast medium by removing the metal band and rubber

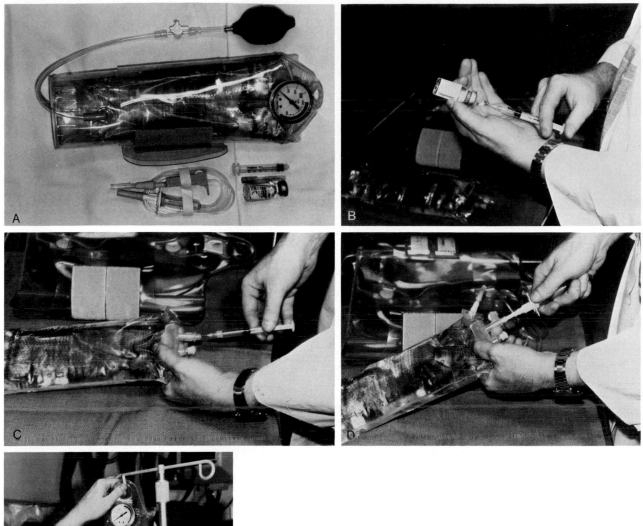

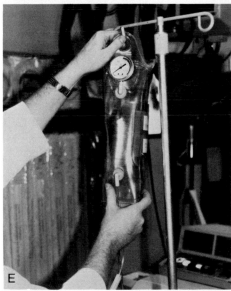

▶ Figure 4–14

A, Components of a constant-pressure pump and heparin bag. B, The technologist is drawing up the heparin. C, Injection of heparin into a wet solution bag of normal saline or dextrose and water. D, Insertion of sterile plastic intravenous tubing into a heparin bag. E, A heparinized solution bag is being hung on an intravenous standard in preparation for use.

stopper (Fig. 4–17A). He or she then carefully pours the contrast medium into a sterile basin (Fig. 4–17B). In a few moments, the radiologist fills a syringe of contrast medium for the purpose of establishing the exact location of the catheter once it is in position, just prior to injection. While the radiologist begins the percutaneous puncture technique, another technolo-

gist team member also dons a gown and gloves and stands ready to assist the radiologist. While this is taking place, another technologist team member loads the contrast medium into the automatic injector (Fig. 4–18). Once the target vessel has been catheterized, the injection parameters are programmed. The patient is once again advised that a certain amount of discom-

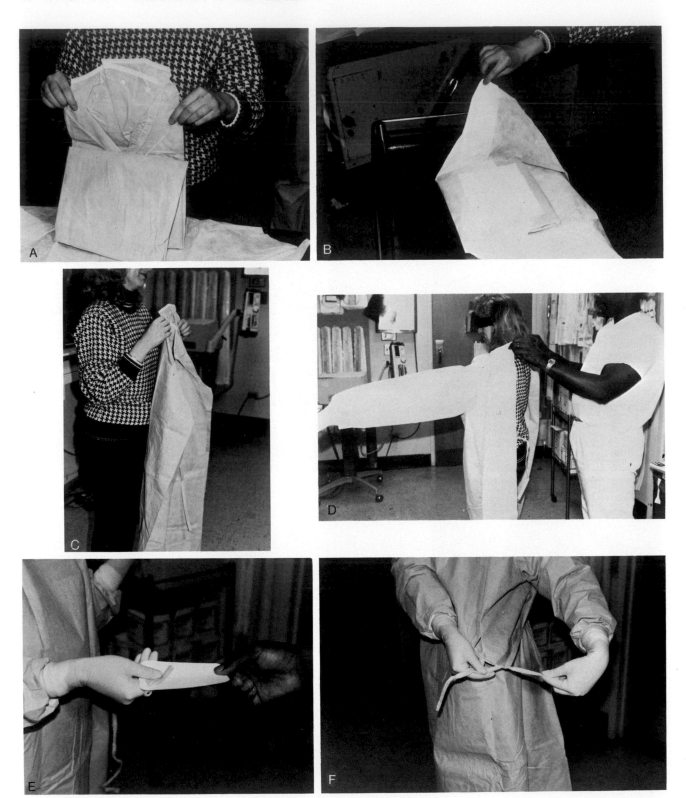

▶ **Figure 4–15**

A, Opening of a sterile gown pack. *B,* The radiologist grasps the inner portion (upper flap) of the gown. *C,* The gown is unfolded to its full length. *D,* The technologist assists the radiologist into a gown. As the arms are thrust into the gown, the technologist pulls the excess material back and secures the gown at the neck. *E,* The unsterile technologist receives a sterile paper waist belt from the gloved radiologist. *F,* The radiologist turns in a circular motion and the waist belt now encompasses the entire waist. The radiologist now secures the waist belt.

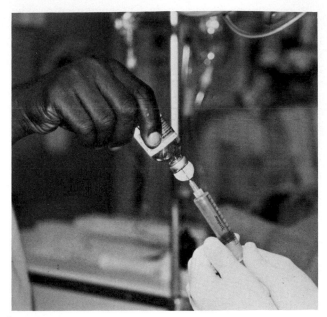

► **Figure 4–16**

The technologist assists the radiologist in loading of a local anesthetic into a syringe.

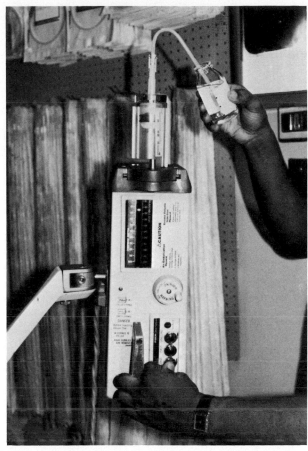

► **Figure 4–18**

The technologist loads the pressure injector with a contrast agent. The vertical position of the injector head allows air bubbles to rise to the top of the syringe.

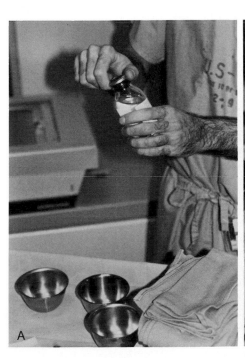

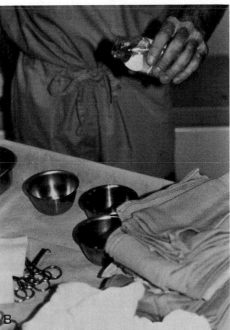

► **Figure 4–17**

A, The technologist carefully removes the metal band and the rubber stopper from a vial of contrast medium. *B,* The technologist carefully pours the contrast medium into the designated sterile basin.

fort will be felt, and the importance of the patient's remaining still during the injection and filming is reiterated.

Specific Site Preparation

Listed below are some methods used to prepare specific sites for invasive/interventional procedures.

Femoral Arteriography. The area over the inguinal crease is shaved from the symphysis pubis (medially) to the lateral border of the hip. Regional preparation extends from the umbilical level to the mid-thigh and includes the perineum. Both sides are prepared in order to give the radiologist a choice of entry.

Axillary Arteriography. The armpit and lateral axillary borders of the chest are shaved. Regional preparation is made to include the dependent side of the chest wall and the shoulder axillary portion to the brachial fossa (elbow).

Translumbar Aortography. The midline and 5″ lateral to the vertebral column should be shaved. Regional preparation should be made from the subscapular area to the top of the buttocks.

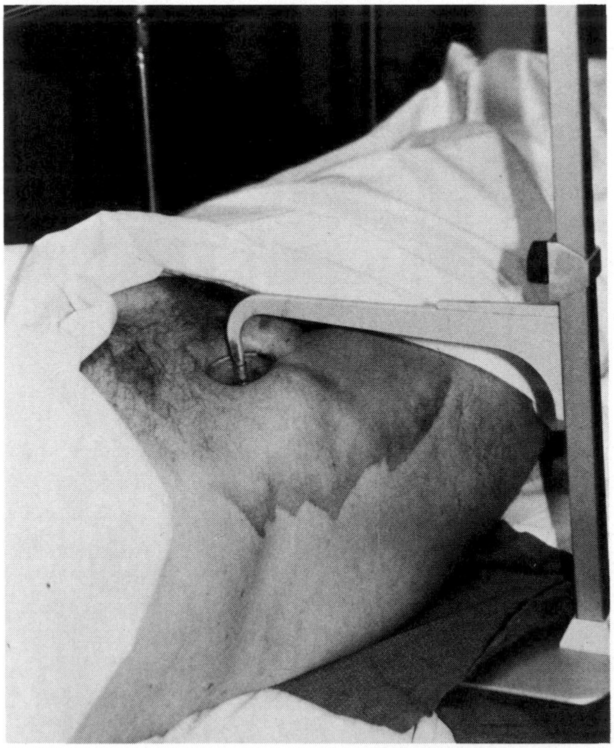

▸ **Figure 4–19**
A C-clamp provides arterial compression to the common femoral artery following the removal of the angiographic needle. This compression is applied while in the angiography suite and is not removed until all bleeding has stopped.

Percutaneous Transhepatic Cholangiography. The right axillary region should be shaved. The area from the axillary plane to the right anterior iliac spine should be prepared. The patient should be placed in an oblique position during the preparation to ensure that the posterior portion of the rib cage is cleansed.

▸ POSTPROCEDURAL ORDERS

Once the angiographic procedure is completed, compression is applied to the injection site immediately after the catheter is removed. This compression is first applied manually with several 4 × 4″ dressings that are held in place by direct pressure of an individual's hand (e.g., by the radiologist or technologist). This compression may be continued with one of many types of devices that secure direct pressure to the injection site. The C-clamp is one type of arterial compression device (Fig. 4–19). The patient is not transported back to his or her room until all bleeding has stopped, compression has been removed, and the site is covered with a bandage.

Postangiographic orders for the completed procedure are included in the patient's chart and include instructions for nursing personnel to follow upon the patient's arrival (Table 4–4).

▸ RADIATION PROTECTION AND SAFETY PROCEDURES

Sources of Scatter and Primary Radiation

In angiography, the potential of increased radiation dosage is significant. Several radiation hazards must be addressed. Scatter radiation is the primary source of exposure to the technologist. The scatter radiation levels off at field sizes greater than 30 × 30 cm^2.[1] The distance from the primary beam is an important consideration for the technologist. The intensity of the beam is inversely proportional to the square of the distance (inverse square law). The scatter radiation intensity is 1 : 1000 of the primary beam 1 meter from the skin entrance site with a 20 × 20 cm field size.[1] The position of the x-ray tube can increase the dose to the technologist by a factor of two. An over-the-table C-arm delivers as much as twice the amount of radiation as an under-patient x-ray tube. When employing cineangiography, scatter radiation accounts for approximately 50% of the total scatter radiation to the primary operator when performing cardiac catheterization. Video recording utilizing a single-frame recording device can significantly reduce the amount of radiation. Precise and expedient use of fluoroscopy (C-arm) by the radiologist or interventional radiologist safeguards both the patient and the technologist from unnecessary radiation.

▶ **Table 4–4**

POSTPROCEDURAL ORDERS ISSUED BY THE RADIOLOGIST
OR ATTENDING PHYSICIAN

1. Complete bed rest ×___16___ hours.
2. Input and output every 6 hours × 24 hours.
3. *Vital Signs:*
   Blood pressure: every 15 minutes × 1 hour, then every hour.
   Pulse: × 4 hours, then every 4 hours × 12 hours.
   Respirations: × 4 hours, then every 4 hours × 12 hours.
4. Check the following:
   ___×___ Groin for hematoma: every 15 minutes × 1 hour, then every hour × 4 hours,
   then every 4 hours × 12 hours.
   ___×___ Dorsalis pedis or posterior tibialis pulses: every 15 minutes × 1 hour, then every
   hour × 4 hours, then every 4 hours × 12 hours.
   ___×___ Leg for warmness and color: every 15 minutes × 1 hour, then every hour × 4
   hours, then every 4 hours ×12 hours.
5. Encourage the patient to take oral fluids.
6. Contact the attending physician for further orders regarding medication and diet
   and for any adverse change in vital signs.

Methods to Reduce Radiation Exposure

Many different types of protective equipment are available for personnel working in the radiation environment of the angiography suite. The Joint Commission on Accreditation of Healthcare Organizations (JCAHO) has published requirements in their rules and regulations that pertain to cardiovascular and invasive/interventional procedures. Many of the following protective devices are a mainstay of those regulations.

All devices should have a required 0.5-mm lead thickness equivalency (NCRP report No. 102 recommends a 0.5-mm lead equivalent). The radiologist and technologist usually wear an apron with a 0.5-mm lead equivalency. All lead aprons must undergo periodic fluoroscopic evaluation, and all tests must be documented in writing with signatures by the appropriate authority. The lead aprons that are now being manufactured include a lead flap that covers and protects the thyroid gland. Lead collars can also be worn to protect the thyroid gland. Thyroid shields (once optional) are now routinely used in the construction of lead aprons. During a typical angiogram, the thyroid dose can be up to 1.7 times that recorded by a radiation badge worn at the collar. Thus, a thyroid shield is a necessity for personnel standing next to the C-arm. Although a pregnancy apron with a 1-mm lead equivalency is available, pregnant personnel should be discouraged from working in the radiation area during the entire gestational period. Specific regulations or recommendations by the State Department of Nuclear Safety, JCAHO, and by the hospital are responsible for determining the standards of practice for pregnant personnel.

Personnel required to have corrected eyewear can choose to purchase leaded eye glasses. Personnel who wear tinted glass lenses gain some benefit from attenuation of the scattered beam. There is a 20-mrem absorption by the lens during a cardiac catheterization. The radiologist or cardiologist should be limited to tending to five patients/wk if lens exposure is not to exceed 5 rem/yr. Leaded eyeglasses absorb at least 70% of scatter exposure. Side shields are mandatory because the primary beam and scatter source are at an angle to the fluoroscopy monitor.[4]

Eye exposure is twice the scatter exposure measured by the collar radiation badge.[3] Leaded shields are usually suspended from the ceiling and are intended to protect the operator's face. These shields absorb approximately 95% of scatter exposure that is received by the head and neck. They also force the primary operator to move away from the primary beam. Ideally, these leaded shields should be wrapped with a sterile transparent plastic. However, they present a major complication, because the leaded shields cannot be used with rotating C-arms and simply get in the way. Leaded shields, which are referred to as "leaves," are usually suspended from the image intensifier, and leaded "curtains," which are located at the side of the fluoroscopy table, are designed to protect the radiologist's legs. Leaded leaves and curtains are mainly relegated to routine diagnostic fluoroscopic procedures, rather than invasive imaging.

Leaded gloves (the heavy, bulky finger or mitt-design types) are used in routine fluoroscopic procedures but are impractical for invasive procedures. In the recent past, radiologists tried wearing an apparatus that was described as a reusable lead-liner that was worn on the hands. The radiologist then placed a sterile pair of plastic gloves over the liner. However, this method did not work well. The gloves were very warm, and the operator's hands perspired heavily. The gloves were cumbersome, and the users complained of a very poor "feel" and difficulty with discrete hand and finger movements. Sterile, lead-

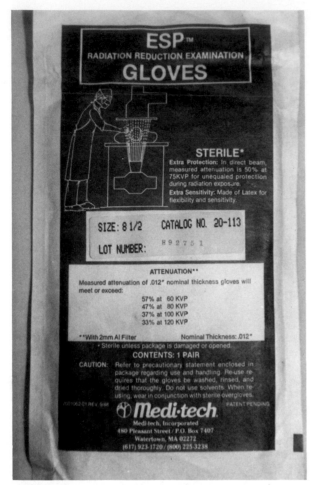

▶ **REFERENCES**

1. Curry TS, Dowdey JE, and Murray RC: Christensen's Introduction to the Physics of Diagnostic Radiology. Philadelphia, Lea & Febiger, 1984.
2. Erlich RA and McCloskey ED: Patient Care in Radiography, 3rd ed. St. Louis, CV Mosby, 1986.
3. Reuter FG: Physician and patient exposure during cardiac catheterization. Circulation 58:134, 1978.
4. Richman AH, Chan B, and Katz M: Effectiveness of lead lenses in reducing radiation exposure. Radiology 121:357, 1976.

▶ **BIBLIOGRAPHY**

Abrams HL: Abrams Angiography: Vascular and Interventional Radiology, 3rd ed. Boston, Little, Brown, 1983.

Hurlbert BJ and Landers DF: Sedation and analgesia for interventional radiologic procedures in adults. Semin Intervent Radiol 4:151, 1987.

Johnsrude IS, Jackson DS, and Dunnick NR: A Practical Approach to Angiography, 2nd ed. Boston, Little, Brown, 1987.

Kadir S: Diagnostic Angiography. Philadelphia, WB Saunders, 1986.

Kandarpa K: Handbook of Cardiovascular and Interventional Radiologic Procedures. Boston, Little, Brown, 1989.

Kee JL: Laboratory and Diagnostic Tests with Nursing Implications. East Norwalk, CT, Appleton-Century-Crofts, 1983.

Larson E: Innovations in health care: Antisepsis as a case study. Am J Public Health 79:92, 1989.

Pagana K and Pagana T: Diagnostic Testing and Nursing: A Case Study Approach. St Louis, CV Mosby, 1982.

Reuter S, Redman H, and Cho K: Gastrointestinal Angiography. Philadelphia, WB Saunders, 1986.

Swamy S, Segal L, and Mouli S: Percutaneous Angiography. Springfield, IL, Charles C Thomas, 1977.

Torres LS: Basic Medical Techniques and Patient Care For Radiologic Technologists, 3rd ed. Philadelphia, JB Lippincott, 1987.

Tortorici MR: Fundamentals of Angiography. St Louis, CV Mosby, 1982.

Watson JC: Patient Care and Special Procedures in Radiologic Technology. St Louis, CV Mosby, 1974.

White RI: Fundamentals of Vascular Radiology. Philadelphia, Lea & Febiger, 1976.

▶ **Figure 4–20**

Radiation-reduction examination gloves worn by the radiologist during an angiogram. The attenuation factors are listed on the packaging.

impregnated surgical gloves are now available. These gloves can be used by the radiologist or cardiologist during a special procedure (Fig. 4–20). Just like other optional items, these lead-impregnated gloves are not for everyone. Although they afford increased protection to the hands of the radiologist, some radiologists indicate that the gloves just don't have a good "feel." Manipulations of guidewires and catheters are delicate maneuvers that may be influenced by the sensitivity of a material and the ease by which the radiologist can manipulate those devices in the arterial system. However, the gloves do provide an 0.38-mm lead equivalent protection to the hands.

The radiologist, hospital physicist, and hospital radiation safety officer are individuals who usually decide which radiation safety devices are purchased for the department of radiology and cardiovascular/interventional technology.

▶ **SELF-ASSESSMENT QUIZ**

1. _____ contact   a. Agents suspended in air or dust
2. _____ indirect contact   b. Transmission via the nose or mouth
3. _____ droplet   c. From one person to another
4. _____ vehicle   d. Infected objects to a host
5. _____ airborne   e. From equipment and blood

6. What specific change took place in hospitals that significantly reduced hospital deaths?
   a. certification of health care workers
   b. employees unionized
   c. all personnel wore white clothing
   d. hand washing and the use of antiseptics before and after patient contact

7. In the vascular suite, the primary source of infections is or are
   1. due to poor patient preparation
   2. the patient's own immune system
   3. angiographic personnel
   4. angiographic equipment and instruments
      a. 1 only
      b. 1 and 2
      c. 3 and 4
      d. 1, 2, 3, and 4

8. If the technologist thinks that his or her surgical gloves are contaminated but is not sure, what should he or she do?
   a. discard them immediately
   b. wash them with soap
   c. pretend it did not happen and tell no one
   d. wash them with alcohol

9. In a sterile field, what happens if a technologist places his or her hands below his or her waist?
   a. they are contaminated and he or she should wash his or her hands
   b. they are contaminated and he or she should change gloves
   c. the technologist is only allowed to prepare the patient but not participate in the procedure
   d. nothing: the technologist can place his or hands anywhere that he or she wishes

10. When opening up a sterile cloth pack, the tray should be positioned with the triangular flap
    a. facing opposite the technologist
    b. facing to the right of the technologist
    c. facing the technologist
    d. facing to the left of the technologist

11. When preparing the patient with iodine or a surgical soap, you use a firm _____ stroke.
    a. front to back
    b. forward
    c. counterclockwise or clockwise
    d. side to side

12. How long should a surgical scrub take to complete?
    a. 1 minute
    b. 2 minutes
    c. 5 to 10 minutes
    d. 5 to 15 minutes

13. Which of the following facts would be part of a patient history?
    1. allergies
    2. hematocrit
    3. prothrombin time
    4. blood pressure
       a. 1 only
       b. 1 and 2
       c. 1, 2, and 3
       d. 1, 2, 3, and 4

14. Which of the following laboratory tests does not determine coagulation time?
    a. PT
    b. PTT
    c. APTT
    d. hematocrit

15. Which of the following tests is the MOST sensitive?
    a. APTT
    b. PTT
    c. Pro-time
    d. PT

16. Meperidine (Demerol) and morphine sulfate are examples of
    a. analgesics
    b. sedatives
    c. antihistamines
    d. anticoagulants

17. Heparin and warfarin (Coumadin) are examples of
    a. analgesics
    b. sedatives
    c. antihistamines
    d. anticoagulants

18. What is povidone-iodine (Betadine)?
    a. an antiseptic
    b. an antiemetic
    c. a narcotic
    d. a sedative

19. Which type of isolation is used to protect the patient from being infected via x-ray equipment?
    a. enteric
    b. respiratory
    c. protective
    d. strict

20. In terms of opportunistic disease, what should the technologist look for in the patient's clinical history?
    1. blood-borne diseases
    2. respiratory infections
    3. antibiotic-resistant infections
    4. organ transplantation
       a. 1 only
       b. 1 and 2
       c. 1, 2, and 3
       d. 1, 2, 3, and 4

▶ STUDY QUESTIONS

1. List and describe three reasons why an arteriogram would be ordered.

2. List the names of three laboratory tests designed to determine blood clotting time.

3. What information is provided by a hematocrit?

4. Describe four or five guidelines for the administration of premedication.

5. List and describe five medications that may be administered prior to a cardiovascular or interventional procedure.

6. Explain why technologist-patient communication has a direct bearing on the success of an invasive procedure.

7. List and describe three methods of transmitting infection.

8. What is meant by "body substance precautions"?

9. List and describe five rules for surgical asepsis.

10. Describe the procedure for preparing the injection site for percutaneous puncture.

▶ SECTION TWO

▶ EQUIPMENT AND IMAGE ENHANCEMENT TECHNIQUES

CHAPTER FIVE

► SELECTION, OPERATION, AND FUNCTION OF ANGIOGRAPHIC EQUIPMENT

► CHAPTER OUTLINE

Basic Suite Design
Optional Suite Considerations
    Storage Space
    Control Area and Equipment Room
    Darkroom Facilities
    Film Viewing
    Tray Set-Up and Disposal Rooms
    Patient Observation and Recovery Area
Imaging Equipment
    Generators
    X-Ray Tubes
    Fluoroscopy Systems

Image Intensifier
Television Monitors
Procedural Tables
Serial Film Changers
Automatic Injectors
Filters, Grids, and Screen-Film Combinations
Guidewires
Catheters
    Criteria for Catheter Selection
Needles
Supplementary Equipment
Systemic Heparinization

► CHAPTER OBJECTIVES

Upon completion of Chapter 5 the technologist will be able to:

1. State a rationale for building and having an angiography suite
2. Draw a floor plan for an angiography suite
3. List the primary pieces of equipment found in an angiography suite
4. Identify the ancillary equipment found in an angiography suite
5. Describe a design model for a control room, film-viewing area, and darkroom facilities

► BASIC SUITE DESIGN

The first consideration in the planning of a cardiovascular (angiography)/interventional suite is to determine the quantity and variety of procedures that will be performed on a monthly basis. Outfitting angiography suites is an expensive process, and it is a waste of money when expensive equipment is underutilized. Consideration must be given to the items that are included with the purchase price of the equipment as well as to options that involve additional costs.

In consideration of the suite design, it is important to note that cardiovascular/interventional procedures are invasive and must be conducted in a sterile environment. The facility must provide for an area to conduct surgical asepsis.

The suite should be large enough to comfortably accommodate all primary equipment and accessories. In addition, there should be enough space to accommodate emergency equipment in the event of life-threatening situations. A special procedures or angiographic suite should be at least twice the size of a standard radiographic and fluoroscopic room.

Ideally, the room should be at least 500 to 600 ft² with a minimal width of 20 ft (not including the observation/control room). The space should be rectangular and should allow for a ceiling height of 9'. This height allows for ceiling-crane suspension of tubes, monitors, injectors, and other equipment so that they will not cause interference if a person walks around the suite. All wiring and transformer cables should be concealed in order to maximize the floor space (Fig. 5–1).

Two types of ceiling illumination are necessary for the angiographic suite. Multiple fluorescent lights serve as the major light source, and incandescent lights provide the "soft" background light source. The latter should be controlled with a rheostat switch to vary the light intensity according to the needs of the radiologist.

Whenever possible, the suite should be equipped with a stainless-steel sink and a standard leg- or foot-activated surgical scrub sink. The scrub sink can be situated anywhere within the procedural suite that does not require the physician and assistants to pass between the sterile tray and the patient in order to wash their hands and don surgical gowns.

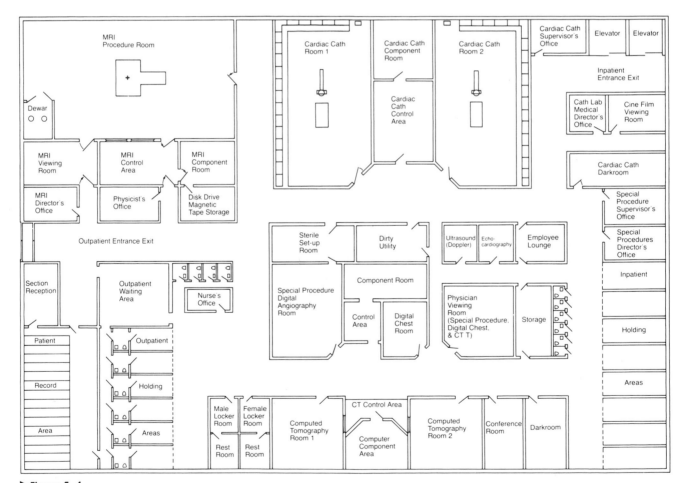

► **Figure 5–1**

This shows a floor plan for a modern, high-technology section of an imaging department. (From Williams CO and Groce KA: The importance of appropriate suite designs in the era of computerized imaging. Radiol Clin North Am 24(3):337, 1986).

▸ OPTIONAL SUITE CONSIDERATIONS

Storage Space

The angiographic suite must have ample storage space. All storage areas should have doors. For easy access, angiographic catheters should be stored in an upright position. The support brackets should be able to support reasonable numbers of each type of catheter that is routinely used. Many storage systems are possible. The type of storage depends on the layout of the physical facilities, the financial considerations, and the preference of the radiology staff (Fig. 5–2).

Control Area and Equipment Room

The control area should be separate from the procedure room and should contain adequate floor space (50 to 75 ft²). This area usually accommodates the x-ray generators, the component modular cabinet racks, and an air conditioner. Most important, the component layout must provide ready access to the cabinets for maintenance and repair.

A separate control room for x-ray and image-recording devices is recommended. Control panels for exposure equipment and programming devices for the rapid film changer should be adjacent to the proce-

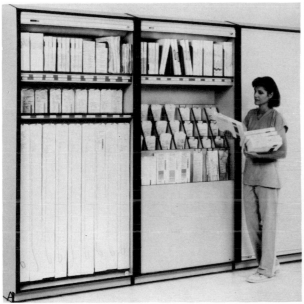
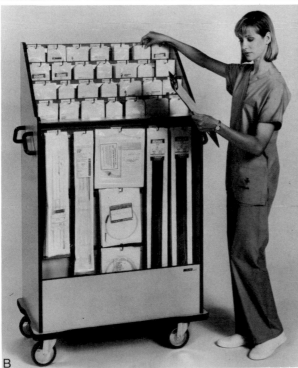
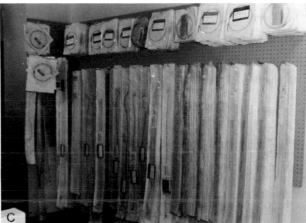
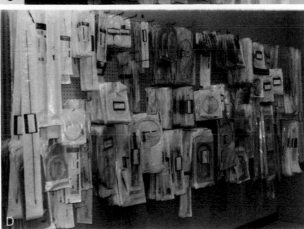

▸ Figure 5–2

A, Examples of commercially prepared storage systems. These are the CS-200 and CS-300 Medical Storage Systems. *B,* An example of a commercially prepared portable storage system. This is an AS-440 Portable Storage System for catheters and accessories. (*A* and *B,* Courtesy of Datel Medical Storage Systems, Grand Rapids, MI.) *C* and *D,* Examples of a simplified and inexpensive storage system constructed by technologists, consisting of a pegboard and assorted hooks for attachment of catheters and assorted accessories and supplies.

dural suite. Holding areas are essential to the needs of a present-day angiographic suite. Patient holding areas serve as an observation/recovery/waiting area for patients who have been examined and who are awaiting transportation back to their rooms and also for patients who are awaiting their scheduled procedures. This area keeps the patients clear of the traffic in the hallway adjacent to the angiographic suite. The holding areas should be equipped with defibrillators with intrapaddle electrocardiographic capacity, an emergency crash cart, electrocardiographic monitors, blood pressure cuffs, stethoscopes, and other life-saving equipment and accessories (Fig. 5–3).

Darkroom Facilities

Planning of the special procedure area should include space for a dedicated darkroom. This darkroom should be well ventilated and should include chemical automixers installed beside the standard replenishment tanks. These devices provide improved quality assurance of the processed radiographs and reduce the hazards of odor and spillage on the personnel who prepare the replenishment chemicals. The darkroom should also contain space for a cine film processor, a radiographic duplicator, and a subtraction unit.

Film Viewing

Film viewing rooms should be located near the darkroom. Adequate viewing and counter spaces are necessary to better review and evaluate the radiographs and comfortably provide space for the radiologist, technologists, and physicians to discuss the next step that will be taken with each patient. Whenever possible, a motorized film viewer should be utilized. This illuminator can accommodate several hundred radiographs. All viewing lamps should be of equal brightness. A counter surface or small table can be provided for the radiologist to interpret the radiographs and dictate the radiologic report after completion of the procedure. This is advantageous for the patient and referring physician as well as for the radiologist. The results of the procedure can be immediately dictated and recorded in the patient's chart. The attending physician or surgeon can then plan the next step in the patient's treatment.

Tray Set-Up and Disposal Rooms

Depending on allocated space, separate areas should be provided for the setting up and tearing down of trays. One designated area will facilitate the set-up of

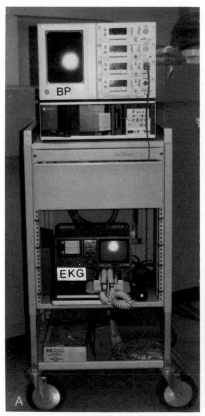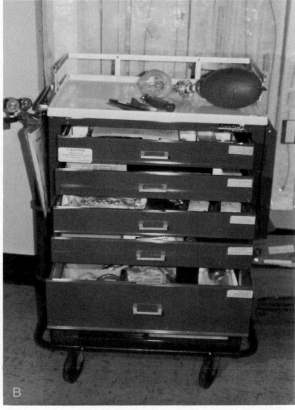

▶ **Figure 5–3**

A, Self-contained unit that includes an electrocardiogram monitor (EKG), defibrillator (DF), and internal blood pressure monitor (BP). B, Mobile emergency crash cart consisting of multiple drawers of varying depths, which make possible the storage of many life-saving implements and life saving drugs. An oxygen tank is mounted on the side of the cart. A spacious countertop and hard rubber wheels complete this essential piece of equipment.

trays for scheduled procedures. Mistakes, unnecessary contamination of items, and equipment omissions can be minimized if the technologist has a reasonable area in which to prepare for a procedure. Another room could serve as a "contaminated instrument room." A separate work area is a necessity for several reasons. When tearing down tray-sets, after the completion of a procedure, it is essential that contaminated articles be disposed of in a proper manner. It is possible that accidental needlesticks could occur when the technologist is distracted during tray disassembly. The contaminated instrument area should have floor-mounted cabinets to store cleaning supplies that are used frequently. An "aseptic" work sink is necessary to wash away contaminated solutions. Both rooms should have large trash receptacles that are plainly marked in order to reduce cross-contamination from biohazardous materials (see Fig. 4–3).

Patient Observation and Recovery Area

Patients awaiting their procedures and patients waiting to be transported back to their rooms should be placed in a designated observation or recovery room, rather than in an area in public view. Patients awaiting their procedures will be understandably anxious, and patients who have had their examinations may have some form of discomfort. Thus, it is essential that both types of patients be held in an area that can be observed by the technical staff. The observation/recovery area should be equipped with emergency life-saving equipment as well as with necessary items used to monitor the patients' vital signs.

► IMAGING EQUIPMENT

Generators

In modern angiographic and interventional suites, high-performance equipment should be selected. When vascular procedures are performed, minimum ratings of 700 and 1000 mA are recommended because of the short exposure frequency that is required. In departments in which many cardiovascular procedures are performed, a constant potential generator is preferred. A constant potential generator is capable of producing ratings up to 3000 mA and has exposure times as short as 0.001 sec.[1] However, a three-phase 12-pulse generator with a power rating of 85 to 100 kilowatts (kW) at 100 kilovolts (kV) is a very expensive component and must be justified according to the number and quantity of procedures to be performed. The control panel should provide the highest possible current (in milliamperes [MA]) at the shortest possible exposure times. This ensures the best diagnostic quality while minimizing the radiation exposure to the patient.

X-Ray Tubes

When choosing x-ray tubes, their intended application is very important. The smaller the focal spot, the better the image resolution, but the smaller the size of the exposure field. In angiography, it is desirable to produce sharp images of vascular structures. To accomplish this, small focal spots are used. For most nonmagnification studies, a 0.6-mm focal spot does nicely. A 0.6-mm focal spot yields sharper vessel borders compared with a 1- or 1.2-mm focal spot. However, for lateral abdominal studies, it may be advantageous to utilize a 1- to 1.2-mm focal spot.

For magnification angiography, a 0.3-mm focal spot is required. Magnification radiography is discussed in Chapter 6. X-ray tubes with focal spots smaller than 0.3 mm are available to give increased sharpness; however, many factors must be considered when selecting tubes with fractional focal spots (focal spots <1 mm in size). Generally, the smaller the focal spot, the lesser the tube-target-angle, the smaller the field size, and the more expensive the tube. Additionally, when the actual focal spot is smaller, a greater amount of heat is generated on the anode. Anode heat is actually infrared radiation that builds up within the tungsten target when it is struck by the focused electron beam that comes from the filament. With fractional focus tubes, the beam is focused to smaller areas on the target, making it necessary to find a way to quickly dissipate the increased heat. In order to compensate for this increase, the rate of revolutions of the anode is substantially increased. A tube with a 0.3-mm focal spot contains an anode that will rotate about 10,000 revolutions/min. An x-ray tube with a 0.1-mm focal spot rotates about 20,000 times/min. A second factor that affects the temperature of the anode is the angle of the anode. For angiography, the angle of the anode is usually set between 10 and 12 degrees. This reduction in the angle of the anode accounts for the reduced size of the exposed field. Each focal spot has its own tube rating. In the past, the angiographer had to refer to a chart that was supplied by the tube manufacturer for the calculation of anode heat units. However, in most angiographic suites, mechanical devices are built in or connected to the control panel to calculate heat units automatically. Audible and visual indications of tube overload take place if heat unit capacity is reached. In many cases, when heat unit capacity is reached, the rotor does not activate.

Fluoroscopy Systems

The usual system for fluoroscopy is a C- or U-arm. This arrangement permits fluoroscopy in many planes without having to move the patient. Two current examples of fluoroscopic equipment are the Toshiba Model CAS-210B C-Arm Support with Double-Track Ceiling Rail (Fig. 5–4A), and the Picker Cardicon-L Cardiovascular/Interventional Imaging System (Fig.

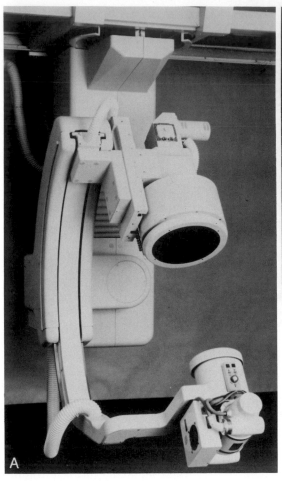

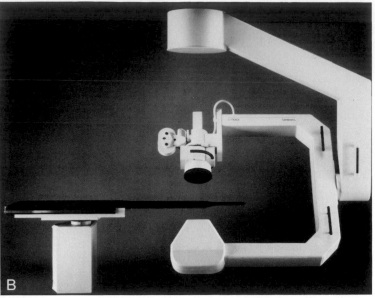

► **Figure 5–4**

A, Toshiba Model CAS-210B C-Arm Support with Double-Track Ceiling Rail. (Courtesy of Toshiba America Medical Systems, Rolling Meadows, IL) *B*, Picker Cardicon-L Cardiovascular/Interventional Imaging System. (Courtesy of Picker International, Inc., Highland Heights, OH.)

5–4*B*). Both systems are designed for cardiovascular, angiographic, and interventional procedures and can efficiently perform head-to-toe fluoroscopy, radiography, and digital fluorography.

Image Intensifier

The purpose of an image intensifier is to convert the x-ray image to a brighter but smaller image on the output phosphor. The specific type of intensifier selected depends on the sophistication of the procedures to be performed. Image intensifiers are available in many different sizes. The diameter of the input screen is determined during the manufacturing process. Common diameters are 6″ and 9″. However, the diameter may be as large as 12″ or 14.″[2] A video or cine camera can be attached to the image intensifier. Many special procedure suites have a high-resolution image intensifier and television with the capability for magnification fluoroscopy that is necessary for small vessel arteriography and interventional procedures. The system can be expanded further to include a 105-mm rapid-sequence spot-film device and video recording system. This equipment is standard in cardiac catheterization laboratories.

Television Monitors

The standard resolution of the television monitor is 525 lines/frame. The primary fluoroscopic television monitor should be positioned in such a way that it does not require the operators to continually rotate their heads for viewing. It is common for the monitors to be mounted on the ceiling and placed across the table from the point where the physician or radiologist is standing. An example of monitor placement is seen in Figure 5–5, which describes the Integris V 3000 Vascular Imaging System by Phillips Medical X-Ray Systems. Note that the video screen on the right is utilized for dynamic DSA imaging, and the monitor on the left is utilized for conventional fluoroscopic imaging and viewing.

Procedural Tables

The angiographic table should be made from a low-absorption material with minimal beam attenuation. The table should be situated in the center of the suite to facilitate free movement by personnel around the table. The table may be mounted off center to be certain that the lateral overhead x-ray tube can be

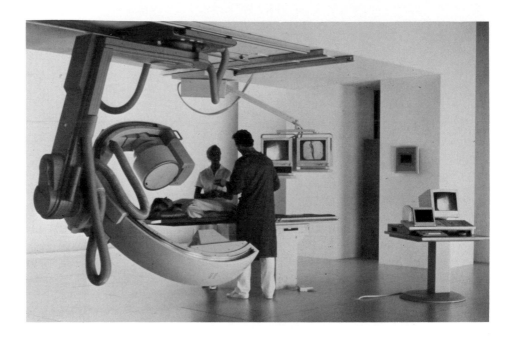

▶ **Figure 5–5**

Phillips Integris V 3000 Vascular Imaging System. (Courtesy of Phillips Medical X-Ray Systems, Shelton, CT.)

adjusted to produce a radiograph with a linear enlargement factor of two. The angiographic table should be of the pedestal type with a free-floating tabletop that can be adjusted to match the height of the radiologist and to perform magnification radiography. For peripheral angiography, a stepping-table is essential. A stepping table will shift the patient over the exposure field (e.g., during the runoff portion of an aortogram). After a flush injection of the abdominal vessels, the table will shift, and subsequent injections and exposures will take place over the pelvis, thighs, legs, and feet. In some situations a cradle-top table is useful (as is a tilt-table) for occasions when the patient is to be placed in an oblique position without being moved; however, the C-arm has eliminated the need for a cradle.

Serial Film Changers

Many types of film changers are available. Film changers are of either the cut-film or the roll-film variety. The cut-film changer is currently being used as the primary film changer in most hospital angiography departments. Some film changers have film supply magazines and receivers that can be used for both anteroposterior and lateral filming. Other magazines can be used in only one projection. Thus, a separate film changer is necessary for each projection. Differences exist in changer magazine capacity (quantity of film) as well as in maximum filming rate. Some film changers contain a keyboard-operated α-numeric film-marking labeling system, and others utilize the standard removable flashcard system. The AOT-S film changer, manufactured by Elema-Schonander, Inc., has a cassette that holds up to 30 single sheets of unexposed 14 × 14″ film. The

AOT-S free-standing rapid film changers can permit up to 6 exposures/sec. For peripheral angiography, either a stepping-table or an extra large field changer using cassettes can be employed. This technique is advantageous for arteriography and venography of the lower extremities.

Figure 5–6 will probably bring back a few memories to the technologist who was practicing biplane angi-

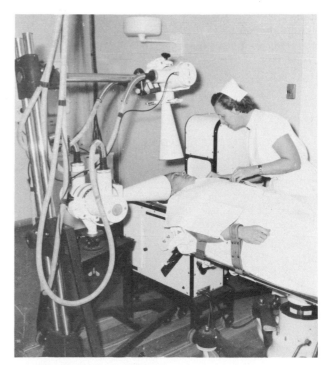

▶ **Figure 5–6**

1950s-era biplane angiography set-up. (Courtesy of Elema-Schonander, Inc., Schaumburg, IL.)

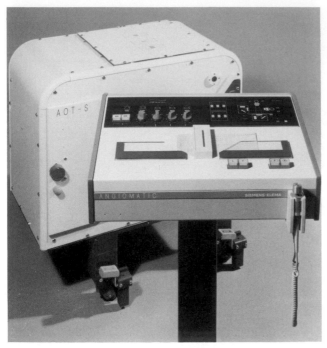

▶ **Figure 5–7**
AP AOT-S Cut-Film Changer with Angiomatic Programmer. (Courtesy of Elema-Schonander, Inc., Schaumburg, IL.)

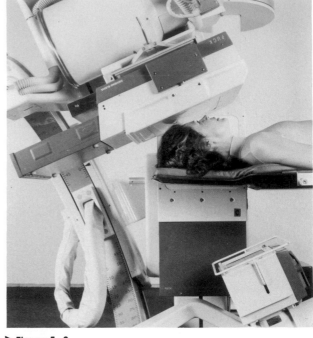

▶ **Figure 5–8**
PUCK Film Changer in biplane format. (Courtesy of Elema-Schonander, Inc., Schaumburg, IL.)

ography in the 1950s. Note that the biplane x-ray tube arrangement is floor-mounted. Figure 5–7 shows an anteroposterior AOT-S cut-film changer with an automatic card-generated serial film control. Figure 5–8 shows how PUCK film changers are arranged in a biplane format. Figure 5–9*A* and *B* shows the most current model SEP 90/PUCK 90M cut-film changer and programmer. Figure 5–10*A* through *F* demonstrates the loading and unloading of the receiver of a PUCK cut-film changer. In Figure 5–10*F* the technologist has grasped the exposed films as he removes them from the receiver and is about to "flip" them so that they will be processed sequentially according to arterial, capillary, and venous phases of circulation. The PUCK cassette holds 20 individual sheets of 14 × 14″ film. Figure 5–11*A* through *F*

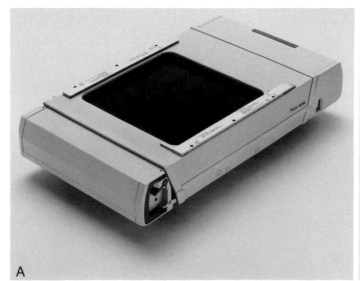

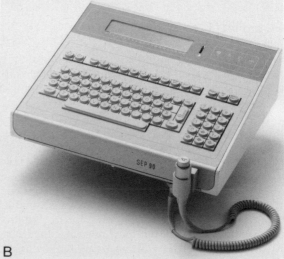

A   B

▶ **Figure 5–9**
A, SEP 90/PUCK 90M Cut-Film Changer. *B,* SEP 90/PUCK Programmer. (*A* and *B,* Courtesy of Elema-Schonander, Inc., Schaumburg, IL.)

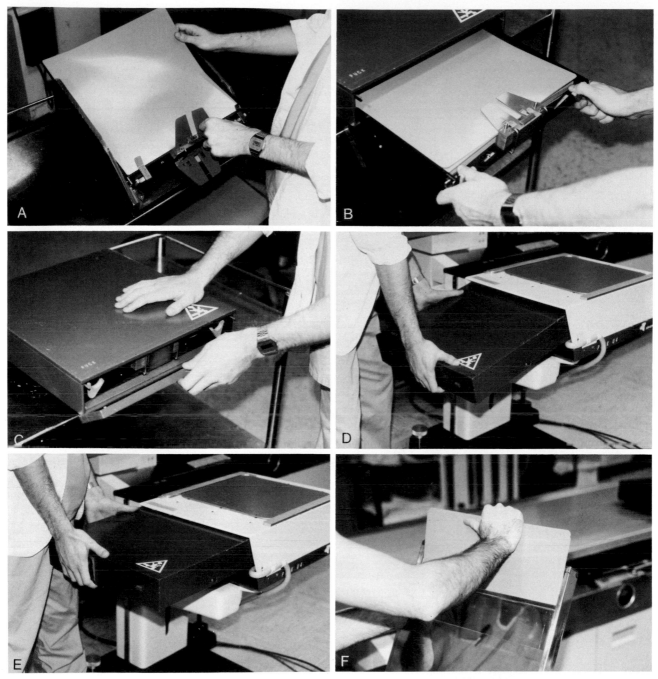

► **Figure 5–10**

A, Darkroom loading of PUCK cassette. *B,* PUCK cassette containing 20 sheets of 14 × 14″ film is loaded into a storage magazine. *C,* The storage magazine is loaded and secured for use. *D* and *E,* Following darkroom loading, the technologist inserts the loaded storage magazine into the PUCK changer. *F,* Following the angiographic run, the technologist in the darkroom removes exposed film from the cassette-film-receiver for processing and development.

demonstrates the sequential loading and unloading of an AOT-S cut-film changer. Notice how the film is guided by the technologist into the storage magazine, and note also the metal spacers that separate each film. The AOT-S storage cassette/magazine can accommodate 30 single 14 × 14″ sheets of film.

Automatic Injectors

Many excellent angiographic injectors are available. One of the more recent innovations is the ceiling-suspended contrast media injector. The ceiling-mounted injector should be part of the initial room design, rather than included as an afterthought. Its

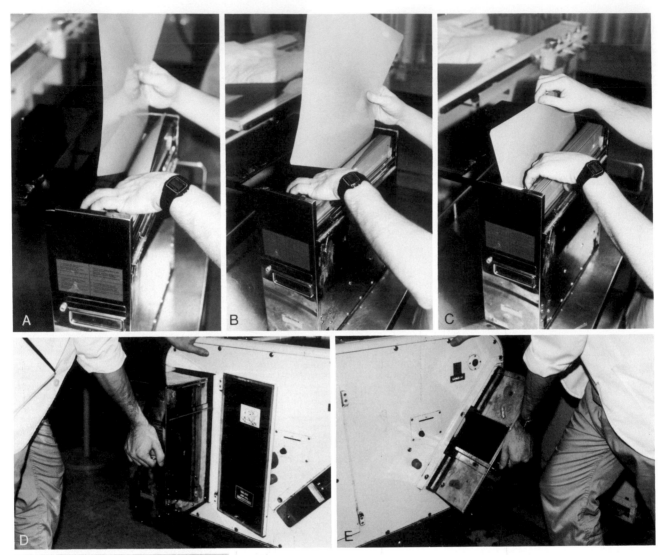

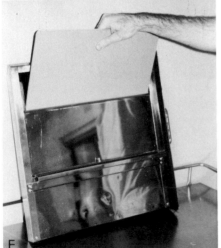

▶ **Figure 5–11**

A to *C,* The technologist is in the darkroom inserting unexposed film into an AOT-S loading cassette. Notice that each film is inserted into a slot that is separated by two metal spacers. *D,* The loading cassette containing 30 individual sheets of 14 × 14" film is inserted into the loading slot of the AOT-S Cut-Film Changer. *E,* After the exposure run, the exposed films are sent sequentially to a receiver cassette. The receiver cassette is then brought to the darkroom. *F,* The exposed films are removed from the receiver cassette and processed so that they will exit the film processor in the correct sequence of circulation. Note that the receiver door locks in the open position.

location must be chosen carefully so that it is not a hazard to other equipment mounted on the ceiling. Figure 5–12*A* and *B* represents two possible configurations of a Medrad OCS 115 Ceiling-Mounted Overhead Counterpoise System. This particular injector head can be positioned exactly at the elevation and angle desired. It swivels horizontally a full 360 degrees and up to $4\frac{1}{2}''$ laterally. This injector can be positioned well out of the way after the injection has been completed. The injector control unit can be either mounted on a rack or placed in a remote location. The injector arm for most injectors can be attached to the table in close proximity to the patient, where it will move with the table during panning or stepping that takes place during a runoff (Fig. 5–13). Injection volume, peak injection rate, and acceleration to peak rate are adjustable. Injection pressure is selected by a switch. Most injectors contain safety features that prevent injection when incorrect variables are established. Flow-rate–guided mechanical injectors with a pressure limiting device are frequently employed. Most injector functions are synchronized with the movement of the angiographic table and serial film changer. Two commonly used injectors include the

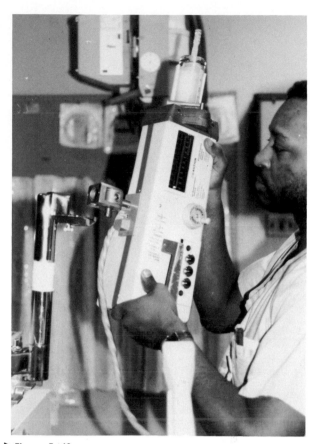

▶ Figure 5–13

The technologist has detached the Viamonte-Hobbs injector head from the console, and he is attaching the injector head to the examination table in preparation for stepping.

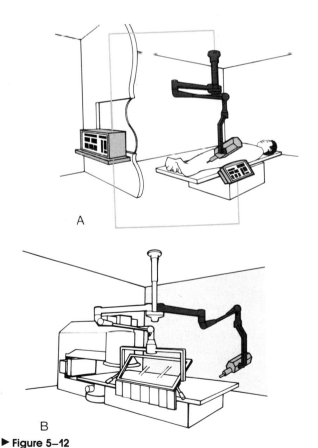

▶ Figure 5–12

A, Medrad OCS 115 Ceiling-Mounted Overhead Counterpoise Injector System. *B,* Alternate Ceiling Mount for Medrad OCS 115 Injector System. (*A* and *B,* Courtesy of Medrad, Inc., Pittsburgh, PA.)

Medrad Mark V system (Fig. 5–14*A* and *B*) and the Viamonte-Hobbs Angiomat 6000 digital injector, manufactured by Liebel-Flarsheim (Fig. 5–15*A* and *B*), which contains a powerful injector head and an advanced microprocessor control console that are mounted on an easily maneuvered mobile stand.

Figure 5–16*A* shows the disposable syringe that is used with the Angiomat 6000 Injector, and in Figure 5–16*B* the technologist is inserting a disposable syringe into the syringe sleeve. Figure 5–16*C* shows the disposable syringe fully inserted into the sleeve, in a locked position. The base of the syringe sleeve is then moved forward, and the syringe is then locked into the vertical (loading) position. Useful features of these injectors include (1) a heating device, which heats the contrast medium to body temperature and reduces viscosity (Fig. 5–16*D*); (2) mechanical injection-limiting capability; (3) flow rates of up to 40 ml/sec; (4) linear acceleration (gradual increase in contrast delivery to prevent catheter recoil); and (5) the capability for injector or film changer delay. Figure 5–16*E* shows the technologist filling the injector syringe. A sterile connector tubing with a Luer-Lok adapter is attached to the injector, while the

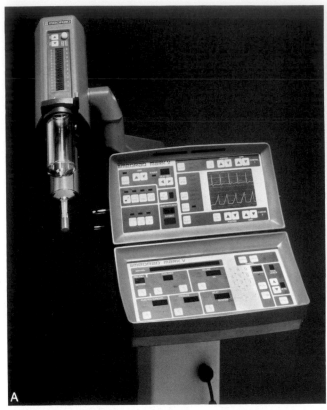

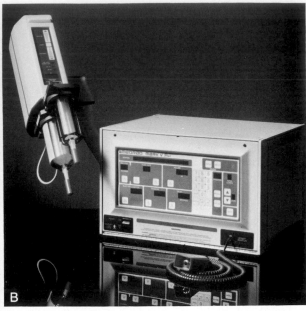

▶ **Figure 5–14**

A, Medrad Mark V Injection System with electrocardiogram trigger. *B,* Mark V Plus, with console. (*A* and *B,* Courtesy of Medrad, Inc., Pittsburgh, PA.)

other end of the tubing is located within an open bottle of contrast medium. The technologist is activating a switch that directs the piston-driven barrel forward and backward until the syringe is full and devoid of any air bubbles.

Filters, Grids, and Screen-Film Combinations

Please refer to Chapter 6 for a discussion of the angiographic applications of filters, grids, screens, and film.

Guidewires

Stainless-steel wires function to provide a guide for the angiographic catheter. The guidewire is most often used in conjunction with the Seldinger technique for percutaneous arterial puncture and catheterization. Current literature states that the average length of a guidewire varies; however, the length of a guidewire is usually twice that of a catheter. Wires can be as short as 30 cm and as long as 260 cm. For most routine angiography (using the Seldinger technique), the guidewire length varies between 50 and 145 cm.

Guidewires can be coated or impregnated with heparin to help prevent clot formation and may also be coated with Teflon to reduce the coefficient of friction. The coefficient of friction refers to the movement of a guidewire within a catheter and the resistance it creates. A Teflon-coated guidewire can advance more smoothly within a catheter compared with a guidewire that is not coated with Teflon. Teflon guidewires less frequently result in sloughing off of the inner catheter wall when the guidewire is advanced. Guidewires that are not coated with Teflon have a greater chance of sloughing off the inner catheter wall and increase the chance for injecting foreign material into the vascular system.

The guidewire basically consists of an outer case of tightly wound stainless-steel, which encloses a wire core that may be either fixed or movable. The inner core is a straight piece of stainless-steel wire. If the inner core is fixed, it is usually secured a short distance from the distal tip of the guidewire. This provides a flexible spring-wire tip that facilitates passage of the guide through sclerotic or tortuous vessels. The length of the standard length flexible guide tip is 3 cm, but 7.5-cm flexible distal-tipped guide tips are also available.

The movable-core spring guide has a movable inner part that can be used to vary the length of the flexible tip. When fully inserted, the inner core is used to straighten guides that have a floppy distal tip. When the inner core is withdrawn, the curve returns.[5] The characteristics of a guidewire are described in Figure 5–17.

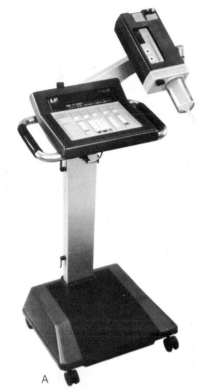

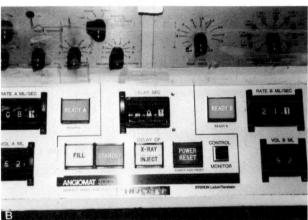

▶ **Figure 5–15**

A, Viamonte-Hobbs Angiomat 6000 Digital Injection System. The compact, powerful injector head and advanced dual processor control console are mounted on an easily maneuvered mobile stand. *B*, Angiomat 3000 Control Panel. (*A* and *B*, Courtesy of Liebel-Flarsheim, Cincinnati, OH.)

Guidewires can be classified into the following categories: introducing; exchange; long, floppy-tipped; deflecting; torque; and open-ended.

The *introducing guidewire* is typically 0.035" or 0.038" in diameter and has a straight or flexible J tip (Fig. 5–18). These wires are coated in Teflon. *Exchange guidewires* (180- to 260-cm lengths) allow for the replacement of catheters (Fig. 5–19). They usually have a relatively stiff body to provide stability and a soft, flexible J tip. *Long, floppy-tipped guide-*

wires are commonly used to bypass severe vascular atherosclerotic plaques and to allow catheters to reach a selective or superselective position (Fig. 5–20). The terms selective and superselective refer to blood vessel branches that extend beyond the trunk or main artery and that are entered by a catheter. For example, the celiac axis/trunk artery is an artery that arises off the abdominal aorta. Following the placement of a guidewire into the aorta and selection of the celiac trunk, a catheter is advanced over the wire until it enters the celiac artery. If an injection is made into the celiac trunk, a selective injection has taken place. If the catheter is advanced further into either the gastric, splenic, or hepatic artery, followed by injection of contrast media, a superselective injection has taken place.

Deflecting guidewires are useful for bending straight catheters, recurving C-shaped or sidewinder catheters, advancing catheters selectively, and retrieving intravascular foreign bodies (Fig. 5–21). *Torque guidewires* offer more control of catheter manipulation and are designed for safe, selective, and subselective catheterization of cardiac vessels and vessels of the brain, abdominal viscera, and extremities. These guidewires are very expensive and are easily damaged. The dedicated tips can easily be kinked by any forceful manipulation (Fig. 5–22). The multipurpose *open-ended guidewire* is water-proofed with Teflon tubing and is open at both ends so that it can be used as a sliding core guidewire, as a fine, injectable catheter, or as a probe for measuring intra-arterial blood pressures (Fig. 5–23). It is especially useful for injecting contrast during angioplasty procedures to document proper positioning and for infusing thrombolytic agents.

Guidewire tips may be straight (Fig. 5–24) or they may be J-shaped with a gentle or tight radius (Fig. 5–25). Straight wires are indicated when the patient's condition is not complicated by atherosclerosis, intraluminal narrowing, or tortuosity. J-shaped wires permit increased maneuverability through tortuous vessels with increased safety. Some J-wires are equipped with a variable stiffness so that, when flexible, they can be safely advanced through eccentrically and concentrically stenosed vessels. When firmness is required for advancing an overlying catheter, this can be imposed on the guidewire by an external manipulator.

Flexible-tipped guidewires can loosen, unravel, or break with repeated sterilization. This can cause damage to the blood vessel. In addition to structural changes occurring in reusable guidewires after repeated sterilization, reusable products have more of a chance of causing blood remnants to be passed from one patient to another (cross-contamination), even with good cleaning and sterilization techniques. Guidewires, catheters, and other angiographic supplies are now manufactured for one-time use and are then discarded. The use of disposable products for cardiovascular and interventional procedures has significantly reduced the chance of cross-contamination.

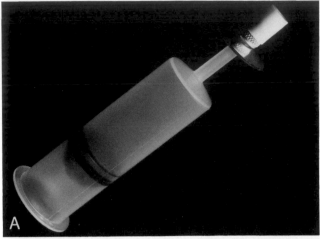

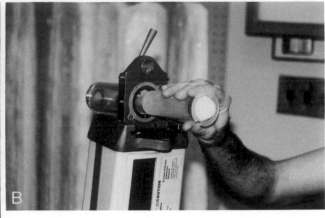

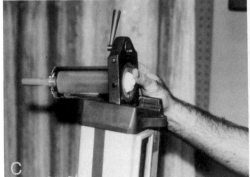

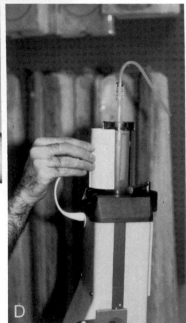

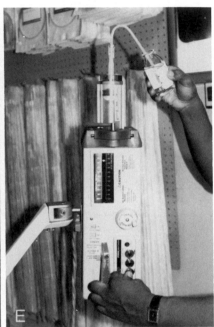

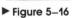

▶ **Figure 5–16**

A, Viamonte-Hobbs Injector Disposable Syringe. (Courtesy of Liebel-Flarsheim, Cincinnati, OH.) *B,* The technologist is inserting a disposable syringe into the syringe sleeve of the Viamonte-Hobbs 3000 Injector. *C,* The disposable syringe is fully inserted and prepared for locking. *D,* The heating device is affixed to the syringe sleeve. The contrast medium should be heated and injected at body temperature. *E,* The technologist is filling the injector syringe with contrast medium.

Catheters

Catheters serve as pipelines for the delivery of a contrast medium from an external source to a specific location within the human body. Catheters are manufactured for diagnostic and therapeutic angiography as well as for other interventional and noninvasive procedures. Many materials are used in the manufacture of catheters. For the most part, catheters are made of polyethylene, Teflon, polyurethane, Dacron, or nylon. Catheters are of varying lengths and diameters. For practical purposes, discussion of the manual or "custom" shaping of catheters, punching in side holes, and so forth is omitted because this practice is antiquated and impractical today. The only benefit of manual catheter construction is lower cost. Polyethylene catheter material on a spool can be purchased less expensively than can catheters sold individually.

Although catheter surfaces may vary, a smooth outer surface decreases arterial trauma. Catheters also vary in the thickness of their inner and outer walls. The catheter's size is determined by the outer diameter. The diameter of the catheter should be the smallest size that allows adequate delivery of a given dose of contrast medium. The inner lumen of a catheter (which is determined by French number and by the thickness of the catheter wall) and the length of the catheter determine the maximal flow rate through the catheter. The system that was devised to determine catheter size, diameter, number, and needle size was created by Charrière, a French surgical instrument maker. This system is called the *French scale* (Fig. 5–26*A* and *B*). With this system, one (each)

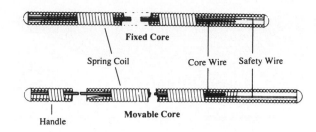

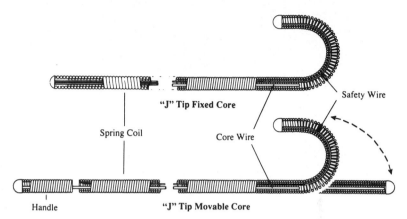

► **Figure 5–17**

A sample catalog page describing the characteristics of guidewires. (From USCI Division, C. R. Bard, Inc., Billerica, MA.)

Charrière unit is equal to $\frac{1}{3}$ mm (0.33 mm), which is also equal to one French number. For example, a 1-mm outer diameter is equal to a No. 3 French catheter. If the diameter is expressed in inches, it is necessary to know that 1″ = 25.4 mm. To convert from inches to millimeters, simply multiply the number of inches by 25.4.

The size of the catheter is especially important when dealing with children. For pediatric patients, sizes No. 3 to 6 French are indicated. In adults, one usually uses French No. 4 to 7. A No. 30 French catheter would be used for intravascular insertion of special instruments or manipulative devices, whereas smaller catheters are used for interarterial digital sub-

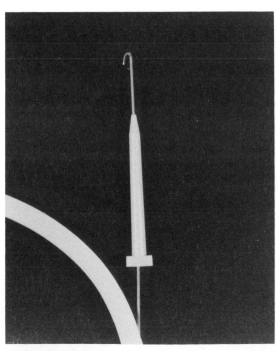

► **Figure 5–18**

Introducing guidewire 0.038″ with flexible J tip.

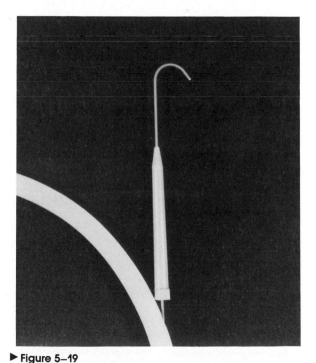

► **Figure 5–19**

An example of an exchange guidewire. This is a TSCF type, 1-mm, with an 0.035″ diameter, 260-cm-long, curved (Amplatz), heparinized guidewire used in catheter exchange. (Courtesy of Cook, Inc., Bloomington, IN.)

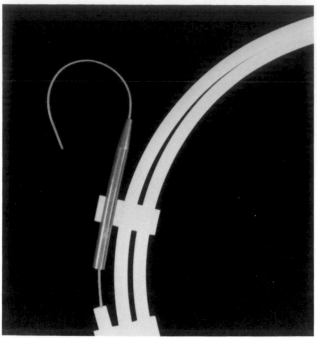

▶ **Figure 5–20**

An example of a long, floppy-tipped guidewire. This has a 15-mm "J," fixed core; flexible distal tip; tapered fixed core; 0.035" diameter; 145 cm in length. This is one of the "floppiest" "J" guidewires. (Courtesy of USCI Division of C. R. Bard, Inc., Billerica, MA.)

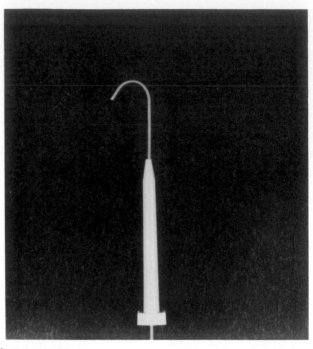

▶ **Figure 5–21**

An example of a deflecting guidewire. This is a TSCF type, Teflon coated, 3-mm curved, fixed core guidewire with a 6-cm, flexible tip. (Courtesy of Cook, Inc., Bloomington, IN.)

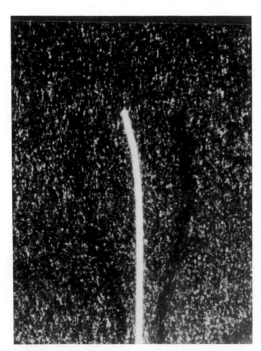

▶ **Figure 5–22**

Example of a torque guidewire. This is an HSF type with a diameter of 0.038", length of 125 cm, and a Lunderquist-Ring Torque guidewire that is indicated for nonvascular interventional studies. This wire is so stiff that it could puncture an arterial or venous wall. Thus, it is not indicated for vascular angiography. (Courtesy of Cook, Inc., Bloomington, IN.)

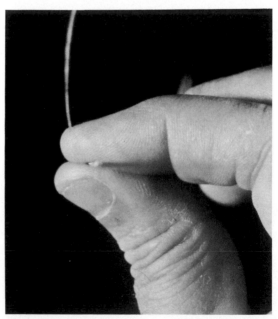

▶ **Figure 5–23**

An example of an open-ended guidewire as seen from above.

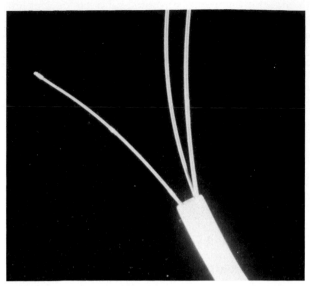

▶ **Figure 5–24**

An example of a straight guidewire.

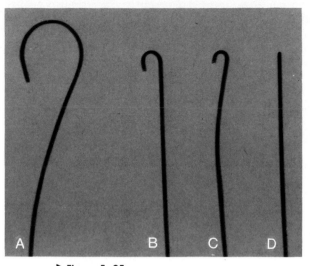

▶ **Figure 5–25**

An example of J wires of different sizes.

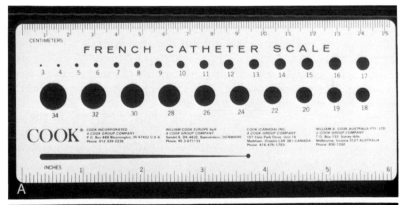

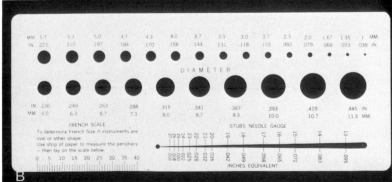

▶ **Figure 5–26**

A, Front surface of a French catheter scale card developed by the French instrument maker Charrière. Each unit or French number is approximately equal to 0.33 mm. *B,* Back surface of a French catheter scale card. (*A* and *B,* Courtesy of Cook, Inc., Bloomington, IN.)

traction angiography. Currently, the trend is to use smaller diameter, thin-walled catheters because improvement in catheter technology and design has made possible the reduction in the amount of contrast medium needed for most procedures.

As described earlier in this chapter, torque refers to the ability of the radiologist to manipulate the catheter within the vascular system. High-torque catheters usually have a reinforced wall to permit the catheter to be maneuvered in a desired fashion. The thin-walled, high-flow catheters do not have braided walls and thus have poorer torque control.

Commercially available catheters are radiopaque, because they are impregnated with barium, bismuth, lead, or other radiopaque material. Many synthetics are currently used in the manufacture of catheters. All catheters used in cardiovascular and interventional procedures are disposable. *Polyethylene* is a catheter material selected by many radiologists. *Polyurethane* catheters have a softer tip and are, therefore, safer for selective placement into aortic branches. This material is rubber-like and is manufactured with a wire mesh within the walls of the catheter shaft. This mesh increases torque control, which is essential for selective catheterization. Catheters made from *Teflon* are useful for mid-stream injections, in which high pressures are necessary for rapid delivery of a contrast medium. When they are used in conjunction with Teflon-coated guidewires, the lowest coefficient of friction is achieved. Teflon catheters have an excellent memory. "Memory" refers to the shaped end of the catheter tip. When a selective catheter is advanced over a guidewire, the catheter tip straightens slightly. When the guidewire is withdrawn from the catheter, the catheter tip should reassume its original shape. A *preformed* catheter is a type of catheter whose tip reassumes its exact shape once the wire is withdrawn.

Dacron catheters accommodate many combinations of catheter tips. The National Institutes of Health (NIH) Gensini, Lehman, and Sones catheters are usually made of Dacron and are used in pulmonary and cardiac angiography and in obtaining cardiac pressures. These catheters are available in both reusable and disposable forms. As described earlier in this chapter, the use of disposable products practically eliminates all possibilities of cross-contamination. Like guidewires, catheters undergo changes with repeated sterilization. Catheters can become brittle and eventually break with repeated use.

Catheters are usually coated with Teflon and are frequently associated with Teflon-coated–heparin-impregnated guidewires. This makes possible the lowest coefficient of friction. All foreign substances, including catheters and guidewires, are thrombogenic (i.e., allow the formation of a blood clot). Blood clots form and adhere to the surface of these foreign objects. Clots commonly form in the side holes and catheter tip. For this reason, catheters are impregnated with heparin when manufactured. Even with

this anticlotting agent, thrombi and fibrin collect and adhere to the surface of the catheter. Catheters as well as guidewires should be irrigated with a heparinized solution and should be placed within a heparin bath when they are not used. The cellular proteins of the blood can aggregate or clump together on a catheter, forming a *thrombus*. If this thrombus breaks off, it will enter the vascular system as a thromboembolism (a moving blood clot) and may result in potentially life-threatening situations, such as stroke (a cerebrovascular accident or a myocardial infarction). To minimize the formation of blood clots, careful attention is directed to flushing catheters and avoiding arterial trauma, spasm, and wedged positioning of the catheter tip. (During a selective or superselective procedure, the catheter tip is located inside the vessel lumen. Usually, this presents a tight fit or "wedged" position.)

There are four basic catheter shapes: (1) straight (Fig. 5–27A), (2) single curve (Fig. 5–27B), (3) double or multiple curve (Fig. 5–27C), and (4) pigtail (Fig. 5–27D and E). Most catheters used for adult angiography are between No. 5 and 7 French in the outer diameter. Straight catheters (with no curve) are used for nonselective arteriography (flush), have an open end, and may or may not have side holes. When present, side holes are placed symmetrically about the circumference of the catheter tip. The side holes help distribute the contrast medium evenly while minimizing catheter whip (recoil). With catheter side holes, flow rate is increased from 15 to 20%. Catheters with side holes (but with a closed end) are useful for intracardiac right heart and pulmonary artery injections. There is no jet effect and minimal recoil with the use of such catheters. Because there is a closed end, these catheters cannot be introduced percutaneously, except through a paper-thin Mylar or Teflon sheath. Percutaneous puncture of the femoral artery with the Seldinger technique is employed with most routine angiography (Fig. 5–28). If a patient has had femoral graft surgery, the axillary artery provides an alternative site for percutaneous puncture (Fig. 5–29).

Catheters can be placed almost anywhere in the body. Catheters that are placed within "trunk" arteries (e.g., the inferior vena cava and abdominal aorta) facilitate a "flush" injection of contrast medium from the trunk vessel to its branches. For example, a straight-tipped catheter placed in the aorta, infrarenally, will demonstrate the visceral branches of the aorta, including the celiac trunk or axis, superior and inferior mesenteric arteries, and renal arteries and their respective branches. Another site for a flush injection is the aortic arch. A pigtail catheter is frequently placed at the aortic arch. An injection at this location demonstrates the primary vessels that arise off of the arch, namely the innominate artery on the right side and the left common carotid and left subclavian arteries on the left side. Pigtail catheters are usually made specifically of polyethylene and Teflon. The pigtail catheter was created to permit an even

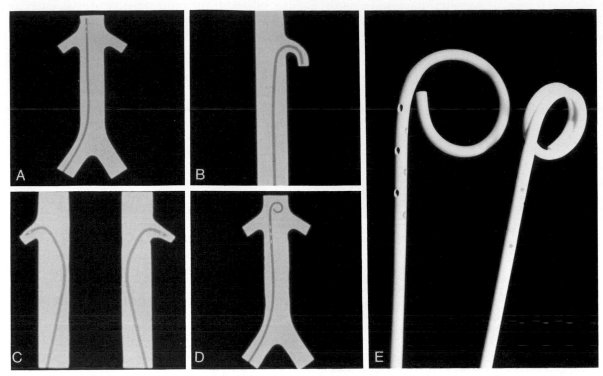

▶ **Figure 5–27**

A, A straight femoral-aortic flush catheter, with an open end and six side holes. *B,* Single J curve–visceral selective catheter, with an open end with no side holes. *C,* Double or multiple curve–visceral selective catheter, with an open end with two side holes. *D,* Pigtail femoral-aortic flush catheter, with an open end and 12 side holes. (*A to D,* Courtesy of Cordis, Inc., Miami, FL.) *E,* Close-up of two different-sized pigtail catheters, revealing symmetrically spaced side holes.

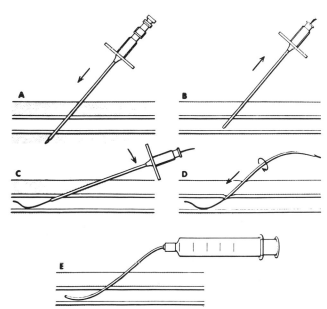

▶ **Figure 5–28**

Application of the Seldinger technique of arterial puncture. *A,* Puncture of both walls of the vessel. *B,* Retraction of the tip of the cannula into the arterial lumen after withdrawal of the needle insert. *C,* Passage of the guidewire through the cannula into the artery. *D,* Passage of a smoothly tapered catheter tip over the guidewire into the artery. *E,* The catheter in the lumen of the artery after withdrawal of the guidewire. (From Curry JL and Howland WJ: Arteriography. Philadelphia, WB Saunders, 1966.)

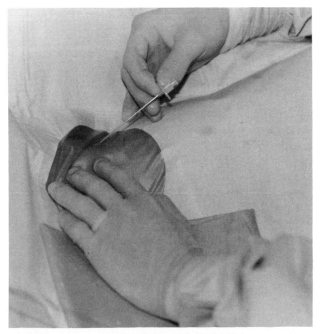

▶ **Figure 5–29**

Application of percutaneous axillary artery needle puncture.

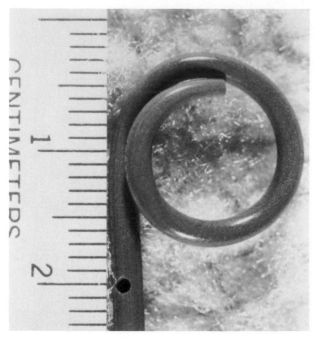

▶ **Figure 5–30**

An example of a pigtail catheter.

distribution or "flush" of rapidly injected contrast medium in large vessels, to allow homogeneous opacification, and to prevent whiplash or catheter tip recoil. The pigtail catheter becomes straight when coupled with an internal guidewire and resumes its shape when the guidewire is withdrawn (Fig. 5–30). The image presented with a flush study identifies the anatomic and pathologic details of the vasculature and determines the next step for the radiologist.

After the vasculature is viewed from the flush approach, other catheters may be used to visualize smaller branches of the arteries. Arteries that bifurcate or branch off from their points of origin may do so in an unpredictable manner. In order to "selectively" enter these irregular and sometimes tortuous pathways, special catheters are employed. Catheters that are used to enter small branches of trunk vessels are referred to as preformed, preshaped, or selective catheters. When attempting to demonstrate a branch of an artery, it is necessary to exchange that catheter with a selective catheter. A guidewire is reinserted into the flush catheter; the catheter is removed; and the selective catheter is then fed over the guidewire. Together, the guidewire and the catheter are advanced to the desired location, where the guidewire is then removed. After removal of the guidewire, the catheter resumes its original shape and a second injection is given into that selected site.

Some vessels have unique variances. Such is the case of the celiac trunk or axis. This trunk vessel has three primary branches that feed the stomach, liver,

and spleen. If the radiologist desires to enter any of those three arteries, he or she must exchange the selective catheter with one that is even smaller. This is referred to as a superselective approach. As described earlier in this chapter, selective catheters with preformed tips should resume their original shape following retraction of the guidewire. Multiple curve catheters are almost always used for selective angiography. Figure 5–31 *A* and *B* shows a wide variety of flush and selective catheters and their specifications, which are manufactured by two major producers of angiographic equipment.

Multiple-curve catheters are especially suited for catheterization of caudal- and cranial-directed vessels. Selective catheters have tips that are usually tapered, resulting in a reduction of the cross-sectional inner catheter diameter and a reduction in flow rate. Adjustments are made in the (flow rate) injection of contrast media when catheter tips are altered. In most selective catheters, only an end hole is present (with no side holes). A high-pressure injection through an end-hole catheter creates a dangerous jet effect, which may cause laceration and perforation of the arterial intima or endothelium.

Criteria for Catheter Selection

Good memory is one of the criteria that are used for selecting a catheter. Other factors include good torque control, low thrombogenicity, low coefficient of friction, low degree of radio-opacification, and low cost. Selection of the catheter is also subjective, based on the radiologist's preference, experience, and previous contact with a manufacturer's representative.

Needles

Currently, there is a wide range of needle assemblies for percutaneous arterial needle puncture. The needles are available in various sizes and are identified by gauge number. The smaller the gauge number, the bigger the bore of the needle. Needles are also described by length and cannula thickness. Needle length is measured in inches. A thin-walled, 18-gauge needle, 2 to 3″ in length is an example of a simple format that is very popular. The needle is a sharply beveled (for single use) metal needle that easily accommodates a 0.035″ or 0.038″ guidewire. Needle assemblies with Teflon sleeves are also available. The Teflon sleeve is antithrombogenic and reduces the complication of hematoma, vessel dissection, and other complications of needle failure. Once the injection is completed and the sleeve is within the artery, catheter exchange may be performed more easily. Figure 5–32 *A* through *C* shows three of the most commonly employed arterial needles that are used for percutaneous puncture.

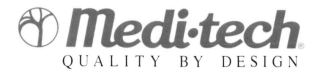

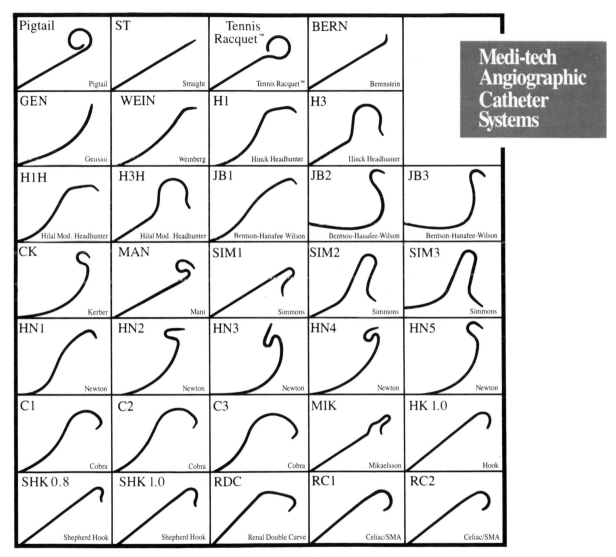

Technical Specifications and Ordering Information

A

► **Figure 5-31**

A and B, Medi-tech Angiographic Catheter Systems technical specification and ordering information. This shows a wide range of flush catheters and selective catheters for vascular use. (Courtesy of Medi-tech/Boston Scientific Corporation, Watertown, MA.)

Figure continued on next page

Angiographic Products

Flush Catheters

Digiflex® High Flow Catheters

Order Number	French Size	Tip Shape	Length (cm)	Compatible Guidewire	Flow Rate[1] cc/sec.
30-150	4	Pigtail	65	.035	19
30-151	4	Straight	65	.035	19
30-152	4	Pigtail	90	.035	16
30-153	4	Straight	90	.035	16
30-154	5	Pigtail	65	.038	34
30-155	5	Pigtail	90	.038	29
30-156	5	Pigtail	100	.038	27
30-157	5	Straight	65	.038	34
30-158	5	Straight	90	.038	29
30-159	5	Straight	100	.038	27
30-160	5	Pigtail	65	.035	34
30-161	5	Straight	65	.035	34
30-162	5	Pigtail	90	.035	29
30-163	5	Straight	90	.035	29
30-164	5	Pigtail	100	.035	27
30-165	5	Straight	100	.035	27
30-170	6	Pigtail	65	.035	40 +
30-171	6	Straight	65	.035	40 +
30-172	6	Pigtail	90	.035	38
30-173	6	Straight	90	.035	38
30-174	6	Pigtail	100	.035	37
30-175	6	Straight	100	.035	37
30-176	6	Pigtail	65	.038	40 +
30-177	6	Straight	65	.038	40 +
30-178	6	Pigtail	90	.038	38
30-179	6	Straight	90	.038	38
30-180	6	Pigtail	100	.038	37
30-181	6	Straight	100	.038	37

Imager™ Flush Catheters

Tennis Racquet™

Order Number	French Size	Tip Shape	Length (cm)	Compatible Guidewire	Flow Rate[1] cc/sec.
34-201	5	Ten. Racq.	65	.035	34
34-203	5	Ten. Racq.	90	.035	29
34-205	5	Ten. Racq.	100	.035	27
34-207	5	Ten. Racq.	65	.038	34
34-209	5	Ten. Racq.	90	.038	29
34-211	5	Ten. Racq.	100	.038	27

[1] All measurements are at 1,050 psi and 37°C with Renografin® 76.
Packaged 10 catheters per box. All catheters have eight side holes.
Renografin is a registered trademark of E.R. Squibb and Sons Inc.

Selective Catheters

Imager™ Torque Catheters (braided)

Order Number	French Size	Tip Shape	Length (cm)	Compatible Guidewire	Flow Rate[1] cc/sec.
35-102	5	ST	65	.038	19
35-103	5	ST	100	.038	17
35-105	5	ST	65	.035	19
35-106	5	ST	100	.035	17
35-107	6	ST	65	.038	35
35-108	6	ST	100	.038	30
35-132	5	BERN	100	.038	17
35-133	5	BERN	100	.035	17
35-134	6	BERN	100	.038	30
35-142	5	WEIN	100	.038	17
35-143	5	WEIN	100	.035	17
35-144	6	WEIN	100	.038	30
35-212	5	H1	100	.038	17
35-213	5	H1	100	.035	17
35-214	6	H1	100	.038	30
35-232	5	H3	100	.038	17
35-233	5	H3	100	.035	17
35-234	6	H3	100	.038	30
35-312	5	H1H	100	.038	17
35-313	5	H1H	100	.035	17
35-314	6	H1H	100	.038	30
35-412	5	JB1	100	.038	17
35-413	5	JB1	100	.035	17
35-414	6	JB1	100	.038	30
35-422	5	JB2	100	.038	17
35-423	5	JB2	100	.035	17
35-424	6	JB2	100	.038	30
35-432	5	JB3	100	.038	17
35-433	5	JB3	100	.035	17
35-434	6	JB3	100	.038	30
35-482	5	MAN	100	.038	17
35-483	5	MAN	100	.035	17
35-484	6	MAN	100	.038	30
35-510	5	SIM1	65	.038	19
35-511	5	SIM1	65	.035	19
35-515	6	SIM1	65	.038	35
35-512	5	SIM1	100	.038	17
35-513	5	SIM1	100	.035	17
35-514	6	SIM1	100	.038	30
35-522	5	SIM2	100	.038	17
35-523	5	SIM2	100	.035	17
35-524	6	SIM2	100	.038	30
35-532	5	SIM3	100	.038	17
35-533	5	SIM3	100	.035	17
35-534	6	SIM3	100	.038	30
35-612	5	HN1	100	.038	17
35-613	5	HN1	100	.035	17
35-614	6	HN1	100	.038	30

Maximum Flow Rate Guidelines (cc per second)

	4 French			5 French			6 French		
	65cm	90cm	100cm	65cm	90cm	100cm	65cm	90cm	100cm
Digiflex High Flow — Pigtail — Straight	19	16		34	29	27	40 +	38	37
Imager Flush — Tennis Racquet				34	29	27			
Digiflex Non-Braided — Selectives	14*		10*	26		19			
Imager Torque — Selectives				19		17	35		30

The above table is provided as an example and should be used only as a guide.   All measurements made at 1,050 psi and 37°C using Renografin® 76.   *Do not exceed 750 psi.

B **Medi-Tech Customer Service/Ordering Information (800) 225-3238**

► **Figure 5–31** Continued

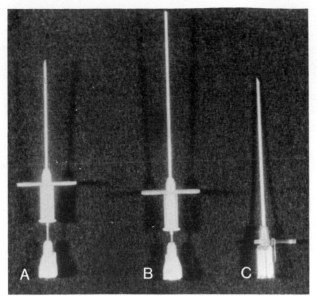

▶ Figure 5–32

Arterial needles. *A,* Potts-Cournand needle; *B,* Amplatz needle;
C, Seldinger single-wall needle.

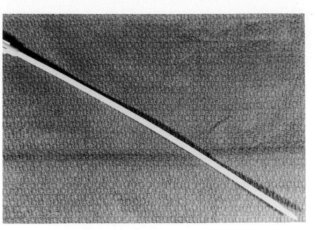

▶ Figure 5–33

An example of a vessel dilator.

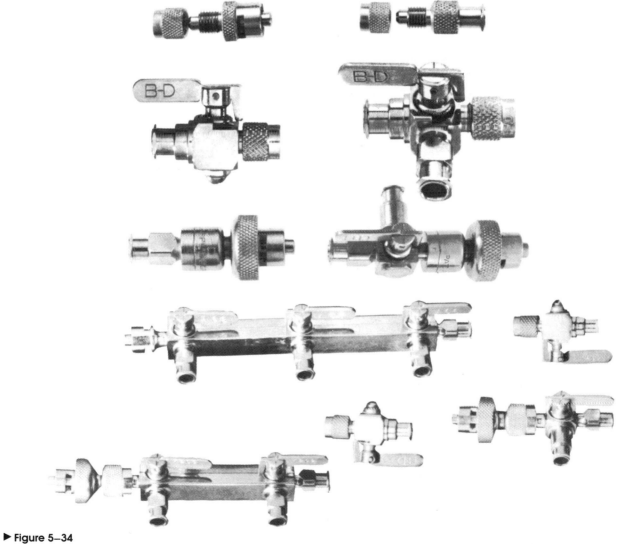

▶ Figure 5–34

Various adapters, connectors, and stopcocks. (From Snopek A: Fundamentals of Special Radiographic Procedures, 3rd ed.
Philadelphia, WB Saunders, 1992, p 92.)

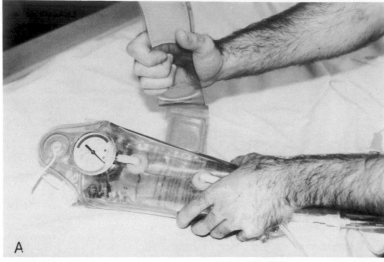

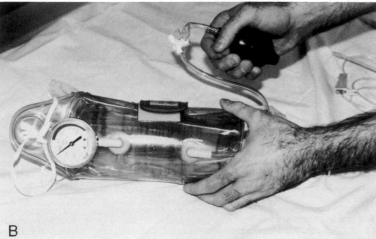

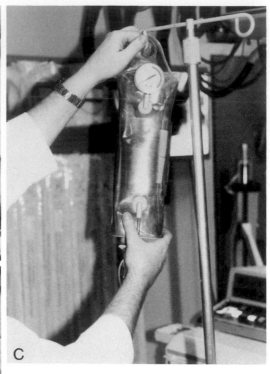

▶ **Figure 5–35**

A, The technologist places the heparinized solution bag into the pressure pouch. *B,* The heparin pouch is inflated to a pressure of 300 mm. *C,* The technologist attaches the pressurized heparin pouch to the vertical intravenous stand and prepares for systemic heparinization.

Supplementary Equipment

Vessel dilators are used to stretch or expand the needle hole to the French size of the catheter. This prevents damage or tearing of an artery. This process is repeated until the catheter can be passed comfortably into the vessel (Fig. 5–33).

Adapters (usually the Luer-Lok type) are utilized to connect syringes and accessories to catheters or other miscellaneous items. The ends of the adapters must be compatible. A variety of adapters should be available, such as male to female, female to female, with and without rotating capabilities, tapered and nontapered, and with and without sidearms to be used for flushing. Adapters are used to connect plastic and rubber tubing of all sizes, and like most angiographic equipment, adapters can be metal and designed for reuse, or plastic and disposed of after use.

Stopcocks direct the flow of fluid from one place to another. The stopcocks are used most frequently to direct the flow of fluids between two (two-way) or three (three-way) items. Stopcocks have male-female connections just like the adapters.

Manifolds are simply several stopcocks or adapters that are connected in a linear or "Y" pattern. The primary difference is that the linear arrangement provides for individual adjustment of each stopcock, whereas the Y configuration does not permit individual adjustment of the stopcock (Fig. 5–34).

Systemic Heparinization

During angiography, blood clot formation poses a hazard for the patient. All instruments are considered to be thrombogenic, and blood adheres to the tips of catheters and to the surface of guidewires. Blood clots that break free have the capacity to travel throughout the vascular pathways (as emboli), resulting in potentially life-threatening complications. In order to reduce the chances of clot formation, heparin is continually infused through the vascular system. This is referred to as systemic heparinization. Heparin is added to a unit of normal saline or dextrose and water solution. In Figure 5–35A the technologist places the heparin bag into a pressure pouch and then inflates it to 300 mm of pressure (Fig. 5–35B). The last step in preparation is achieved when the technologist attaches the pressurized heparin bag to an elevated intravenous stand (Fig. 5–35C). For further discussion regarding systemic heparinization, please refer to the preprocedure process described in Chapter 4.

► REFERENCES

1. Damiano MM and Kandarpa K: Basics of Angiographic Equipment. *In* Handbook of Cardiovascular and Interventional Procedures. Boston, Little, Brown, 1989.
2. Kadir S: Diagnostic Angiography. Philadelphia, WB Saunders, 1986.

► BIBLIOGRAPHY

Abrams H: Abrams Angiography, Vol 1, 3rd ed. Boston, Little, Brown, 1983, pp 105–185.
Athanasoulis C: Interventional Radiology. Philadelphia, WB Saunders, 1982.
Cope C, Burke D, and Meranze S: Interarterial Catheterization Techniques. Bloomington, IN, Cook, Inc., 1992.
Curry JL and Holland WJ: Arteriography. Philadelphia, WB Saunders, 1966.
Johnsrude IS, Jackson DS, and Dunnick NR: A Practical Approach to Angiography, 2nd ed. Boston, Little, Brown, 1984.
Snopek AM: Fundamentals of Special Radiographic Procedures, 3rd ed. Philadelphia, WB Saunders, 1992.
Tortorici MR: Fundamentals of Angiography. St. Louis, CV Mosby, 1982.
Tortorici MR: Concepts in Medical Radiographic Imaging, Circuitry, Exposure, and Quality Control. Philadelphia, WB Saunders, 1992.
Williams CO and Groce KA: Photo of Importance of Appropriate Suite Designs in the Era of Computerized Imaging. Philadelphia, WB Saunders, 1986, p 340.

► SELF-ASSESSMENT QUIZ

1. How large should an angiographic suite be?
   a. 50 to 100 ft²
   b. 150 to 300 ft²
   c. 300 to 500 ft²
   d. 500 to 600 ft²

2. The control area should
   a. be separate from the procedure room
   b. be located within the procedure room
   c. be located next to the light room in diagnostic radiology
   d. also be used as a patient holding area

3. What viewing device is preferred in angiography?
   a. a single-bank view box
   b. a double-bank view box
   c. a motorized film viewer
   d. a four- to eight-bank view box

4. Where vascular procedures are performed, minimum ratings of _____ and _____ mA are recommended.
   a. 300 and 500
   b. 500 and 600

c. 600 and 800
   d. 700 and 1000

5. What is the average focal spot range for routine angiography?
   a. 0.1 to 0.3 mm
   b. 0.3 to 0.6 mm
   c. 0.6 to 1.0 mm
   d. 0.6 to 1.2 mm

6. In order to produce a magnification film, the focal spot can be no larger than
   a. 0.1 mm
   b. 0.3 mm
   c. 0.6 mm
   d. 1.2 mm

7. For routine angiography, the average anode target angle is
   a. perpendicular to the film
   b. 3 to 6 degrees
   c. 5 to 10 degrees
   d. 10 to 12 degrees

8. What piece of equipment converts the x-ray image to a brighter but smaller image?
   a. generator
   b. image intensifier
   c. fractional focus x-ray tube
   d. television monitor

9. All of the following terms represent serial film changers, except
   a. Angiomat 6000
   b. Elema-Schonander
   c. AOT-S
   d. cartridges or magazines

10. Viamonte-Hobbs, Liebel-Flarsheim, and Angiomat 6000 are examples of
    a. serial film changers
    b. automatic contrast media injectors
    c. angiographic procedural tables
    d. C- and U-arms

11. The process that results in the removal of structures that interfere with anatomic and pathologic details is called
    a. magnification
    b. contrast enhancement
    c. subtraction
    d. coefficient of friction

12. The name "Seldinger" is associated with
    a. a type of film changer
    b. a type of subtraction unit
    c. percutaneous arterial needle puncture
    d. a constant pulsing generator

13. Guidewires may be coated or impregnated with
    a. heparin
    b. platelets
    c. saline
    d. plasma

14. The term "movable core" pertains to
    a. catheters
    b. guidewires
    c. adapters
    d. manifolds

15. Which guidewires are useful for recurving C-shaped or sidewinder catheters?
    a. exchange
    b. long, floppy-tipped
    c. deflecting
    d. torque

16. Which catheters are used for measuring intra-arterial blood pressures?
    a. exchange
    b. open-ended
    c. deflecting
    d. long, floppy-tipped

17. It is permissible for disposable catheters and guide-wires to be sterilized after use and then reused.
    a. true
    b. false

18. What instruments serve as pipelines for the delivery of contrast media?
    a. needles
    b. guidewires
    c. automatic injectors
    d. catheters

19. Catheters can be used for therapeutic as well as diagnostic procedures.
    a. true
    b. false

20. The French scale was devised by
    a. Roentgen
    b. Seldinger
    c. Chevalier
    d. Charrière

21. A No. 6 French catheter has an outer diameter of
    a. 0.3 mm
    b. 2.0 mm
    c. 3.0 mm
    d. 5.0 mm

22. Which of the following are examples of catheter material?
    1. stainless steel
    2. polyurethane
    3. Dacron
    4. polyethylene
       a. 1 only
       b. 1, 3, and 4

c. 1, 2, and 3
d. 2, 3, and 4

23. Modern catheters are usually coated in Teflon.
    a. true
    b. false

24. Which of the following represent catheter shapes?
    1. straight
    2. single-curve
    3. double-curve
    4. pigtail
       a. 1 only
       b. 1 and 2
       c. 1, 2, and 3
       d. 1, 2, 3, and 4

25. Single- and double-curved catheters are designed for selective injection.
    a. true
    b. false

▶ STUDY QUESTIONS

1. You are responsible for designing a cardiovascular, angiographic, or interventional suite. For this room, you have unlimited funds. Describe the characteristics of the room design, and list all the equipment that you would need to perform all desired procedures. Please include a schematic diagram of the floor plan.

2. How do the x-ray tubes used in angiography differ from those used in conventional angiography?

3. List three types of guidewires and explain their uses.

4. Any material placed within the vascular system is considered to be thrombogenic. In what ways can we minimize the formation of blood clots on catheters and guidewires?

5. What are the primary differences between a roll-film changer and a cut-film changer?

6. List three types of catheters and explain their uses.

7. What is meant by the term cross-contamination, and how can it be minimized?

8. Describe the criteria used in the selection of a catheter.

► CHAPTER SIX

► IMAGE ENHANCEMENT TECHNIQUES

► CHAPTER OUTLINE

Direct Serial Magnification Angiography
Angiographic Tubes
Subtraction Technique
Production of the Subtraction Print

Digital Subtraction Angiography
Basic Concepts
Equipment

► CHAPTER OBJECTIVES

Upon completion of Chapter 6 the technologist will be able to:

1. List the two primary factors that affect the size of the image
2. Explain the purpose of direct serial magnification radiography
3. Explain the characteristics of an angiographic x-ray tube
4. Produce a magnification radiograph
5. Explain the line-focus principle
6. Explain the purpose of film subtraction
7. Define what is meant by film subtraction
8. List and describe the four steps in production of a subtraction print
9. Demonstrate how to produce a subtraction print
10. Explain the basic concept of digital subtraction angiography (DSA)

In Chapter 5, the physical aspects of outfitting an interventional vascular or nonvascular imaging suite were discussed. This equipment allows performance of a wide variety of interventional procedures. High-capacity generators (with constant potential) should be capable of delivering at least 1000 milliamperes (mA) for conventional angiography and up to 1500 mA for cardiovascular studies. Motion artifacts are almost eliminated with these constant potential generators. However, in Chapter 6, this process is carried one step further, and the equipment as it relates to the enhancement of the finished image is discussed. This chapter includes a description of direct serial magnification angiography, subtraction technique, and digital subtraction angiography (DSA).

▸ DIRECT SERIAL MAGNIFICATION ANGIOGRAPHY

Magnification usually does not contribute to the visible accuracy of the radiographic image. Thus, in most cases, great pains are taken to avoid or eliminate it. However, almost every body structure is enlarged geometrically on the finished radiograph. For example, if a patient is lying supine on the radiographic table to have a flat-plate abdominal film taken, the kidneys (although lying as close as possible to the radiographic table) are actually magnified because of the distance of the organs from the film, which is placed at least 4″ lower in the Bucky tray (Potter-Bucky diaphragm). Thus, as long as there is an interval distance between the object and the film, there will be magnification. In most general radiographic suites, this magnification is limited because of the usual 40″ source-image distance (SID). In chest radiography, a standard distance of 72″ is used to minimize the magnification of the heart. On the horizon for general radiography is the potential usage of a 60″ SID. This increased distance significantly increases film sharpness. To offset this increase in SID, the sensitivity of the intensifying screens is increased. Thus, the loss of image intensity or density as a result of the increased SID (according to the inverse square law) is offset by increasing the speed (response) of the screen phosphors. Time will determine how this new technique will affect interventional radiography.

The two primary factors that affect the size of the image are object-image distance (OID) and SID. An increase in OID or a decrease in SID (in relation to the object) produces magnification. From a practical standpoint, an increase in the OID has greater influence on magnification, because there is a limit as to how short the SID can be decreased and still cover the film area.

If one wishes to determine the degree of magnification, one would simply divide the source-image-receptor distance (SIRD) by the target-object distance (TOD):

$$\text{Magnification} = \frac{\text{SIRD}}{\text{TOD}}$$

If one wishes to determine the object-image-receptor distance (OIRD), one would simply subtract the TOD from the SIRD:

$$\text{OIRD} = \text{SIRD} - \text{TOD}$$

Magnification technique as applied to angiography can be described as a process that intentionally enlarges the image, without producing any loss of recorded detail.

Imaging systems in present-day angiographic suites are capable of magnifying images many times over. However, additional consideration must be given to the purchase of specialized equipment that usually complements this enhancement technique. This equipment (e.g., fractional-focus x-ray tubes) substantially increases the costs of the equipment. Fractional-focus x-ray tubes can cost three times more than conventional radiographic tubes. Because of increased temperatures produced by the anode, tube life can be shorter than with conventional x-ray tubes.

For the typical angiographic department, 2 to $2\frac{1}{2}$ times magnification is usually adequate for direct serial magnification angiography. A 0.3-mm focal spot or less is required for magnification, and most radiologists find the two times magnification adequate.

If enlargement of three times or greater is sought, then a 0.1-mm focal spot is necessary; however, these tubes are much more expensive. The radiologist and radiology administration must consider the efficacy of purchasing fractional-focus x-ray tubes that are smaller than 0.3 mm.

Two times magnification is created when the TOD and OID are equal. A separation of 15″ or more between the object and the film permits the use of the "air-gap" principle (dissipation of x-ray scatter in the air) and eliminates the need for a grid. This makes for a better use of the x-ray beam (Fig. 6–1). Modern rare-earth systems are also used to further aid in the reduction of milliamperes. High kilovoltage techniques serve to lengthen the scale of contrast while reducing the dose of radiation to the patient. Several factors for serial magnification are listed in Table 6–1. Two times linear magnification is the most frequently used magnification ratio. If one wishes to calculate area magnification, all one has to do is square the linear magnification. For example, a two times linear magnification would equal a four times area magnification.

$$\text{Area of magnification} = \text{square of linear magnification}$$

Direct serial magnification has value in many, but not all, anatomic areas. Perhaps the greatest use of serial magnification is in neuroangiography. Many radiologists routinely do lateral cerebral angiograms with direct magnification. Direct serial magnification can be applied in selected situations in visceral angiography, particularly when combined with subselective injection of a contrast medium into the organ that is being evaluated. This is especially true with the

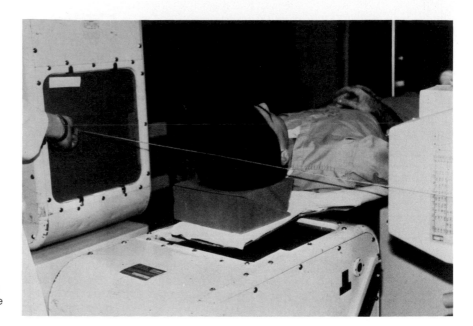

▶ **Figure 6-1**

The technologist is measuring the source-image distance (SID) to ensure that it is 40". The target-object distance (TOD) is 20".

pancreas and the liver; however, the limiting feature of visceral magnification lies within the x-ray tube. The fractional-focal spot (0.3 mm) used in conventional angiography usually has an oval configuration. For visceral angiography, a round configuration is preferred. When considering the purchase of a fractional-focus x-ray tube for visceral angiography, one has to test the focal spot at practical clinical milliampere stations to ensure that the milliampere levels required to attain the fractional focus are not below the clinical range. Focal spots enlarge with increasing current. This is called blooming. Indications for serial magnification are shown in Table 6-2.

Angiographic Tubes

X-ray tubes used in magnification radiography are very different from the x-ray tubes used in conventional diagnostic radiology. The conventional x-ray tube can sustain complete heat loading of the anode with one exposure because there is generally time for the anode to cool between exposures. In angiography and interventional radiology, several exposures are made within short time intervals, and there is practically no time for the anode to cool between exposures. Each angiographic "run" consists of a series of exposures made so rapidly that the anode loading and cooling is considered as a single exposure.

Maximum heat loading of the anode is referred to in units called kilowatt-seconds (anode heat units, or ahu) and is calculated by multiplying kVp × mA × time × 1.41 (three-phase 12-pulse). Modern angiographic tubes include a tungsten-rhenium anode. This innovation drastically reduced aging of the highly stressed focal spot track. Each x-ray tube has its own unique tube rating. For example, an angiographic tube with a 0.3-mm focal spot, 12-degree target angle with an anode rotation of 10,000 rpm and powered by a three-phase 12-pulse generator must coincide with that specific tube rating chart.

The x-ray tubes used in diagnostic and interventional radiology present focal spot sizes that are quite variable. Careful consideration must be given to selecting the proper focal spot, because it affects not only the image but also the kilowatt ratings and the effective field area covered (effective focal area) (Ta-

▶ **Table 6-1**

FACTORS SUGGESTED TO PERFORM SERIAL MAGNIFICATION

1. Fast exposure time (in milliseconds)
2. High kilovoltage (80–110 kVp)
3. Air-gap principle
4. 100 mA
5. Tight collimation
6. Ultrafast screens (rare earth)
7. High-speed film

▶ **Table 6-2**

INDICATIONS FOR SERIAL MAGNIFICATION

1. To better determine the vascular anatomy
2. To examine posterior fossa vasculature
3. To further evaluate suspicious defects as seen on a routine angiogram
4. To evaluate lenticuostriate arteries
5. To further evaluate a patient with a neurologic deficit and a negative result on an angiogram
6. To better observe components (in a vascular strain) to suggest a histologic diagnosis
7. To observe vascular defects within an intracranial lesion
8. To observe the structure of a mass lesion

ble 6–3). The *fractional* or *microfocus* x-ray tube is necessary if magnification is to be performed. This means that the focal spot can be larger than 0.3 mm. In general terms, the smaller the focal spot, the sharper the image. The major advantage of a small focal spot is that the spatial resolution is increased. However, with small focal spot tubes, the amount of heat loading of the anode increases. As a result, the kilovolt peak and milliamperes per exposure, as well as the total number of exposures, are limited, rendering them unacceptable for use in routine angiographic examinations. Small focal spots are constructed by decreasing the incident angle of the anode. As the incident angle decreases, the heel effect becomes a major factor affecting uniform field density. The size of the field covered must be reduced to have an acceptable uniform density. This is a major problem in routine angiography but offers no barrier in magnification radiography, because small fields coned to the area of interest are used. For routine angiography, focal spots ranging from 0.6 to 1.2 mm are utilized.

Rotating anodes are constructed on the basis of the *line-focus principle*, which serves to provide a focus that, when projected toward the film, is smaller than its actual area on the target. This principle is accentuated in angiography and especially in magnification radiography, because the focal spot is between 0.1 and 0.3 mm, and the effective focal area is reduced substantially. In addition, the anode angle (face) is also reduced. Most radiographic x-ray tube anodes are placed at an angle. The range of the angle is 10 to 20 degrees for diagnostic studies.[1] Because greater details are desired in angiography, smaller anode angles are utilized (10 to 13 degrees) (Table 6–4).

In the fractional focus x-ray tube, the electron stream is focused toward the rotating anode. This highly intense electron stream strikes the focal tract of the rotating anode and places severe stress on the anode structure. In conventional diagnostic x-ray tubes, the anode is struck by a larger focus that distributes the heat throughout the focal tract while the anode rotates about 3300 revolutions per minute (rpm). As a result of the increased heat absorbed by

▶ **Table 6–3**

COMPROMISES BETWEEN MAGNIFICATION AND NONMAGNIFICATION FOCAL SPOTS

Effects	Magnification Focal Spot	Nonmagnification Focal Spot
Penumbra	Decreased	Increased
Unsharpness	Decreased	Increased
Resolution	Increased	Decreased
Tube rating	Decreased	Increased
Anode rotation speed	Increased	Decreased
Target angle	Decreased	Increased
Field coverage	Decreased	Increased
Stop-motion sharpness	Decreased	Increased
Exposure time	Increased	Decreased

▶ **Table 6–4**

ANODE ANGLE/FORMAT COVERAGE*

Anode Angle (Degrees)	Field Coverage (cm)
6	20 × 20
9	30 × 30
10	33 × 33
12	41 × 41
15	51 × 51
16	54 × 54
17.5	58 × 58

* (cm × cm) — SID = 100 cm.
SID = Source-image distance.

the target in fractional focus tubes, manufacturers have increased the anode's revolutions per minute to between 10,000 and 20,000 rpm, thus further distributing the heat of the anode over a greater area of the focal tract. Fractional-focus x-ray tubes permit placing the film at a distance from the body part to permit direct magnification of the radiographic image, without sacrificing image sharpness.

▶ SUBTRACTION TECHNIQUE

The technique of subtraction was first introduced in 1961 and makes possible the clear visualization of certain information on an angiogram by the removal of nonessential structures. The procedure does not add new information but enhances patterns of radiopaque contrast material. It is used sometimes in conjunction with direct magnification radiography. Subtraction has the ability to eliminate structures that overlie the vascular anatomy that is filled with contrast, thus making the obscured vascular anatomy visible (Table 6–5).

Production of the Subtraction Print

There are four essential steps in the production of a subtraction image, as shown in Table 6–6. The first step is to select a scout film for the creation of a diapositive mask. The scout film can be defined as a selected serial film in the angiographic run that has no visible contrast material. In other words, the scout film is a film that is exposed just before the arrival of the contrast bolus. Depending on the selected injec-

▶ **Table 6–5**

ADVANTAGES OF SUBTRACTION

1. Image enhancement
2. Ability to improve and enhance visible details
3. Ability to produce a subtraction print even when original image is suboptimal

► **Table 6–6**

TECHNIQUE FOR SUBTRACTION

1. Take a scout film
2. Prepare a diapositive mask
3. Registration: superimpose contrast-filled angiogram film over the mask
4. Create the final subtraction print

tion delay, it is usually one of the first four films in the serial run.

The second step is to prepare the diapositive mask. The mask film produced will be the exact copy of the scout film, but with the densities reversed. Thus, from a conventional negative radiograph, a positive radiograph or mask is produced. The black areas are changed to white ones, and the white areas or the attenuated areas of the scout are changed to black ones.

The subtraction mask is created by taking a sheet of mask film, superimposing it on the scout film, and then exposing it for a selected timed interval to white frosted light (Fig. 6–2*A* and *B*).

Next, one should select one of the contrast-filled angiogram films and superimpose that film over the mask—a process that is called registration. Thus, when the (diapositive) mask is superimposed over the contrast-filled angiogram film, the positive and negative images of the bones tend to negate each other, and only the added contrast vasculature is visualized. This film is known as the subtraction mask (Fig. 6–3*A* and *B*).

The last step is to make the subtraction print. To obtain a subtraction print, the subtraction mask is placed over the angiogram as in step 3; a subtraction print film is placed on top of these; and another exposure is made. The subtraction print film is then processed, and an image of only the contrast-filled vessels is visible.

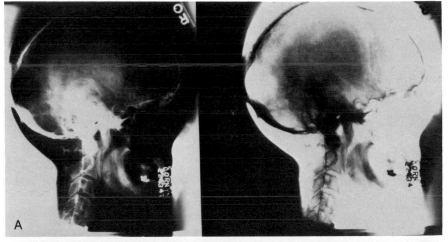
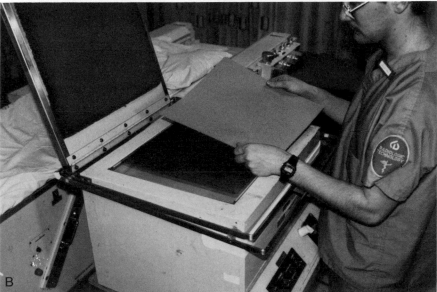

► **Figure 6–2**

A, A side-by-side display of the scout film on the left and the subtracted diapositive mask on the right. *B*, The technologist is preparing to create the subtraction mask by superimposing a sheet of mask film on the scout film.

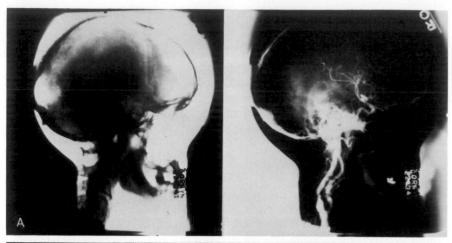

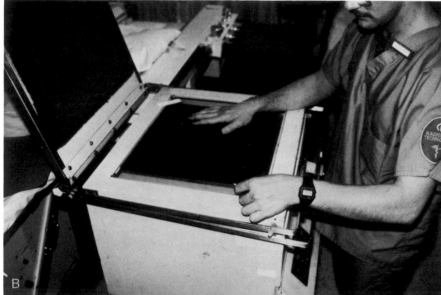

► **Figure 6–3**

A, A side-by-side display of the subtraction mask film and the contrast-filled angiogram film. *B,* The technologist is preparing to superimpose the subtraction mask film and contrast-filled angiogram film. This critical process is called registration.

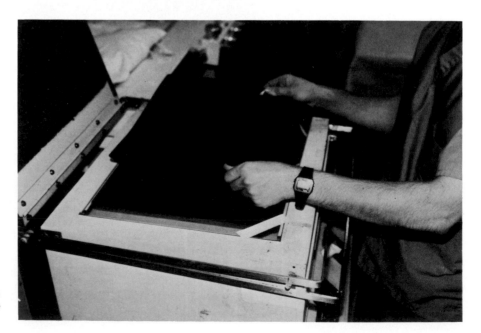

► **Figure 6–4**

The technologist is completing the subtraction process by making the subtraction print.

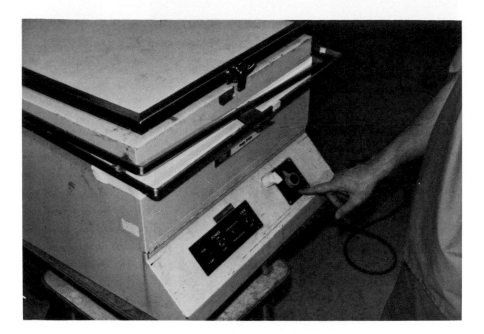

▶ **Figure 6–5**

The technologist is setting the timer for the subtraction print.

Subtraction print film has a one-sided emulsion. It is better to place the subtraction print film over the angiogram with the emulsion side up rather than down, as with duplicating film. The emulsion side is placed in the upright position because the light source must pass through the base before striking the subtraction film (Fig. 6–4).

Figure 6–5 is one type of subtraction unit, the DuPont Cronex duplicator-subtractor. A 25-watt, frosted white light bulb is contained within the unit. This light source is approximately 15″ from the print-ing frame. The usual time of exposure is about 3 seconds for a mask and 6 to 8 seconds for the finished subtraction point.

Notice, in Figure 6–3, the use of keyhole colli-mation. Additional collimation serves to further en-hance film contrast. These devices can be made rather cheaply, and they slide easily into the collimator head (Fig. 6–6).

Some examples of applications of subtraction tech-nique follow. Figure 6–7A shows peripheral vascular disease involving a large part of the pelvic vasculature in a 67-year-old man. An abdominal aortogram and runoff (demonstration of abdominal and peripheral vessel branches) were performed. Figure 6–7B re-veals a subtracted study following left iliac angio-plasty. Note the improved blood flow on the left side, which is emphasized by subtraction.

In Figure 6–8, subtraction successfully eliminates adjacent structures while revealing the "ragged," plaque-laden appearance of the distal aorta and com-mon iliac regions in this 62-year-old man.

Subtraction helps to reveal the presence or absence of normal vasculature as seen on this normal arch study in a 55-year-old man (Fig. 6–9).

In the evaluation of carotid disease and reduced blood flow in a 56-year-old man (with the head turned away from the injected side), a subtraction study clearly demonstrates a 95% stenosis of the left inter-nal carotid artery (Fig. 6–10).

Figure 6–11 demonstrates a subtracted right lateral view of the anterior cerebral circulation in a 64-year-old man who had an acute myocardial infarction. This patient suffered a stroke within hours of the infarc-tion. Note how subtraction clearly demonstrates the presence of an embolus of the internal carotid artery, just in front of the bifurcation of the anterior and

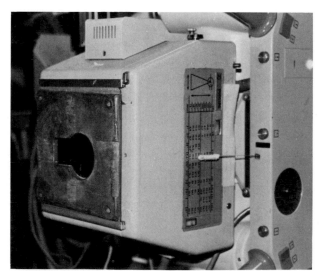

▶ **Figure 6–6**

The keyhole collimator is a means of attaining tight collimation and enhancement of subject contrast.

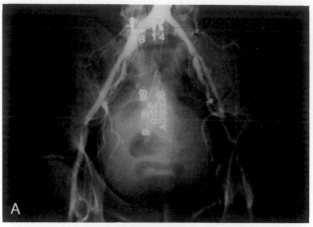

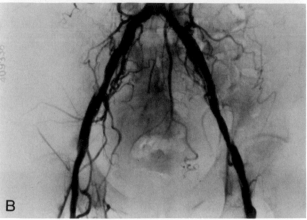

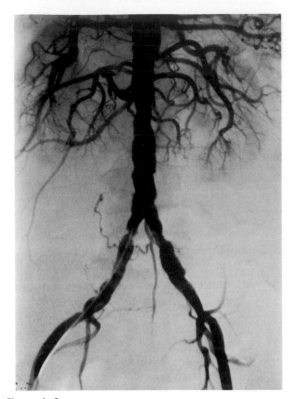

▶ **Figure 6–8**

A 62-year-old man with advanced atherosclerosis of the distal aorta and common iliac arteries.

▶ **Figure 6–7**

A, A 67-year-old man with atherosclerotic disease of the pelvic vasculature. *B,* Subtraction study following iliac angioplasty.

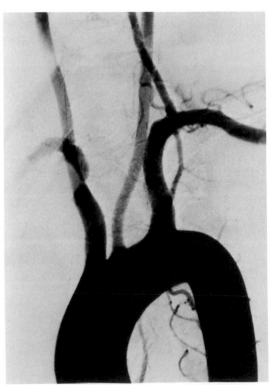

▶ **Figure 6–9**

Subtraction study delineating a normal aortic arch.

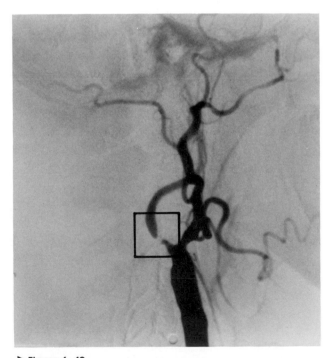

▶ **Figure 6–10**

Subtraction study delineating 95% stenosis of the left internal carotid artery.

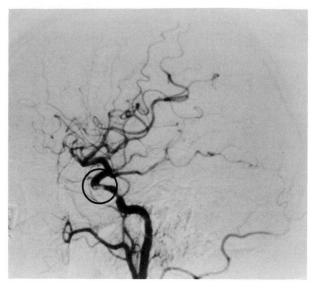

▶ **Figure 6–11**

Subtraction study of the anterior cerebral circulation of a 64-year-old man after an episodic myocardial infarction.

middle cerebral arteries. Note also how subtraction demonstrates reduced blood flow to the middle cerebral artery (which is a direct continuation of the internal carotid artery).

The advantages of subtraction imaging are also noted in a patient who had a giant cell tumor of the

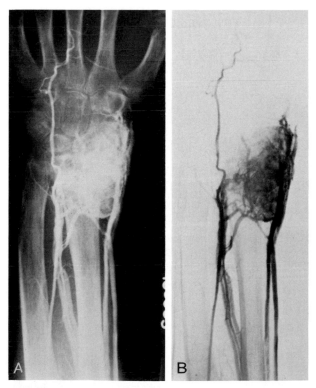

▶ **Figure 6–12**

A and B, Two subtraction studies of a patient with a giant cell tumor of the distal forearm.

distal forearm (Fig. 6–12). Note the increased visualization of the vascular tumor when the bone is subtracted out of the image.

In conclusion, the subtraction technique can be employed to further enhance many forms of contrast vascular pathology as well as delineate the presence or absence of normal vascular anatomy.

▶ DIGITAL SUBTRACTION ANGIOGRAPHY

Perhaps one of the greatest impacts on diagnostic radiology during the last 2 decades has been the introduction of digital computers to radiology and their application in computed tomography (CT), DSA, and magnetic resonance imaging (MRI).

From its beginning in the early 1970s, CT has served as the springboard for computer application in diagnostic and therapeutic angiography.

DSA at its inception was presented as a possible replacement for intra-arterial studies. There was an initial belief that venous procedures would significantly reduce the inherent risks that are common to invasive arterial studies. It was envisioned that DSA would result in reduced hospital stays, shorter examination times, reduced film exposure, and less cost to the patient.

Radiologists quickly found that there were many problems related to DSA imaging via the intravenous route of contrast medium administration.

Like conventional film subtraction, patient motion between exposure of the mask or scout image and the contrast-filled image degrades the subtraction print. Cardiac motion, respiratory motion, and peristalsis present major problems in an evaluation of DSA.

Venous injections in the superior vena cava and peripheral veins present problems in timing. The cardiac output of patients varies greatly. A patient who has a poor output per cardiac cycle will not pump enough blood containing a contrast medium to provide an adequate diagnostic study. These patients are difficult to time-sequence for digital vascular timing.

The amount of contrast medium used in each intravenous injection is much greater than that used in each intra-arterial injection. This becomes a concern in patients whose cardiac condition and renal status are questionable.

Intra-arterial DSA can be utilized by using less or diluted contrast material. The timing in intra-arterial DSA studies is the same as for conventional film angiography. The "real-time" dynamic presentation is much shorter than in conventional film processing and can significantly reduce the examination time.

Major improvements in digital technology were apparent in the early 1980s. Improvements in imaging quality were the greatest achievement of that period. Larger pixel matrices became available and were combined with further refinement of the image intensifier and viewing monitor systems.

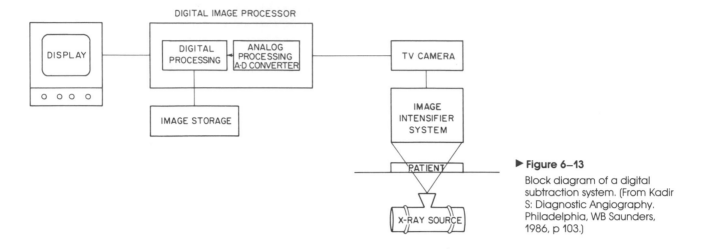

▶ **Figure 6–13**

Block diagram of a digital subtraction system. (From Kadir S: Diagnostic Angiography. Philadelphia, WB Saunders, 1986, p 103.)

Basic Concepts

The term *analog* describes a physical quantity (e.g., x-ray intensity, light, voltage) that operates in a continuous fashion. Many things in life operate continuously—for example, a baseball dropped from a tall building falls continuously; tap water running from a faucet runs continuously until turned off. The velocity of the baseball and water are continuous or analog quantities.

Digital computers are organized to utilize discrete quantities rather than analog information. In order for a computer to use an analog signal, the information must be converted to a digital format. This requires the use of a device called an analog-to-digital converter (ADC), as shown in Figure 6–13.

The analog image has continuous information without discrete areas or steps. If one were to examine the optical density presented on a film-screen analog image, one would see that the image varies from one point to another according to the change in x-ray intensity. The voltage of this image in a video signal would vary continuously on a monitor.

In the conversion from analog to digital, a number value is assigned to each area of the image that is sampled. This sampling gives a two-dimensional table of values called a *matrix*. The matrix would resemble a grid-like crossword puzzle; each number or integer assigned to the matrix is termed a *pixel* or picture element. Generally, the pixels that make up the image matrix are of equal size.

Each pixel has its own density, thus rendering many shades of gray and enabling one to enhance the image to the level of one's satisfaction. The electronic signal of each pixel is *digitized* and stored in memory. Stored memory contains line pairs that are divided into 512 or 1024 pixels. Digitized gray levels are assigned to each pixel in a scale from black to white. The black represents 0, and white represents 1024. Thus, the image (memory or number of pixels) can be stored for later recall and evaluation.

Equipment

In order for the image to be viewed on the monitor, there must be special equipment that is capable of performing all the various tasks, ending with the observed image.

The image processor is the central processing unit (CPU). This unit consists of a computer and image-producing hardware that controls all functions. The

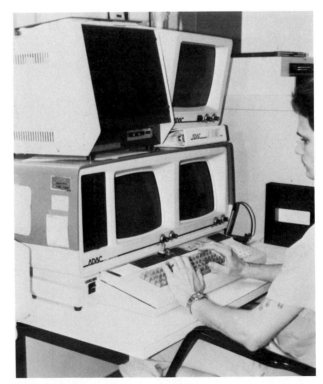

▶ **Figure 6–14**

The technologist is accessing stored data from the image processing unit by way of the keyboard. The selected images are then displayed on a video monitor.

technologist operates all functions regarding image processing.

In a special imaging department, the control room that contains the DSA system is separated from the procedure suite. Overhead monitors are placed strategically in the procedure suite so that the radiologist can observe the dynamics of the study while the technologist in the control area operates the computer and observes the same image on another monitor. A leaded glass window facilitates observation as well as communication between the technologist and the radiologist (Fig. 6–14).

In the DSA system, the television monitors receive a converted light-to-electrical signal that ultimately forms an image. Photosensitive semiconductors can detect minute changes of focused light, and these changes are interpreted by the television camera.

In conventional fluoroscopy, the processed image appears on a television monitor. The rate of scanning is so rapid that the human eye cannot detect the scanning process but sees a two-dimensional image on the monitor. These images are referred to as *frames* and are produced at a rate of 30 frames/sec.

The video monitors reveal the subtracted images in real time as the selected images are being obtained.

This processing occurs at such a rapid rate that, to the observer, it seems to occur instantaneously.

Hard copies of a study can be obtained at any time by the use of a multiformat camera or laser imager.

Figure 6–15 is an example of a negative aortic arch arteriogram on a 57-year-old man. Note that three different images were selected for a permanent record.

Figure 6–16 demonstrates two different images of a left renal thrombus in a 62-year-old male patient. Note the differences between the renal vessels and how the diagnostic visible quality of the images can be changed to yield a different pattern of contrast. The arrows on both images indicate the site of the thrombus.

Figure 6–17A demonstrates a large plaque-like lesion in the distal aorta, just above the iliac bifurcation on a 72-year-old man. Balloon angioplasty was performed, and a digital subtraction image reveals that the diameter of the aorta has been increased and, presumably, blood flow to the right iliac artery was improved. The clarity of the image of this examination was enhanced by subtracting out the superimposed bony details of the lumbar spine and pelvis (see Fig. 6–17B).

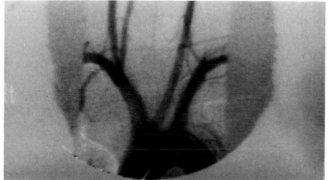

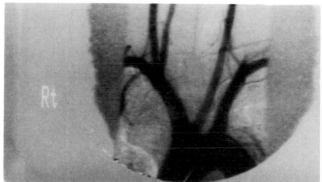

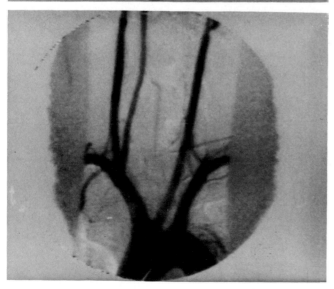

▶ **Figure 6–15**

An example of a negative result from an aortic arch arteriogram on a 57-year-old man. Note that three different digital images were selected for a permanent record.

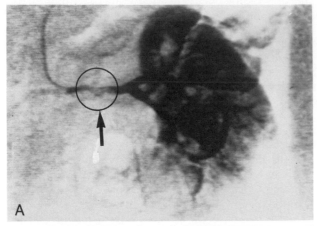

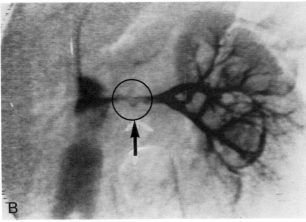

▶ **Figure 6–16**

A and B, Two images of a 62-year-old man with a left renal thrombus.

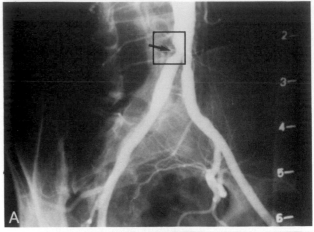

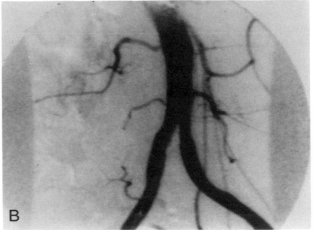

▶ **Figure 6–17**

A, A large plaque-like lesion in the distal aorta of a 72-year-old man. B, A subtraction image of the same patient shown in A. The image is enhanced by subtraction of superimposed bony details.

From our experience, conventional serial film angiography and intra-arterial DSA have progressed as partners in the diagnostic evaluation of patients with peripheral vascular disease.

▶ REFERENCE

1. Tortorici MR: Concepts in Medical Radiographic Imaging: Circuitry, Exposure and Quality Control. Philadelphia, WB Saunders, 1992.

▶ BIBLIOGRAPHY

Brody WR: Digital Radiography. New York, Raven Press, 1984.
Christensen EE, Curry TS III, and Dowdey JE: An Introduction to the Physics of Diagnostic Radiology, 3rd ed. Philadelphia, Lea & Febiger, 1985.
Greenfield GB and Hubbard LB: Computers in Radiology. New York, Churchill Livingstone, 1984.
Reuter S, Redman H, and Cho K: Gastrointestinal Angiography. Philadelphia, WB Saunders, 1986.
Selman J: The Fundamentals of X-Ray and Radium Physics, 8th ed. Springfield, IL, Charles C Thomas.
Thompson TT: A Practical Approach to Modern X-ray Equipment. Boston, Little, Brown, 1978.

▶ SELF-ASSESSMENT QUIZ

1. What are the two primary factors affecting magnification?
   1. SID
   2. OID
   3. focal spot size
   4. screen speed
      a. 1 only
      b. 1 and 2
      c. 1, 2, and 3
      d. 1, 2, 3, and 4

2. When SID is increased, magnification
   a. increases

b. decreases
c. is not affected

3. When OID is increased, magnification
   a. increases
   b. decreases
   c. is not affected

4. Which factor has the greatest effect on magnification?
   a. OID
   b. SID
   c. focal spot size
   d. size of the object

5. In order to minimize magnification
   a. use the longest possible SID
   b. use the shortest possible SID
   c. increase OID
   d. always use fast screens

6. Which of the following is a fractional focal spot?
   a. 0.6 mm
   b. 1.0 mm
   c. 1.2 mm
   d. 2.0 mm

7. In order to perform serial magnification, the focal spot can be no larger than
   a. 0.1 mm
   b. 0.3 mm
   c. 0.6 mm
   d. 1.2 mm

8. Which of the following terms relates to "clean up of scattered radiation"?
   a. subtraction technique
   b. stereoscopic technique
   c. high-speed screen technique
   d. air-gap technique

9. If the TOD is 20″, the OID is 20″, and the SID is 40″, what magnification ratio exists?
   a. 1 : 1
   b. 1.5 : 1
   c. 1 : 2
   d. 2 : 3

10. The maximum heat loading of the anode is referred to in units called
    a. eddy currents
    b. space charge
    c. hysteresis loss
    d. kilowatt-seconds

11. A 0.3-mm angiographic tube will have an anode rpm of
    a. 3300
    b. 10,000
    c. 20,000
    d. 50,000

12. The smaller the anode angle, the
    a. more heat is absorbed by the anode
    b. less heat is absorbed by the anode
    c. faster the anode rotates
    d. slower the anode rotates

13. The smaller the actual focal spot,
    a. the larger the effective focal area
    b. the smaller the effective focal area
    c. the less the visible detail

14. What is the focal spot range for angiography?
    a. 0.1 to 0.3 mm

b. 0.3 to 0.6 mm
c. 0.6 to 1.2 mm
d. 1 to 2 mm

15. In what year was the subtraction technique first performed?
    a. 1921
    b. 1954
    c. 1961
    d. 1974

16. What is the subtraction mask film?
    a. another type of scout film
    b. the final print film
    c. the opposite of the scout film
    d. the contrast-filled angiogram

17. What is the proper sequence of subtraction angiography?
    1. taking of a scout film
    2. registration
    3. making the subtraction mask
    4. making the subtraction print
       a. 1, 2, 3, and 4
       b. 4, 2, 1, and 3
       c. 1, 3, 2, and 4
       d. 4, 1, 3, and 2

18. The contact film subtraction unit contains what kind of light source?
    a. fluorescent vapor bulb
    b. sodium vapor crystal
    c. plain 25-watt light bulb
    d. frosted white light bulb

19. Subtraction film contains only a single sided emulsion.
    a. true
    b. false

20. Which method of angiography gives the greatest vessel opacification?
    a. digital vascular imaging by intra-arterial injection
    b. digital vascular imaging by intravenous injection

21. The amount of contrast medium utilized in the intravenous method is _____ than the amount used in the intra-arterial method
    a. much less
    b. less
    c. much greater
    d. greater

22. Photosensitive semiconductors are used with
    a. digital subtraction angiography
    b. magnification radiography
    c. first-order subtraction
    d. minification radiography

23. A two-dimensional array of pixel values that make up an image is called a
    a. mask
    b. matrix
    c. digiter
    d. semiconductor

24. What unit consists of a computer and image-producing hardware?
    a. matrix
    b. pixel
    c. television monitor
    d. image processor

25. Hard copies are actually
    a. outdated pixels
    b. worn-out memory banks
    c. memory disks that are filled with data
    d. permanent records of imaging data

26. The enemy of subtraction is
    a. fog
    b. grid cut-off
    c. excess radiation
    d. motion

▶ STUDY QUESTIONS

1. Explain three differences between x-ray tubes utilized in conventional radiography and those utilized in cardiovascular/interventional procedures.

2. Describe the four sequential steps in the production of a subtraction radiograph.

3. Describe the line-focus principle.

4. Define "magnification radiography" and list the factors that affect it.

5. How does focal spot size influence image quality?

6. What x-ray target (anode) angles are utilized when serial magnification is desired?

7. What is the "subtraction mask" film?

8. What are the indications for DSA?

9. Explain what is meant by the term "analogy"

10. How is analog data converted to digital data?

▶ SECTION THREE

▶ PROCEDURAL ANGIOGRAPHY

► CHAPTER SEVEN

► IMAGING OF THE HEART, PULMONARY VASCULAR SYSTEM, AND THORACIC AORTA

► CHAPTER OUTLINE

Cardiac Catheterization
  Indications
  Approaches
  Contrast Material
  Equipment
    Table and Auxiliary Equipment
Coronary Angiography
  Anatomy
  Coronary Arteries
  Coronary Veins
  Catheters
  Guidewires
  Auxiliary Equipment
Ventriculography
  Catheters
  Injection Rate
  Film Technique
Pulmonary Angiography
  Approaches
    Transfemoral
    Brachial
    Internal Jugular Vein
  Catheters
  Injection Rate
  Imaging

  Serial Film Changers
  Film Rate
  Cineangiography
Pulmonary Hemodynamic Evaluation
Cardiac Hemodynamics and Pressures
  Pressure Measurements
Terminology
Congenital Disorders
  Congenital Heart Disease
    Ventricular Septal Defect
    Tetralogy of Fallot
    Aortic Stenosis
    Pulmonary Stenosis
    Transposition of the Great Vessels
  Malformation of the Aorta
    Coartation
Atherosclerotic Heart Disease
Pulmonary Vascular System
  Pulmonary Emboli
  Arteriovenous Malformation
Thoracic Aorta
  Aneurysms
  Aortic Dissection
  Atherosclerotic Aneurysms

► CHAPTER OBJECTIVES

Upon completion of Chapter 7 the technologist will be able to:

1. Describe the indications and contraindications for cardiac catheterization
2. Describe the types of equipment used with cardiac catheterization and coronary arteriography
3. List the main anatomy of the heart
4. List the branches of the coronary arteries
5. Explain pulmonary and systemic circulation
6. Explain some of the criteria used to determine the selection of contrast media
7. Describe the unique characteristics of catheters and guidewires used in coronary and pulmonary arteriography
8. Describe the three approaches to pulmonary arteriography
9. Describe the purposes of pulmonary hemodynamic evaluation
10. Explain the differences between the various types of pressure measurements
11. Describe from a given list, five common congenital defects affecting the heart and great vessels
12. Describe atherosclerosis and its implications
13. Describe balloon angioplasty
14. Describe the radiologic methods used in the detection of pulmonary emboli
15. Explain the application and function of a caval filter
16. List two fibrinolytic agents

▶ CARDIAC CATHETERIZATION

Cardiac catheterization was first accomplished by Bernard in 1844. Using a horse as a subject, Bernard entered the right and left ventricles of the heart using a retrograde catheter placed in the jugular vein and carotid artery.

The first human to be catheterized was Forssmann. In 1929 at the age of 25, Forssmann was serving a residency at the August Victoria Hospital at Eberswold near Berlin. While in training, Forssmann had been exposed to the use of intracardiac injections of epinephrine (Adrenalin) during anesthetic arrests. He perceived that it might be safer and more effective if epinephrine could be injected directly into the heart by way of a catheter passed via a vein in the arm into the heart chamber.

To prove the safety of the procedure, Forssmann proceeded to perform a cut-down on himself and passed a 65-cm catheter through his left antecubital vein into the right atrium. This remarkable feat was accomplished with the help of a technologist holding a mirror in front of the intensified fluoroscopic image so that he could guide the catheter.

During the next 2 years, Forssmann catheterized himself another six times. His research resulted in criticism from the medical community. Most considered his research to be "folly" and dangerous. The lack of acceptance of his research led Forssmann to redirect his attention to other medical concerns, including his interest in urology.

Perhaps the greatest advancements began to emerge in the middle 1950s following Seldinger's introduction of his percutaneous technique in 1953.

In 1959, Sones described a technique for selective coronary arteriography using a brachial approach. Subsequently, Ricketts, Abrams, Amplatz, and Judkins developed widely used techniques, variations of which are still used today.

In 1966, Amplatz began using a technique via the transfemoral route, utilizing selective catheters with slightly varied shapes and curves for each coronary artery.

In 1970, Swan and Ganz introduced a flow-guided balloon-tipped catheter that allowed for bedside introduction of a cardiac catheter for diagnosis and heart monitoring.

In the 1970s and 1980s a new era began, when therapeutic applications of cardiac catheterization were introduced. In 1977, Gruntzig introduced a technique for coronary angioplasty. This new therapeutic treatment in certain clinical indications became an alternative to coronary artery bypass graft surgery.

Perhaps the most exciting domain that is being explored in the 1990s is the intracoronary application of thrombolytic agents for the treatment of patients with acute myocardial infarction. In addition, the sophistication of hemodynamic diagnosis and the evaluation of myocardial function utilizing catheters has settled on an interesting plateau.

Indications

The indications for cardiac catheterization take into account the hemodynamic, diagnostic, and therapeutic information and its possible use in the management of patients (Table 7–1).

Each patient is evaluated by the cardiologist. As with all invasive procedures, the risk must be weighed against the importance or the benefit of the expected results of the clinical procedure.

Approaches

Perhaps one of the reasons the percutaneous femoral approach is preferred is that it negates the use of a cut-down and postprocedural surgical repair.

It would be the method of approach if there is either reduced radial or a reduced brachial pulse or if a previous brachial puncture has been attempted.

▶ **Table 7–1**

INDICATIONS AND CONTRAINDICATIONS FOR CARDIAC CATHETERIZATION

Indications	Contraindications
Coronary atherosclerosis	Ventricular tachycardia/fibrillation (uncontrolled)
Angina pectoris	
Myocardial infarction	Renal failure
Preassessment in thrombolytic therapy	Sensitivity to contrast
	Acute pulmonary edema
Coronary angioplasty	Uncontrolled hypertension
Noninvasive test results that are nondiagnostic	Anticoagulation (heparin/warfarin treatment)
Congenital coronary defects	Fever/infection
Valvular disease	Acute myocardial ischemia
Preoperative evaluation for cardiac arterial bypass graft	
Roadmap coronary collaterals	
Pharmacologic intervention	

Contrast Material

The choice of contrast material resides with the cardiologist or radiologist performing the procedure. Water-soluble, nonionic contrast compounds are used widely in coronary angiography today. We have discussed in previous chapters that methylglucamine (meglumine) salts tend to be better tolerated than are sodium salts.

From our experience, the most widely used ionic contrast materials employed as an alternative to the nonionic agents include Renografin-76 (Squibb) and Angiovist 370 (Berlex Imaging, Inc.). The chemical formulations of Renografin and Angiovist result in reduced calcium binding.

As with all intra-arterial contrast procedures, patients with sensitivity to iodine, renal insufficiency, diabetes mellitus, multiple myeloma, sickle cell anemia, and impaired renal and liver function are at increased risk.

Equipment

Image intensification was first introduced into radiology in the 1950s. The image intensifier has become an important piece of equipment in radiographic procedures such as coronary arteriography, in which the dynamic motion picture needs to be observed during imaging.

Image intensifiers are available in different sizes. With intensifier systems, the trade-off in size is always resolution and gain. Thus, in angiography, the smallest usable input diameter would be recommended. For coronary arteriography, a small image intensifier with an input diameter of from 12 to 17 cm (5 to 7") would be preferred.

For clinical examinations, 35-mm cameras are widely used today. These cameras can be programmed to operate at speeds of up to 80 frames/sec. In conjunction with cineradiography, videotape recording and digital subtraction angiography (DSA) storage and manipulation are widely used.

Table and Auxiliary Equipment

The "cradle table" was the preferred system for many years in coronary angiography. This system left much to be desired. One of the primary problems with this system was the inability to project certain parts of cardiac anatomy without severely foreshortened anatomy when the patient was in the oblique position.

Today, carbon fiber tables provide a strong light table that is easily controlled in all directions with very little beam attenuation. The modern x-ray equipment support stand, whether it is a C-arm or U-arm, should have an isocentered x-ray tube and image intensifier. This allows for both caudocranial and craniocaudal angulation while the patient remains in a basic flat recumbent position. Figures 7–1 to 7–9 demonstrate several equipment-patient configurations.

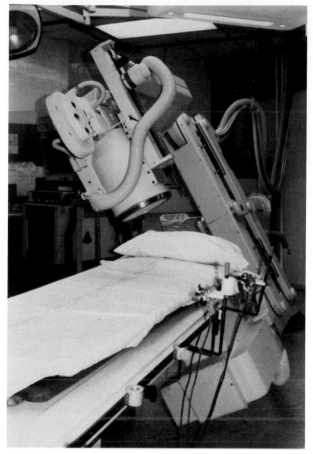

▶ Figure 7–1
60-degree right anterior oblique configuration.

▶ CORONARY ANGIOGRAPHY

The early attempts at coronary angiography were performed with flush injections of the aortic root with simultaneous biplane film angiography of the right and left coronary arteries on regular serial films.

In the early 1960s, Amplatz and Judkins developed preformed catheters that increased the ease and reliability of the procedure and resulted in lower mortality rates (Figs. 7–10 and 7–11).

Anatomy

The heart functions as a muscular pump, circulating blood throughout the body. The heart lies in the center of the chest behind the sternum, and the greater bulk lies slightly to the left of the midline and posteriorly. The heart is protected within the chest cavity by the vertebral column and rib cage posteriorly and by the rib cage and sternum anteriorly. With this oblique placement in the chest cavity, the right heart chambers lie anteriorly in the chest and the left heart chambers lie posteriorly.

The heart consists of three layers. The outermost layer, the *epicardium* (visceral pericardium), is in contact with a protective fibrous sac called the peri-

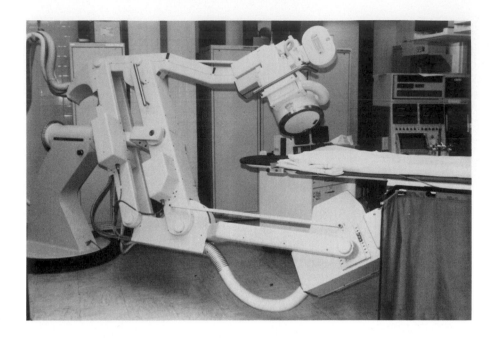

▶ **Figure 7–2**
Left anterior oblique configuration with caudocranial angulation.

cardium or pericardial sac (parietal pericardium). The second or middle layer, the *myocardium*, consists of layers of muscle that surround the heart in a circular fashion. The innermost layer is the *endocardium*, which lines the cardiac chambers and covers the valves. This smooth endocardial surface serves to reduce friction on the fragile red blood cells as well as to decrease and prevent clot formation within the heart chambers.

On the outer surface of the epicardium are the small arteries and veins that supply blood to the heart muscle. These *coronary* arteries and veins penetrate the

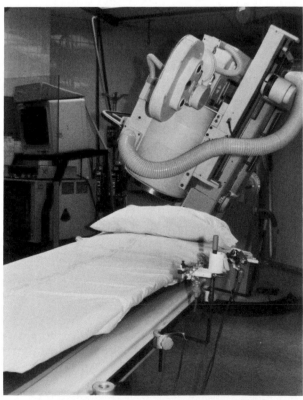

▶ **Figure 7–3**
Forty-degree left anterior oblique configuration.

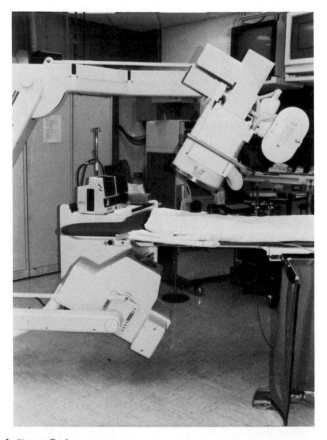

▶ **Figure 7–4**
Craniocaudal configuration. This angulation is in relation to the patient's long axis.

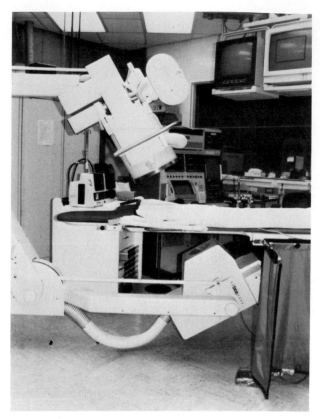

▶ **Figure 7–5**

Caudocranial configuration. This angulation is in relation to the patient's long axis.

myocardium in order to provide oxygen and nutrients to the heart muscle.

Two primary blood vessels supply the heart—the *right* and *left coronary arteries*. Their origin is at the root of the ascending aorta (Fig. 7–12).

Coronary Arteries

At the origin of the aorta just outside of the aortic valve, there is a slight dilatation of the aorta called the *sinuses of Valsalva*. These sinuses are close to the three cusps of the aortic valve and are called the right, left, and posterior sinuses.

Arising from the right and left sinuses of Valsalva are the origins of the right and left coronary arteries.

The *right coronary artery* (RCA) originates in the right sinus of Valsalva, courses anteriorly and to the right between the pulmonary artery and the right atrium, and enters the right atrioventricular (AV) sulcus. It then turns posteriorly and inferiorly to descend in the posterior interventricular groove (sulcus) to provide blood to this region of the heart. In approximately 55% of hearts the next major branch is the sinus node artery, which passes posteriorly and proceeds toward the junction of the *superior vena cava* (SVC) and the right atrium.

The RCA has several major branches. The *acute marginal branch* is the largest branch of the RCA and runs along the acute margin of the right ventricle. It supplies the anterior and diaphragmatic walls of the right ventricle. Two or more muscular branches arise from the RCA to the wall of the right ventricle and also the inferior wall of the right ventricle.

Generally, the RCA terminates by dividing into two branches, the *posterior descending* and the *posterior lateral ventricular branches* (Fig. 7–13).

The *left coronary artery* (LCA) originates from the left sinus of Valsalva and courses toward the left around the anterior and lateral aspects of the aorta. It divides immediately into two major branches. The first branch is called the *left anterior descending* (LAD) *artery* and the second branch is the *circumflex artery*.

The LAD artery passes downward into the anterior interventricular sulcus. This branch gives off smaller

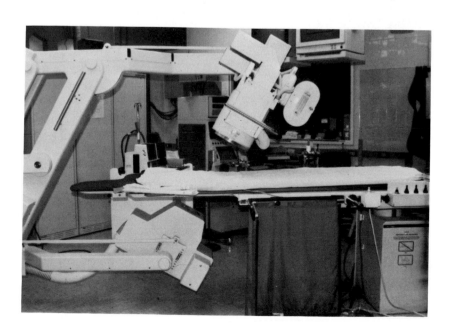

▶ **Figure 7–6**

Craniocaudal configuration showing the relationship with the pedestal type of angiographic table.

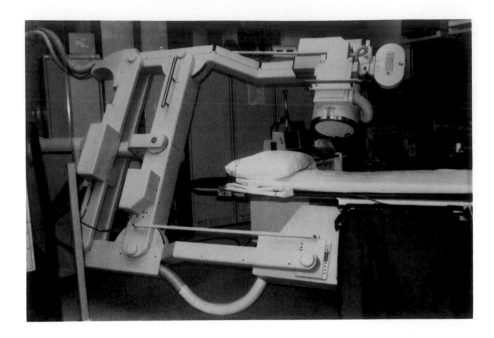

▶ **Figure 7–7**

Left anterior oblique configuration with a floor-mounted parallelogram U-arm.

branches to the interventricular septum anteriorly and one or more diagonal branches.

The *circumflex artery* has a course that may vary. The circumflex artery runs in the left AV sulcus around the left atrium and circles behind the heart. It then supplies branches that travel down the posterior wall of the left ventricle and also provides blood to the posterior and lateral walls of the left ventricle (Fig. 7–14).

Coronary Veins

There are two major groups of coronary veins. The *epicardial veins* are those that accompany the major

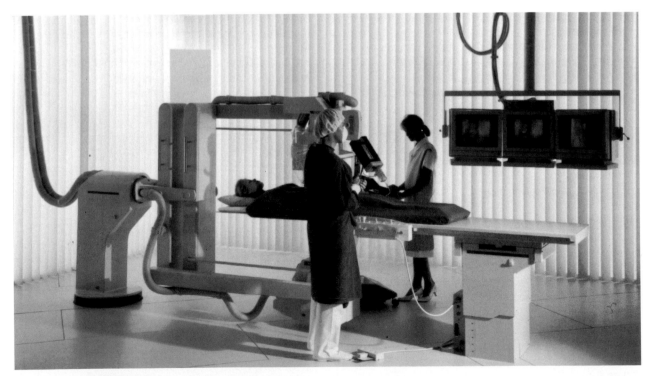

▶ **Figure 7–8**

Philips INTEGRIS cardiovascular imaging system. (Courtesy of Philips Medical Systems, Shelton, CT.)

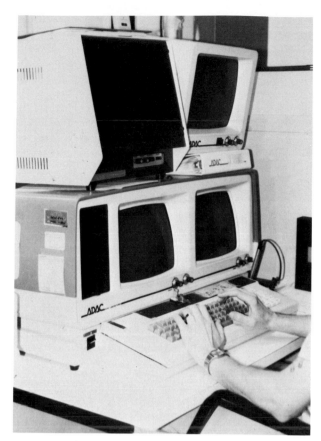

► **Figure 7–9**

ADAC Digital Radiography System.

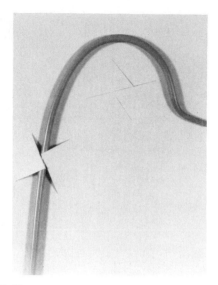

► **Figure 7–10**

AL-III left coronary (Judkins) catheter; No. 8 French 100 cm; used with the Amplatz technique.

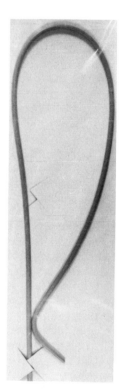

► **Figure 7–11**

AR-I right coronary (Judkins) catheter; No. 8 French 100 cm; used with the Amplatz technique.

arteries. They drain into the coronary sinuses. The second group is known as the *thebesian system* and consists of a variable number of small veins that drain directly into the atria.

The path of the coronary sinus lies in the left AV sulcus and parallels the route of the circumflex artery. The coronary sinus enters the right atrium posteriorly. These epicardial veins can be observed angiographically in the later phases of circulation in coronary arteriography.

If we examine the heart from the anteroposterior (AP) position, we can see that the right atrium lies anteriorly and is the right border of the heart. The right atrium receives deoxygenated blood from the upper chest, head, and lower extremities. This blood is returned through the SVC and the *inferior vena cava* (IVC). This blood enters the right atrium and is circulated through to the right ventricle. The right ventricle pumps the blood into the pulmonary arterial system, where it is reoxygenated. This blood, which has a high oxygen content, enters the left atrium and is then perfused into the left ventricle, where it is pumped into the aorta to oxygenate the body tissues.

The *atria* are chambers for receiving returning blood from the body and lungs. These atrial chambers hold the blood until the pumping chambers of the right and left ventricles have relaxed and are ready to ac-

cept a new volume for ejection to the lungs and body (Fig. 7–15).

Catheters

The choice of a catheter for coronary arteriography depends on a cardiologist's or radiologist's personal taste and past experience.

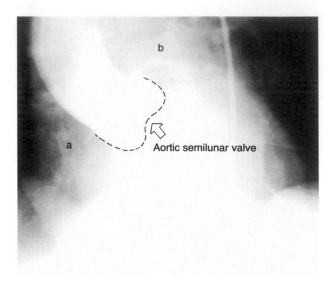

► **Figure 7–12**

Demonstration of the aortic root. (a = right coronary artery; b = left coronary artery; open arrow = aortic semilunar valve.)

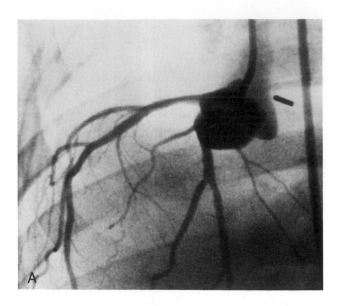

Coronary selective catheters are available in a No. 7 or No. 8 French external diameter with an end shaft that tapers to a No. 5 French diameter at the distal tip. The catheters can be made either from polyethylene (Cook, Inc., Bloomington, IN), polyurethane (Cordis, Miami, FL), or woven Dacron. These standard catheters are available in lengths of 80, 100, and 125 cm.

The controllable stiffness or torque in these preformed catheters is enhanced by the use of steel wire braid or nylon encasement along the shaft of the catheter.

The sizing of coronary catheters is graduated to match the differing diameter of the human aortic root. If the aorta is not dilated or elongated, most angiographers prefer to start with a small secondary curve. The preformed *Judkins left coronary catheter* series is available in three sizes —the JL4, JL5, and the JL6. The J signifies Judkins; the L designates the catheter as a left coronary; and the numbers, 4, 5, and 6 are the length in centimeters of the secondary curve. The distal tapered tip remains in the coronary ostium, and essentially the secondary curve anchors the catheter in the vessel origin.

If the aorta is not dilated or is of average size, many angiographers prefer to start with a 4-cm curve (JL4). If the patient is tall with an elongated or tortuous aorta, a longer secondary curve might be utilized (JL5 or JL6).

The Judkins right coronary catheters are available in similar designations—JR4, JR5, and JR6. The secondary curve in the right preformed catheters is noticeably less than the acute curve found in the left preformed catheters. Generally speaking, the selective catheterization of the RCA is often technically easier than is the catheterization of the LCA (Fig. 7–16A and B).

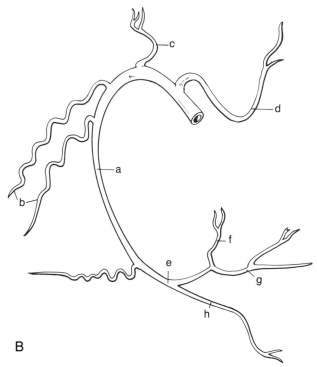

► **Figure 7–13**

A, Selective injection and demonstration of a normal right coronary artery. *B*, The right coronary artery in the left anterior oblique (LAO) position with cephalad angulation. (a = right coronary artery; b = acute marginal branches; c = right canal branch; d = sinoatrial branch; e = crux; f = atrioventricular node artery; g = posterolateral branch; h = posterior descending artery.) (*B*, Redrawn from an illustration by Martha J. Dane.)

The *Amplatz* series of catheters has similar designators. The Amplatz left coronary catheters are sized AL1, AL2, AL3, and AL4. The larger curves are used for patients with dilated roots.

The right Amplatz coronary catheters are designated as AR1 and AR2. The secondary curves of the

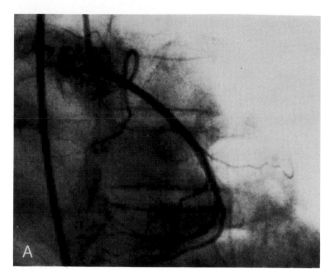

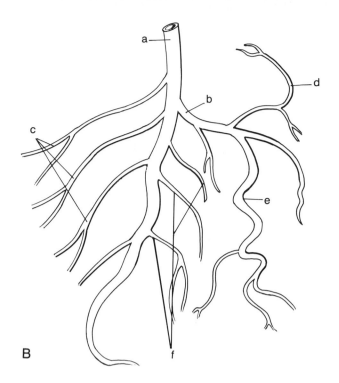

▶ **Figure 7–14**

A, Selective injection and demonstration of a normal left coronary artery. B, The left coronary artery in the left anterior oblique (LAO) position with cephalad angulation. (a = left main coronary artery; b = circumflex artery; c = septal branches; d = atrial circumflex artery; e = obtuse marginal branch; f = diagonal branches.) (B, Redrawn from an illustration by Martha J. Dane.)

Amplatz catheters are considerably less than are those of the Judkins catheters. This often provides a pleasant alternative if the angiographer has trouble placing a given catheter in a patient's anatomy.

The Sones catheter is particularly preferred by many angiographers who use the brachial approach.

This preformed catheter is available in a thin-walled woven Dacron and a polyurethane version (Cordis, Miami, FL). This catheter is well tolerated in the tortuous anatomy of the subclavian system. The Sones unique curve is pressed against the cusp of the aortic valve to push the tip into the coronary ostium.

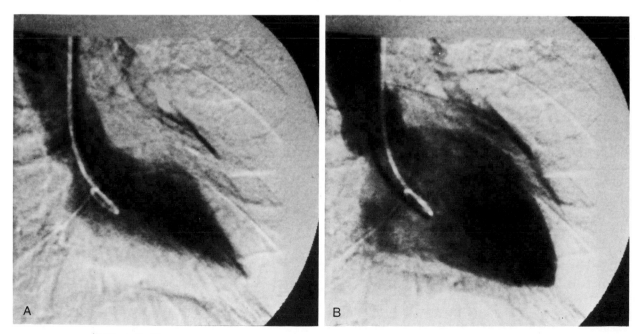

▶ **Figure 7–15**

A, Cardiac ventriculogram; ventricular systole. B, Cardiac ventriculogram; ventricular diastole.

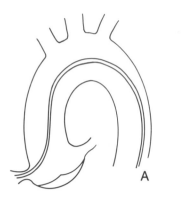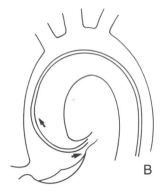

▶ **Figure 7–16**

A, Right coronary artery catheter placement; left anterior oblique (LAO) position. *B,* Left coronary artery catheter placement; slight withdrawal seats the tip in the ostium; left anterior oblique (LAO) position.

This catheter can be used for both the RCA and the LCA (Fig. 7–17*A* and *B*).

Guidewires

The guidewires commonly used are 0.035″ with a "floppy" J tip. The J tip can vary in size, and selection often depends on the tortuosity of the femoral and iliac arteries and also on the degree of atherosclerosis.

Many alternatives are available, including a large selection of curves: 3 mm, 7.5 mm, 15 mm, and also tapered-core, multicurved, and movable-core J-wires (see Fig. 10–32).

Auxiliary Equipment

The three- or four-port stopcock *manifold* has become an integral part of coronary arteriography. This system allows the angiographer to perform several tasks, which are all under the control of a series of stopcocks.

The ports on a stopcock can connect many items, such as syringes and catheters. The side ports can be attached respectively to a pressure transducer, saline flush solution, and contrast medium. The four-port manifold allows for the additional use of a discard port for double flushing (vessel or syringe) or to remove air bubbles from the closed system (Fig. 7–18).

Through the manipulation of these stopcocks the angiographer can instantaneously monitor catheter tip pressure, inject test doses of contrast medium, or flush the catheter with heparinized saline.

Arterial sheaths are used widely during coronary catheterization. Perhaps the primary advantage of a sheath is the ability to exchange and use multiple catheters during a procedure.

The sheath has a manifold hub with a side arm extension. This side arm extension allows for measurement of pressure gradients and the ability to monitor catheter tip pressure through an attached trans-

ducer. The sheath size is generally one French size larger than the catheter being used. Suggested positions for selective coronary arteriography are shown in Table 7–2.

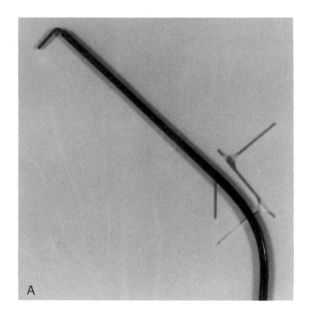

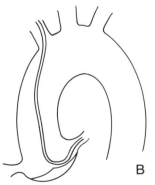

▶ **Figure 7–17**

A, Sones Dacron catheter; No. 7 French; 100 cm with two side holes and an open end. *B,* Sones technique for selective left coronary arteriography via the right subclavian approach. (*B,* Redrawn from an illustration by Martha J. Dane.)

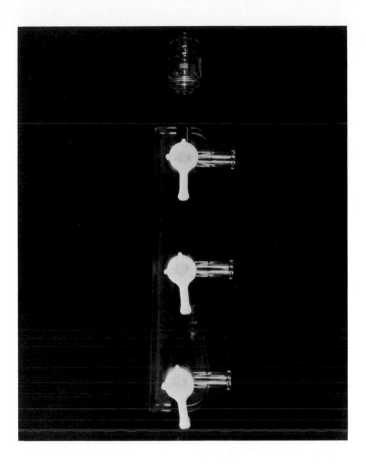

▶ Figure 7–18
Three-post/gauge manifold with rotator open handle.

▶ VENTRICULOGRAPHY

Cardiac ventriculography is used to visualize and portray the anatomy of the ventricles (Fig. 7–19). Indications for ventriculography are shown in Table 7–3.

Catheters

The primary consideration in choosing a catheter for ventriculography is the large amount of contrast material needed to optimally opacify the ventricles.

Cardiologists prefer catheters that can accomplish this rapid delivery while also remaining in a safe, stable position with as little interruption as possible to the normal cardiac rhythm.

Catheters with end-holes are generally deemed unsatisfactory by experienced angiographers. These end-hole catheters often recoil and whip during high-pressure contrast medium injection. This phenomenon may cause a disturbance of the cardiac rhythm or an increased possibility of myocardial injury or suboptimal opacification.

Many cardiologists prefer the *pigtail* catheters for both right and left ventriculography. The No. 7 or No. 8 French pigtail catheter has several distinct advantages. Safety and contrast delivery are often deciding factors.

The pigtail catheter can be introduced percutaneously via the brachial or femoral route with a J-tipped guidewire that is used to straighten the curved "pig end." Many of our colleagues suggest that the pigtail configuration significantly reduces the chance of ventricular ectopic beats (heart beats that do not originate in the sinoatrial [SA] node) and is maneuvered more easily through the valve cusps.

When the catheter enters the ventricle, there is often irritation of the ventricular wall. This can be noted on electrocardiographic tracings and on pressure monitorings. The ideal catheter placement is in the mid-ventricle area or near the apex (Fig. 7–20A and B).

Injection Rate

The injection rate and volume depend on the catheter selected and also on the patient's physiologic and clinical condition, including the size of the ventricle.

For an average size of ventricle, we could utilize a No. 8 French pigtail catheter and a 40- to 45-ml volume of Angiovist 370 injected at a rate of 12 to 16 ml/sec.

Film Technique

Film technique varies according to the type of equipment utilized.

SUGGESTED POSITIONS FOR SELECTIVE CORONARY ARTERIOGRAPHY

Left Coronary Artery *Anteroposterior Position*	The AP position is excellent for views of the left main coronary artery. This projection is also acceptable for portrayal of the middle and distal segments of the left anterior descending and the diagonal arteries.
Anteroposterior Position with Caudal Angulation	This position demonstrates the left main coronary artery and its branches and also the left anterior descending and circumflex arteries.
Right Anterior Oblique Position with Caudal Angulation	The right anterior oblique, at 5 to 15 degrees with a 15- to 20-degree caudal angle, provides an excellent demonstration of the bifurcation of the left main coronary artery into the left anterior descending and circumflex arteries. The circumflex artery is generally viewed in its entirety.
Left Anterior Oblique Position with Caudal Angulation	The left anterior oblique has 35 to 50 degrees of rotation with 10 to 15 degrees of caudal angulation. This is the spider view and provides for visualization of the proximal left anterior descending, the left main coronary artery, and the proximal circumflex artery.
Left Anterior Oblique Position with a Steep (60-Degree) Angulation	This position demonstrates the proximal and mid-portions of the mid-circumflex artery and the entire length of the left anterior descending. There is foreshortening of the left coronary artery on this projection.
Lateral Position	This position is useful in obtaining projections of the proximal circumflex artery and the proximal and distal left anterior descending arteries.
Right Coronary Artery *Anteroposterior Position with Cephalic Angulation*	This projection demonstrates the middle and distal segments of the right coronary artery, the crux, the posterior descending, and the posterior borders of the left ventricle.
Left Anterior Oblique Position with Cephalad Angulation	This position (15 to 30 degrees left anterior oblique and 10 to 15 degrees cephalad) provides for a good generalized view of the right coronary artery. The ostium is clearly viewed and also the proximal, medial, posterolateral, and posterodescending arteries.
Right Anterior Oblique Position with Caudal Angulation	This position (5 to 15 degrees right anterior oblique and 10 to 15 degrees caudal) provides for visualization of the crux, posterolateral branches, and the posterior descending artery.

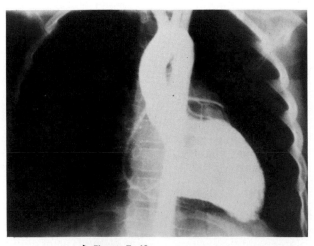

▶ Figure 7–19

A normal left ventriculogram.

Biplane ventriculography for the left ventricle can be viewed optimally with the patient adjusted at a 30-degree right anterior oblique (RAO) position and a corresponding 60-degree left anterior oblique (LAO) position with a 20- to 30-degree cranial angulation to reduce foreshortening of the left ventricle.

If only single-plane cineangiographic equipment is available, a 30-degree RAO position portrays the ventricle in profile and provides a diagnostic view of the mitral valve, the apex, and the anterior and inferior walls.

Cineangiography is performed using a 35-mm camera with a film rate of 50 to 60 frames/sec using a 9″ image intensifier. The large 9″ intensifier provides for complete ventricular field coverage and reduces the magnification factor for diagnosis and assessment of the opacified ventricle.

▶ **Table 7–3**
INDICATIONS FOR VENTRICULOGRAPHY

Left Ventriculography
Left ventricle function
Mitral valve incompetence
Cardiomyopathy
Ventricular septal defects
Congenital heart disease

Right Ventriculography
Right ventricular function
Congenital heart disease
Valvular incompetence
Valvular septal defects

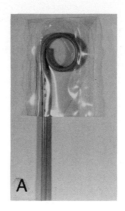

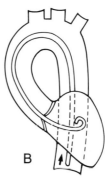

▶ **Figure 7–20**
A, Cordis No. 8 French pigtail cardiac flush catheter; 110 cm with 12 side holes. (Courtesy of Cordis, Inc., Miami, FL.) *B,* A diagram of a retrograde left ventricular catheterization with a pigtail catheter across the aortic valve. (*B,* Redrawn from an illustration by Martha J. Dane.)

▶ PULMONARY ANGIOGRAPHY

In 1931, in Portugal, Moniz and associates published a paper on their success in selectively catheterizing the pulmonary circulation in humans. In essence they followed Forssmann's catheter technique while injecting a contrast material called Uroselectan B. Earlier attempts at pulmonary visualization via a flush of the peripheral veins were unsuccessful, because the contrast agent was low in concentration visibility; the peripheral injections were too slow; and the resultant volumes were too small.

The technical development of catheters along with percutaneous introduction systems (Seldinger), rapid film changers, and pressure-controlled injectors now allow for selective pulmonary arteriography. Indications for pulmonary angiography are shown in Table 7–4.

Approaches

Transfemoral

Many cardiologists or radiologists prefer percutaneous catheter introduction via the femoral vein route. Depending on the catheter used, this approach generally provides for selective and subselective pulmonary arterial catheterization.

From our experience there is often concern when using the femoral approach if the patient exhibits clinical evidence of thrombosis in the femoral or iliac veins or IVC. In this situation, the potential dislodging of thrombi would be a contraindication to the transfemoral approach.

The physician palpates the femoral artery and a puncture is performed approximately 2 to 3 cm medial to the palpated artery into the femoral vein.

Brachial

The brachial or antecubital route by way of cut-down is preferred by many angiographers. The approach,

according to some authors, allows for easier manipulation of the catheter between the left and right pulmonary arteries.

Internal Jugular Vein

The internal jugular vein approach is somewhat more difficult depending on experience. A puncture is made approximately 5 cm below the angle of the mandible between the common carotid artery and the sternocleidomastoid muscle.

Caution should be taken with this technique if the patient is on anticoagulant or thrombolytic therapy.

▶ **Table 7–4**
INDICATIONS FOR PULMONARY ANGIOGRAPHY

Pulmonary embolism
Pulmonary hypertension
Pulmonary artery stenosis
Arteriovenous malformation
Congenital heart disease
Pulmonary tumors
Hemodynamic assessment

Catheters

The *Grollman pigtail* catheter is widely used from the percutaneous femoral route. The Grollman catheter has a "pig" end with an end hole, four side holes, and a 5-cm curve angled at approximately 65 degrees.

The advantage of using an end-hole catheter in the pulmonary system is the ability to use guidewires throughout the procedure. The side holes in this catheter are spiraled around the lumen and are positioned on opposite sides to each other. This provides for less recoil under the high flow rates needed to opacify the pulmonary arterial system (Fig. 7–21).

The *NIH catheter* has a closed end with multiple side holes. The absence of an end hole requires the use of a sheath for venous introduction. A disadvantage of this catheter is the inability to use a guidewire for guidance through difficult passage through the right heart chambers (Fig. 7–22).

Injection Rate

Angiovist 370 and Omnipaque 350 are reasonable choices to visualize the main pulmonary arteries. A typical injection rate would be 20 to 30 ml/sec for a total volume of 45 to 55 ml.

For selective left or right pulmonary arteriography, an injection rate of 15 to 25 ml/sec for a total volume of 20 to 35 ml is recommended.

The angiographer must take into account the patient's pulmonary blood flow, catheter size, and test injections, especially if there is a clinical suspicion of pulmonary emboli.

Imaging

Pulmonary angiography can be performed utilizing biplane serial changers or cineangiographic equipment.

Serial Film Changers

A scout film should be taken in both AP and lateral planes. Chest technique depends on the individual's heart size, vasculature, and pulmonary condition. It is valuable to mark the scout positions in both planes in order to "fine tune" each individual projection prior to contrast injection.

Wedge filters are utilized in certain clinical situations to help optimize diagnostic contrast in the chest area. This can especially help to compensate for a nonattenuated beam in the presence of chronic obstructive pulmonary disease (COPD).

Filming is done during deep inspiration. Good patient communication is important during pulmonary angiography. During injection, the patient's first subjective reaction may be the urge to cough. Communication should let the patient understand what he or she may experience and the importance of holding still in order to reduce motion artifacts.

In selective right or left pulmonary studies, lateral or biplane serial filming is widely employed. For additional views of the selected pulmonary vessels, obliques are commonly utilized, especially where primary vessels may overlap each other.

The right posterior oblique (RPO) position is utilized to best demonstrate the left pulmonary artery. The left posterior pulmonary artery and its branches can best be demonstrated in the left posterior oblique (LPO) position (Fig. 7–23*A*, *B*, and *C*).

Film Rate

Film rate often depends on cardiac output. If cardiac output is limited, circulation time is prolonged. This can require *filming* up to 15 seconds after injection in order to present a complete portrayal of all three phases of circulation.

A suggested filming rate would be 4 films/sec × 3 seconds followed by 2 films/sec × 3 seconds, followed by 1 film/sec for 4 seconds. This sequence results in a film run of 22 films over a time frame of 10 seconds.

The advantage of serial filming over cineangiography is the inherent resolution, vascular detail, and ability to cover the entire thorax and lung area on a single injection.

Cineangiography

The advantage of cineangiography is the dynamic aspect of the equipment. The quality of modern equipment provides the capability for excellent selective diagnosis.

The negative aspect of all image-intensified studies is the small field size available in comparison with the larger serial film format.

▶ PULMONARY HEMODYNAMIC EVALUATION

Pulmonary angiography is often requested to confirm the presence of pulmonary emboli. Current procedural standards are often enhanced by the critical information provided by pressure values in the pulmonary arterial system.

Hemodynamic measurements are established through the catheter preceding the angiographic injection. This information along with the angiographic findings often determines the mode of treatment.

Hemodynamic evaluation may give evidence of left ventricular disease, cardiac tamponade, or cor pulmonale and provide a definitive diagnosis in the absence of pulmonary emboli.

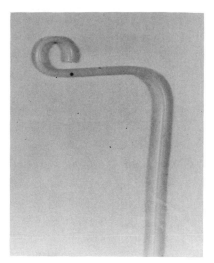

► **Figure 7–21**

Grollman No. 6.7 French pigtail catheter; 100 cm with four side holes.

In the patient with no cardiopulmonary disease and pulmonary hypertension, a mean pressure of greater than 25 mm Hg often indicates obstruction by emboli. As pulmonary artery pressures approach 40 mm Hg, pulmonary obstruction approaches 60 to 70% (Fig. 7–24).

► CARDIAC HEMODYNAMICS AND PRESSURES

We have discussed the indications of cardiac catheterization for establishing a given diagnosis. In addition to the injection of contrast to map and visualize the cardiac chambers and vessels, the measurement of dynamic blood pressure in both *diastole* and *sys-*

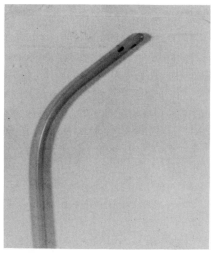

► **Figure 7–22**

NIH No. 7 French catheter; 100 cm with four side holes and a closed end.

tole in the heart chambers and vessels has become an important tool to further evaluate the effects of disease on cardiac circulation.

The systemic veins via the IVC and SVC drain the deoxygenated blood into the thin-walled right atrium.

When contraction (systole) occurs in the right atrium, the deoxygenated blood is pushed through the tricuspid valve into the right ventricle. The tricuspid valve provides for flow in only one direction. When the right ventricle is full, the tricuspid valve closes, and ventricular systole (contraction) pushes the deoxygenated blood through the pulmonary valve into the pulmonary arterial system.

In the pulmonary system there is an exchange of gases. Carbon dioxide is shed during exhalation. The blood is reoxygenated during inspiration and is transferred from the lung capillaries to venules and finally to four distinct veins that emerge from the lungs (two from each) and empty into the left atrium. When the left atrium is full, another contraction takes place and the oxygenated blood is transported to the muscular-walled, high-volume left ventricle (the largest chamber of the heart). As the thick muscular-walled left ventricle contracts, the newly oxygenated blood is pushed through the aortic semilunar valve and then perfused via the aortic arch, thoracic and abdominal aorta, and aortic branches and throughout the entire peripheral arterial system.

The oxygenated blood is directed through the capillary systems (internal respiration) and back into the venous system, where it returns to the heart by way of the peripheral veins to the SVC and IVC and to the right atrium and hence the beginning of another cardiac cycle (Fig. 7–25).

The *cardiac cycle* occurs approximately 75 to 80 times/min, and the time for each cycle is approximately 0.8 second.

Two terms are commonly used to describe the phases of the heart beat. When the atria of the heart are filling, *diastole* describes this period of heart relaxation or rest. Following their filling, the atria and ventricles contract and *systole* begins. Systole is described as the period of heart pumping or work phase. The heart contraction provides a "squeezing" mechanism that forces the flow of blood through the valves and through the cardiac cycle.

The systole phase begins in the atria and then passes into the ventricles. The systole phase results in the familiar "lubb-dubb" sounds that are heard through the stethoscope. The "lubb" sound is caused by the closure of the AV valves (tricuspid and mitral), and the "dubb" sound marks the closure of the semilunar valves (pulmonary and aortic).

The cardiac cycle is under the control of the central nervous system, yet the "beat" originates from a system command in the heart. The heart beat is controlled by a small bundle of muscle tissue located in the posterior wall of the right atrium. This "pacing" area is called the *SA node*. From the right atrium, the electrical impulse travels over the entire atrial muscle, causing the atria to contract. This wave action is

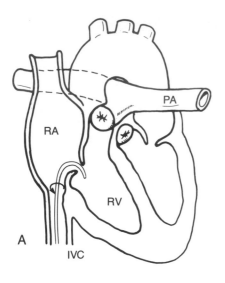

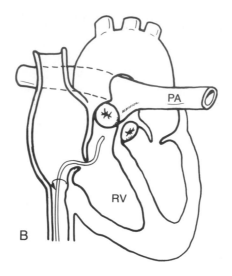

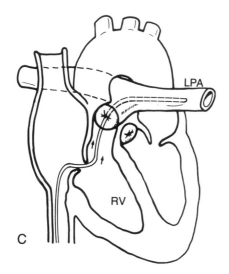

▸ **Figure 7–23**

A, In a right heart catheterization, the catheter is passed via the right femoral vein to the right atrium (RA). Rotation of the catheter orients it toward the right ventricle (RV). (PA = pulmonary artery; IVC = inferior vena cava.) *B,* Further rotation of the catheter causes the catheter to advance vertically, pointing at the right ventricular valve. (PA = pulmonary artery; RV = right ventricle.) *C,* Advancement of the catheter through the right ventricular outflow tract into the main pulmonary artery and selectively directed to the left pulmonary artery. (LPA = left pulmonary artery; RV = right ventricle.) (*A* to *C,* Redrawn from illustrations by Martha J. Dane.)

passed on to a second bundle of nerve tissue called the *AV node,* located in the septum between the right atrium and ventricle. From this area, the wave action and command is transmitted to the *bundle of His,* which consists of a band of specialized cells that pass between the interventricular septum and divide into two main branches called the *Purkinje fibers* (Fig. 7–26).

Thus, the SA node sends an electrical signal to stimulate the atrial walls to contract and push the blood into the ventricles. The AV node then immediately sends an electrical signal to the ventricular walls, triggering contraction of the ventricles and ejection of blood from the heart.

Force is transmitted through fluid as a pressure wave. Thus the essence of cardiac hemodynamic pressure monitoring is to assess the pressure of the blood that is generated during systole and diastole in the chambers of the heart.

The pressure measurement systems used today transform the pressure monitored at the catheter tip into an electrical signal using a *strain-gauge.* The strain-gauge is a transducer. A *transducer* is a device, in this case, that converts a pressure level or change into an electrical resistance. In simple terms, the strain-gauge function depends on the amount of pressure applied across wire sensors. When the variable resistance or hemodynamic pressure increases, the wire is stretched and its electrical resistance increases. This sensing wire (transducer) is connected to a device called a *Wheatstone bridge.*

When the transducer or strain-gauge senses the diastolic or systolic pressure waves through the catheter, the strain-gauge wires are stretched and thus present a changing resistance input signal into the Wheatstone bridge. The Wheatstone bridge assigns an electrical output that is proportional to the pressure applied and sensed on the transducer diaphragm (Fig. 7–27).

A practical system commonly used today is the three-stopcock manifold system. The catheter hub is connected to one side of the manifold, and a small-volume fluid-filled pressure transducer is connected to the other end of the manifold. It is important to

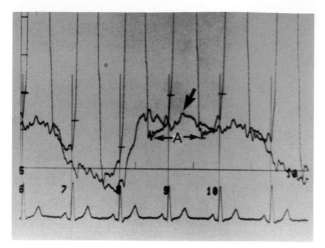

▶ **Figure 7–24**

Pulmonary arterial wedge pressures; the pulmonary arterial wedge pressure is obtained when the catheter interrupts forward blood flow; thus, the catheter is measuring pressure distal to the catheter tip generated by the left atrium (LA). The A wave is the pressure wave caused by atrial systole. The V wave is the pressure fluctuation caused by the atria filling during ventricular systole. The A and V measurements are usually within 1 to 3 mm Hg of each other. The A/V wave sweep above is represented by A, a mean of 7. The normal pulmonary arterial wedge pressure, mean pressure is 4 to 12 mm Hg.

zation). When zeroing the system, the tubing and transducer are flushed with 5% dextrose or normal saline to remove all air. This type of system then requires two pressurized drips—heparin and a plain dextrose with water or normal saline solution. The presence of blood or contrast medium in the catheter during monitoring can provide for false-pressure readings.

Common errors in pressure measurement are shown in Table 7–5.

Pressure Measurements

During catheterization the pressures are measured in each heart chamber and vessel that the catheter enters. The pressure or dynamic force of diastole and systole is monitored from the catheter tip to the transducer. The transducer via the Wheatstone bridge conversion transmits a signal of changing intensity to a cathode-ray terminal (CRT) or monitor, and the pressure levels are presented as varying vertical measurements on a scale measured in conventional blood pressure terminology in millimeters of mercury (mm Hg).

▶ TERMINOLOGY

Systolic pressure is the pressure during ventricular ejection.

Diastolic pressure is the pressure during contraction preceding systole, just before ejection.

Mean pressure is the average pressure in an artery or vein.

End-diastole is the ventricular pressure measured just before contraction (systole).

Right atrial pressure mean is normally less than 8 mm Hg. Elevated pressures can indicate right ventricular failure or tricuspid valve insufficiency.

Right ventricular pressure is normally 15 to 30 mm Hg systolic and less than 7 mm Hg end-diastolic. Systolic pres-

place the transducer and manifold system at the midaxillary level of the right atrium when the system is zeroed to open air. This is very important, because an elevation of the transducer above the heart level can produce a false-negative pressure; conversely, a low-placed transducer can produce an increased positive pressure (see Fig. 7–18).

The stopcocks on the manifold side arms can be manipulated for several different actions. Generally, one of the side arms is connected to a pressurized heparinated saline solution that is used intermittently to flush the catheter of blood (intermittent heparini-

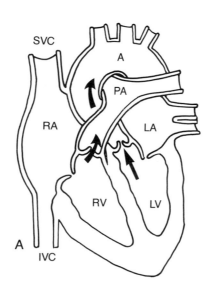
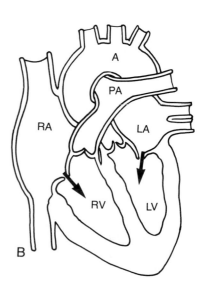

▶ **Figure 7–25**

Ventricular and atrial systole (contraction). A, Contraction of the ventricles; B, Contraction of the atria. (A = artery; PA = pulmonary artery; LA = left atrium; RA = right atrium; RV = right ventricle; LV = left ventricle; SVC = superior vena cava; IVC = inferior vena cava.) (A and B, Redrawn from illustrations by Martha J. Dane.)

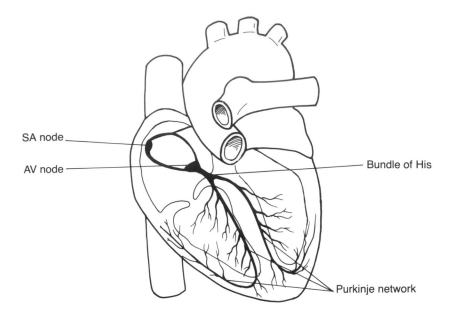

SA node

AV node

Bundle of His

Purkinje network

▸ **Figure 7–26**
The sinoatrial (SA) node, atrioventricular (AV) node, and Purkinje network of the heart. (Redrawn from an illustration by Martha J. Dane.)

sure increases in pulmonary hypertension or pulmonary stenosis. The end-diastolic pressure rises with right ventricular failure and ventricular hypertrophy and fibrosis.

Left ventricular systolic pressure normally ranges from 90 to 150 mm Hg. Elevated systolic pressures can indicate aortic stenosis. Lower-than-normal systolic pressures can indicate shock or severely depressed cardiac output. Left ventricular pressure and diastolic pressure (<10 mm Hg) are elevated in left ventricular failure or can indicate increased ventricular volume.

Pulmonary arterial pressure is normally in the range of 10 to 20 mm Hg. A rise signifies an increase in pulmonary flow that can be an indication of pulmonary vascular disease or an obstruction of pulmonary venous return. The end-diastolic range is 5 to 14 mm Hg (see Fig. 7–24).

Aortic systolic and diastolic pressures vary greatly with age. The systolic mean pressure is in the range of 90 to 150 mm Hg, and the diastolic pressure range is 60 to 90 mm Hg. Increased pressure can indicate aortic insufficiency or patent ductus arteriosus. Reduced aortic pressures are often found in patients with poor left ventricular outflow and low or reduced cardiac output (Figs. 7–28 to 7–33).

▸ CONGENITAL DISORDERS

Congenital Heart Disease

Congenital heart disease most often occurs sporadically, but heredity does appear to play a certain role in families. The incidence of congenital heart disease is higher among the offspring of an affected parent.

Congenital heart disease occurs at a higher frequency when multiple organ defects are present. Pregnant women with viral infections (e.g., rubella) may produce offspring who have congenital heart defects.

There are at least 100 forms or variations of congenital heart disease. Each individual illness often presents different symptoms. Some of the defects undergo correction as the child grows, while in others the problem worsens.

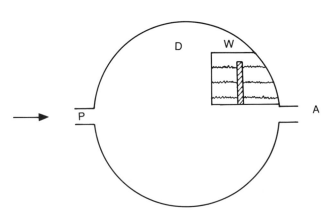

▸ **Figure 7–27**
Strain gauge pressure transducers: Pressure from the catheter into the port (P). The pressure on the diaphragm (D) increases the resistance on the sensing wires (W). The wires are connected electrically to the Wheatstone bridge. *A* represents a vent to atmospheric pressure. (Redrawn from an illustration by Martha J. Dane.)

▸ **Table 7–5**
COMMON SOURCES OF ERROR IN MEASUREMENT OF PRESSURE

Poor frequency response: air bubbles or blood in the system
Catheter whip artifacts: motion of the catheter tip in chambers can provide false readings
End-pressure artifacts: seen in end-hole catheters pointing retrograde (upstream), resulting in elevated pressure levels
Catheter impact artifact: the catheter is struck by heart valves opening or closing
Calibration errors: improper transducer level or air in the transducer or tubing, resulting in false zero levels

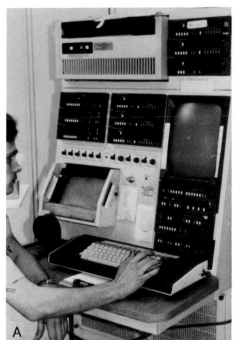

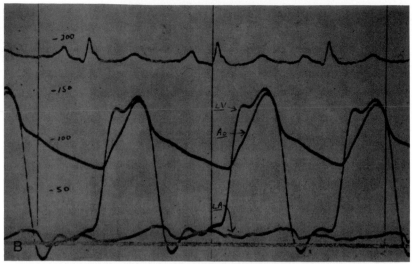

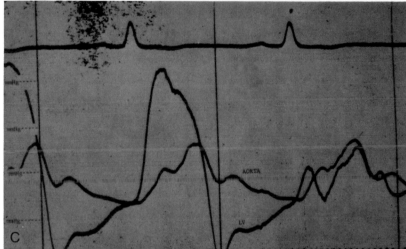

▶ **Figure 7–28**

A, Meddars 300 Modular Physiologic
Display and Recording System. (Courtesy
of PAG Industries, Lenexa, KS.) *B,* No
steep gradient exists between the aorta
(AO) and left ventricular (LV) pressures;
there is a normal gradient. *C,* A steep
gradient exists between the aorta (AO)
and the left ventricle (LV) showing
evidence of aortic stenosis.

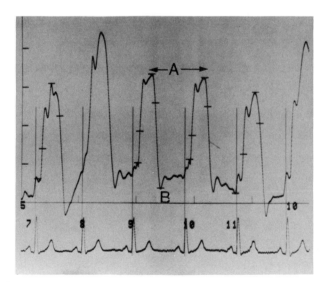

▶ **Figure 7–29**

Right ventricular hemodynamic pressures. The range (*A*) is
representative of the peak systolic pressure measured at
33 mm Hg. The end-diastolic pressure (EDP) is represented by
B and is measured at 2.3/8.2 mm Hg. Normal right ventricle
pressures—systolic: 20 to 35 mm Hg; diastole: 0 to 5 mm Hg;
end-diastole: 2 to 6 mm Hg.

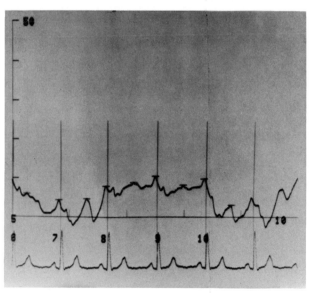

▶ **Figure 7–30**

Right atrial hemodynamic pressures. Because the A wave and
the V wave in the low pressure right atrium is within 1 to 2 mm
Hg, a mean pressure is recorded. The mean (*A*) is measured
at 5 mm Hg. Normal right arterial pressure: 2 to 6 mm Hg
mean.

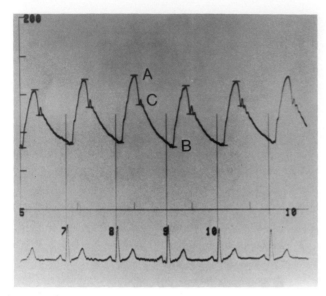

▶ **Figure 7–31**

Intra-arterial hemodynamic pressures monitored by the catheter in the aorta; the arterial waveform consists of systole (A), diastole (B), and the dicrotic notch. Peak systolic pressure measured in this patient is (A) 133 mg Hg. The end-diastolic pressure (B) is measured at 87 mm Hg. The systolic mean is measured at 111 mm Hg. Normal arterial pressures—peak systolic: 100 to 140 mm Hg; end-diastolic: 60 to 80 mm Hg; mean arterial: 70 to 90 mm Hg.

The radiology, cardiology, and medical laboratory departments combine their resources to accurately determine the type of cardiac lesion. Thus, the radiographic studies (cardiac catheterization with angiocardiography) correlate with all clinical and laboratory findings, including echocardiography.

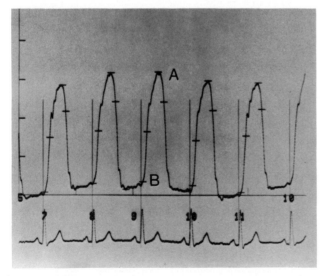

▶ **Figure 7–32**

Left ventricular hemodynamic pressures: systolic pressures are measured at A peaks at 120 mm Hg. The end-diastolic pressure is measured at B with a range of 3.5 to 10.8 mm Hg. Normal left ventricle pressures—systolic peak: 90 to 150 mm Hg; end-diastolic: 3 to 12 mm Hg.

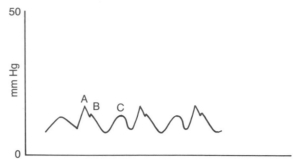

▶ **Figure 7–33**

Right atrial pressure waveform: A wave (A) = atrial systole; C wave (B) = beginning ventricular contraction, closure of valves; V wave (C) = atrial filling during ventricular systole.

Ventricular Septal Defect

Ventricular septal defect (VSD) is the most common congenital cardiac disorder. This abnormality results in a left-to-right shunt because of increased pressure in the right ventricle. The size of the shunt is in direct proportion to the pressures on the two sides of the shunt and the size of the defect.

Although the size of the defect varies, most defects are smaller than the circumference of a pencil. When these defects enlarge in proportion to growth, the child becomes symptomatic because the lungs react to the transmission of high pressure from the left ventricle through the defect on the right side of the heart.

VSDs are usually noted as a loud murmur at an age between 2 weeks and 2 months. Whereas most smaller defects close and require no further intervention, larger defects are usually closed surgically.

Radiographically, infants with left-to-right shunt disease have normal chest x-rays initially, because pulmonary hypertension is the normal state in the newborn. The heart is often enlarged. In the early stages of disease, the ventricles are frequently enlarged, and the left ventricle is more significant then the right ventricle. If the left atrium is enlarged, the esophagus may be displaced. The pulmonary artery is usually dilated and prominent. Angiocardiography is an effective method of demonstrating this defect, and a selective injection will identify the site of the defect and will reveal a shunt of opaque material across the defect from the left ventricle into the right ventricle (Fig. 7–34A to D).

Tetralogy of Fallot

Four individual defects are present with tetralogy of Fallot. Pulmonary stenosis and VSD are the most primary defects, whereas transposition of the aorta and hypertrophy of the right ventricle are considered to be secondary defects.

Pulmonary stenosis results in an increase in the pressure of the right ventricle. The VSD and displaced aorta allow venous blood from the right ventricle to be shunted directly into general circulation. The

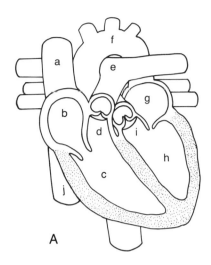

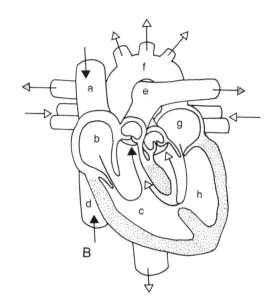

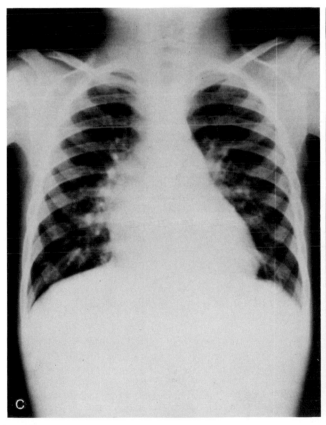

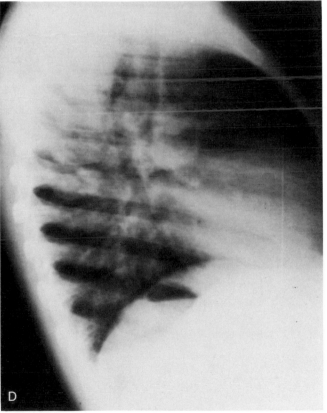

▶ Figure 7–34

A, A normal heart with major chambers and blood vessels. (a = superior vena cava; b = right atrium; c = right ventricle, d = entrance into the pulmonary artery via the pulmonary valve; e = pulmonary artery; f = aortic arch; g = left atrium; h = left ventricle; i = entrance into the ascending aorta via the aortic valve; j = inferior vena cava.) *B,* A ventricular septal defect. In this anomaly there is a hole in the septum separating the left ventricle (h). The deoxygenated blood (*dark arrows*) flows normally through the superior vena cava (a) into the right atrium (b), the right ventricle (c), and the pulmonary artery (e). The oxygen-rich blood returns to the left atrium (g) and flows into the left ventricle (h). Some of the blood from the left ventricle flows normally into the aorta (f), but a portion flows through the defect (*arrow*) and recirculates through the lungs. (*A* and *B,* Redrawn from illustrations by Martha J. Dane.) *C* and *D,* Infant anteroposterior and lateral infant chest with ventricular septal defect.

right-to-left shunt from the right ventricle into the aorta results in cyanosis.

Radiographically, the infant's heart may appear to be smaller than normal. On a chest film taken in the AP position, the pulmonary artery is small, resulting in concavity of the upper cardiac margin in the region of this segment. There is decreased pulmonary vascularity. The right ventricle is enlarged, and the shadow of the transposed aorta is present on the right at the level of the aorta (Fig. 7–35A and B).

Aortic Stenosis

Aortic stenosis refers to a constriction involving blood flow from the left ventricle into the aorta. The aortic valve is the site of this defect, and the condition is often referred to as valvular aortic stenosis.

In the presence of this defect, blood flow from the left ventricle is impeded. The result is increased pressure in the left ventricle. Over a period of time this condition worsens, and the left ventricle undergoes hypertrophy. Symptoms can vary from chest pain, dizziness, or fainting, and some people may suffer heart failure. Most infants and children present no symptoms.

Through cardiac catheterization, we are able to measure the abnormally high pressures of the left ventricle (Fig. 7–36).

Pulmonary Stenosis

Pulmonary stenosis is found most frequently with an intact ventricular septum accompanied by an atrial right-to-left shunt. This is sometimes referred to as the trilogy of Fallot.

Angiocardiography with serial filming usually shows the defect at the atrial level, with a bolus of contrast material propelled throughout the defect rapidly filling the left atrium (Fig. 7–37A and B).

Transposition of the Great Vessels

Transposition of the great vessels occurs in one of every 10 infants born with a heart defect. In this condition the aorta arises from the right ventricle, and the pulmonary artery arises from the left ventricle. As a consequence, two independent circulatory systems exist: In one system, blood circulates between the heart and the lungs, and in the other system, the blood circulates from the heart through systemic circulation but fails to be reoxygenated.

Infants are born with severe cyanosis, and symptoms are usually present within 24 hours after birth. One third of these infants also have a VSD.

Venous angiocardiography demonstrates the contrast material filling the right atrium, right ventricle, and anteriorly placed aorta from the right ventricle. If

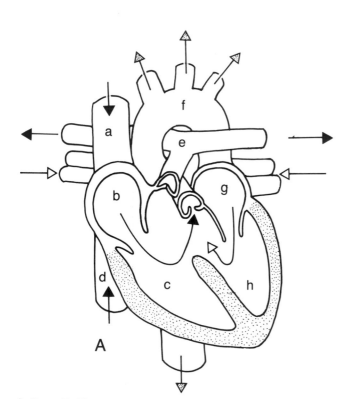

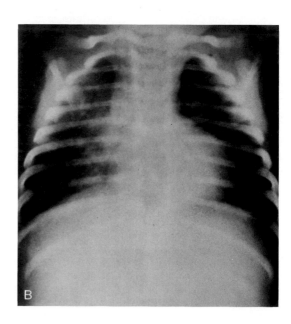

▶ **Figure 7–35**

A, Tetralogy of Fallot—in this anomaly, there are two major problems. The first problem is a hole in the wall separating the right ventricle (c) from the left ventricle (h). The second problem is a narrowing of the entrance into the pulmonary artery (e), which normally takes the deoxygenated blood and sends it to the lungs. Because of this narrowing, some deoxygenated blood flows from the right ventricle, through the defect, and into the aorta (f). (a = superior vena cava; b = right atrium; d = inferior vena cava; g = left atrium.) (Redrawn from an illustration by Martha J. Dane.) *B,* Infant anteroposterior chest with tetralogy of Fallot.

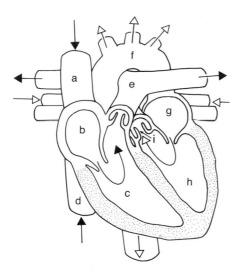

► **Figure 7–36**

Aortic stenosis. Blood flows normally through the right side of the heart and through the lungs. However, the aortic valve (i), which separates the left ventricle (h) from the aorta (f), does not open properly, thus the pressure in the left ventricle rises. (a = superior vena cava; b = right atrium; c = right ventricle; d = inferior vena cava; e = pulmonary artery; g = left atrium.) (Redrawn from an illustration by Martha J. Dane.)

present, the VSD will be noted. The right-sided heart enlargement is also apparent on the angiocardiogram (Fig. 7–38A and B).

Malformation of the Aorta

Coarctation

Coarctation of the aorta is a congenital anomaly that presents as a constriction of an area of the aorta. There are two types of coarctation that differ in their relative location to the ductus arteriosus. In the most common type, the coarctation is distal (postductal) to the ductus. In this type, the proximal blood pressure taken on the arm varies greatly from the pressure taken on the lower legs. The second or "preductal" type occurs proximal of the ductus and is usually associated with other congenital cardiovascular abnormalities.

Angiocardiography is not usually employed in the diagnosis of coarctation; rather, retrograde aortography usually clearly designates the area of coarctation (Fig. 7–39A and B).

► ATHEROSCLEROTIC HEART DISEASE

Coronary artery atherosclerosis is a progressive disease that is characterized by the formation of thickened fatty plaques on the arterial intima. Atherosclerosis produces gradual changes that may lead eventually to a fatal occlusion. The pathogenesis of coronary atherosclerosis is beyond the scope of this text; however, let us say that the accumulation of these fatty deposits eventually produces a narrowing of the arterial lumen. This gradual narrowing brings about ischemia, which is a compromise of blood supply to the cardiac muscle. As this condition worsens, the potential for an infarction increases. An infarct can best be described as an area of ischemic necrosis or, basically, an area of dead heart muscle. Patients with progressive ischemia are often candidates for an acute myocardial infarction, which is the leading cause of death in middle-aged men.

As described earlier, angiocardiography and selective coronary arteriography play an important role in the diagnosis of coronary atherosclerosis. With the addition of balloon angioplasty by way of catheterization, the lives of many patients are being saved every day. Coronary angioplasty is usually performed when the patient is symptomatic (ischemic) and before any permanent damage occurs to the heart muscle. Thus, this treatment is a reasonable alternative to open heart surgery.

Figure 7–40A is a preangioplasty radiograph of a right selective coronary arteriogram of a 56-year-old man who was admitted to the hospital with chest pain. Figure 7–40B is the postangioplasty radiograph of the same patient. The radiograph shows marked improvement of blood flow through the right coronary artery.

Figure 7–41A shows marked stenosis of the anterior descending branch of the LCA in a 44-year-old man just before balloon angioplasty is attempted. Figure 7–41B shows an increase in the diameter of the arterial lumen and a subsequent increase in blood flow after angioplasty is done.

Figure 7–42A reveals an 85% stenosis of the circumflex branch of the LCA (*arrows*) in a 51-year-old man who had pain in the chest, left shoulder, and arm. Figure 7–42B shows the balloon catheter inflated in place (*arrow*). The postangioplasty radiograph (Fig. 7–42C) shows almost a total resumption of blood flow through the previously stenotic area of the artery (*arrow*).

Thrombolysis is often combined with balloon angioplasty to dissolve a clot and recanalize the arterial lumen. Figure 7–43A to F presents a series of six radiographs taken of a 60-year-old man who drove 45 miles to a hospital, only to collapse at the entrance to the emergency room.

► PULMONARY VASCULAR SYSTEM

Pulmonary Emboli

Embolism is a term used to characterize an occlusion of a vessel by the impaction of an embolus. An embolus in most cases is a moving thrombus. Most emboli are created as fragments of a thrombus (a blood clot

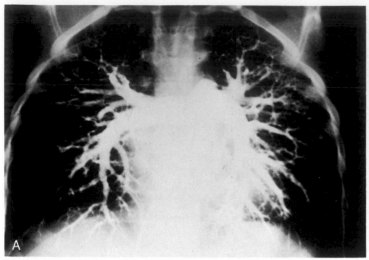

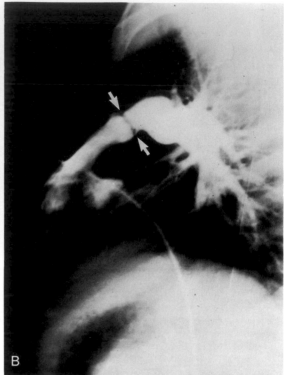

▸ **Figure 7–37**

A, A pulmonary angiogram of a child with pulmonary artery stenosis. Anteroposterior projection. *B*, Right lateral view of pulmonary artery stenosis.

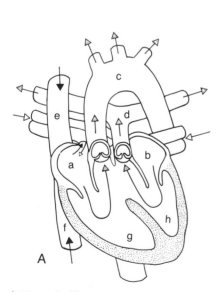

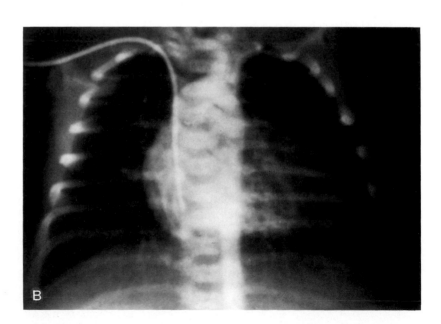

▸ **Figure 7–38**

A, Transposition of great vessels. In this anomaly, the major blood vessels leaving the heart originate from the opposite ventricles than normal. Therefore, the aorta (c) originates from the right ventricle (g), and the pulmonary artery (d) arises from the left ventricle (h). Thus the deoxygenated blood, traveling to the heart through the superior vena cava (e) and inferior vena cava (f), is returned to the body. Oxygenated blood is returned to the left atrium (a) and is pumped by the left ventricle (h) into the lungs again (via the left atrium [b]). (*A,* Redrawn from an illustration by Martha J. Dane.) *B,* Anteroposterior chest radiograph of a child with transposition of the great vessels.

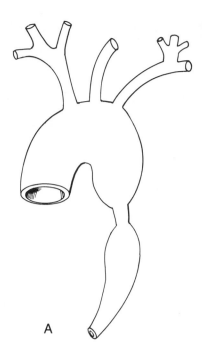

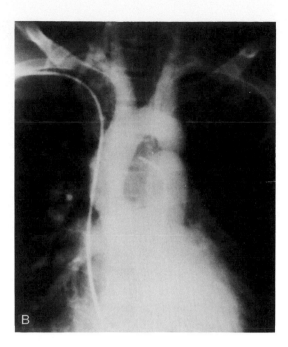

▶ Figure 7–39

A, A diagram of coarctation of the thoracic aorta. (Redrawn from an illustration by Martha J. Dane.) B, A child with coarctation of the proximal (upper) descending thoracic aorta as seen in the anteroposterior position on the aortogram.

lying within a vessel), which can be classed into five main types: (1) disengaged thrombi; (2) gas thrombi; (3) fat thrombi; (4) neoplastic thrombi; and (5) miscellaneous thrombi (e.g., foreign bodies). Most pulmonary emboli originate in the deep venous system of the lower legs.

A thrombus will detach from the vessel wall and follow venous circulation into the right side of the heart, where it enters the pulmonary circulation until the thrombus is unable to pass any further. At this point the thrombus remains fixed in position and blocks blood flow in the distal directions.

Patients suffering from this condition initially expe-rience sudden, severe dyspnea; chest pain; loss of consciousness; and perhaps death. Embolectomy and other surgical procedures are often unsuccessful. The most important factor in reducing mortality is to re-duce the possibility of leg vein thrombosis in high-risk patients.

A procedure that is useful in the diagnosis of pul-monary embolism is a perfusion scan. In a nuclear medicine perfusion scan, radioactive human serum albumin particles are intravenously introduced and perfuse the lung. During perfusion, these particles become trapped in some of the capillary branches of the pulmonary arterial trunk. The radioactive mate-

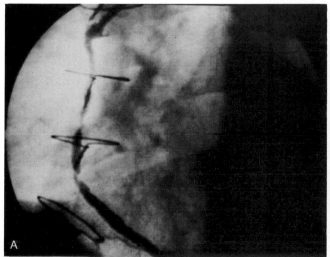

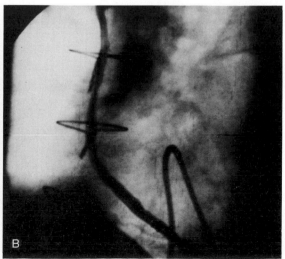

▶ Figure 7–40

Preangioplasty radiograph (A) and postangioplasty radiograph (B) of a right selective coronary arteriogram of a 56-year-old man admitted to the hospital with chest pain.

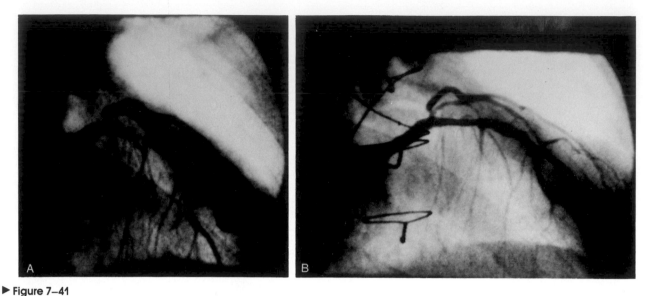

► **Figure 7–41**

A, Marked stenosis of the anterior descending branch of the left coronary artery in a 44-year-old man. B, Postangioplasty of the same patient.

rial emits gamma radiation that is recorded with a scintillation detector (camera).

When a study is normal, the lungs appear as a blackened image, indicating that the distribution of trapped particles (radioactive material) is uniform throughout the lungs. In the presence of an embolism, the affected arterial branch is not perfused with the isotope, and a defect or "cold spot" is noted. This defect is represented as a "nonblackened" area. If no defects are seen on the lung perfusion scan, then we

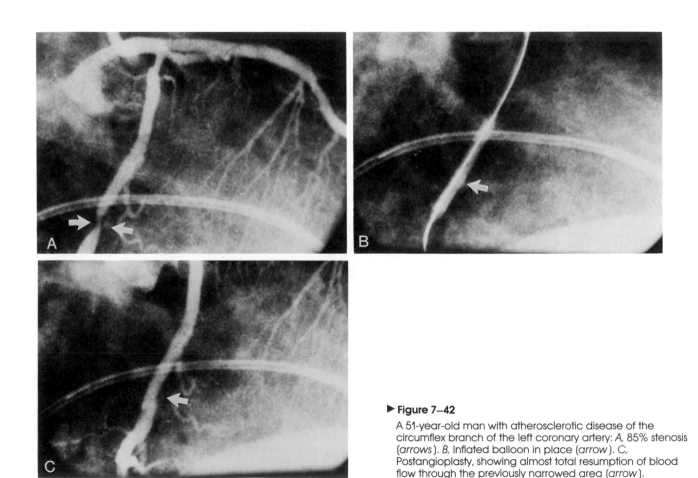

► **Figure 7–42**

A 51-year-old man with atherosclerotic disease of the circumflex branch of the left coronary artery: A, 85% stenosis (arrows). B, Inflated balloon in place (arrow). C, Postangioplasty, showing almost total resumption of blood flow through the previously narrowed area (arrow).

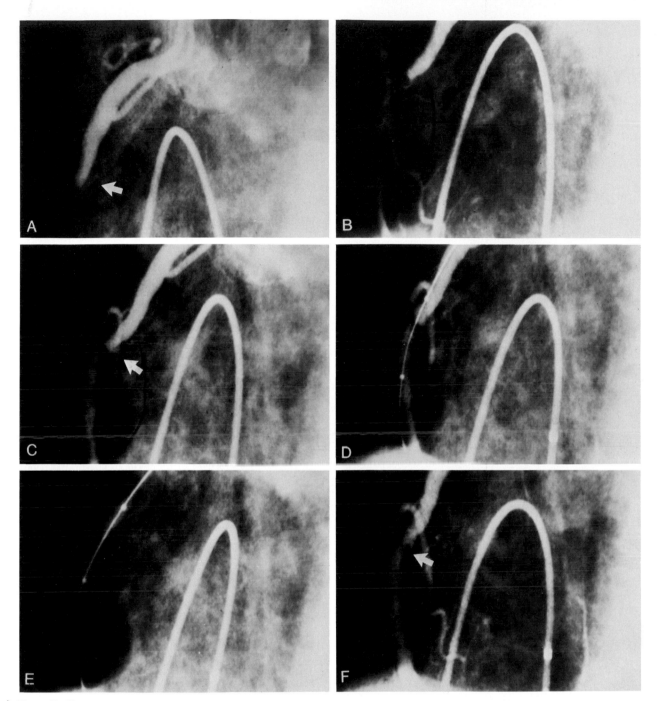

► **Figure 7–43**

A, An initial radiograph showing occlusion of the right coronary artery (*arrow*). *B,* Note the 10-cm clot formation (*brackets*). The radiograph was taken 15 minutes after the administration of streptokinase infusion. *C,* A radiograph taken 60 minutes after streptokinase infusion; again note the clot formation (*brackets*). *D,* A guidewire is in place; a balloon is positioned over the lesion. *E,* Balloon angioplasty; the balloon is inflated. *F,* A postangioplasty radiograph showing recanalization.

can conclude that the patient does not have a pulmonary embolism (Fig. 7–44*A*).

If the perfusion scan reveals a defect, we can be assured that, given the clinical history, the patient has a pulmonary embolism. In the case of an abnormal perfusion scan, we then perform a ventilation scan. This procedure is carried out with the inhalation of xenon, which is a radioactive gas.

Xenon gas determines the amount of ventilation in

the lungs. The xenon scan, in the presence of an embolism, demonstrates all areas of the lung without evidence of defect. Diseases such as emphysema, pneumonia, and metastases produce defects on the ventilation scan; however, this is not the case with a pulmonary embolism. Thus, a normal xenon scan further confirms the diagnosis of a pulmonary embolism (Fig. 7–44*B*).

Pulmonary arteriography is another method of

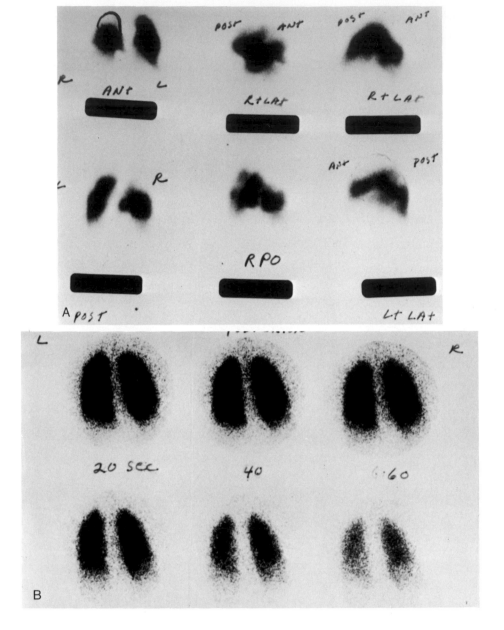

▶ **Figure 7–44**

A, A nuclear medicine lung perfusion scan revealing "cold spots" identified as emboli. B, The xenon lung ventilation scan appears normal.

identifying a pulmonary embolism. Pulmonary arteriography appears to be more accurate compared to radioisotope scanning. However, it is much more invasive and more costly.

Pulmonary arteriography is indicated when the isotope scans are inconclusive, when the lung scan is diagnosed with a positive result in a patient who is at risk for anticoagulation therapy, when the patient exhibits overwhelming evidence of embolism, or when the isotope scans are normal.

The primary contraindications for pulmonary arteriography are severe pulmonary hypertension and sensitivity to the contrast agent. A pigtail catheter is introduced into the pulmonary artery via the right brachial approach. Figure 7–45 shows an example of digital subtraction angiography. Pulmonary angiography is accomplished with digital subtraction as well as with serial cut-filming.

Figure 7–46 is a right pulmonary arteriogram of a 77-year-old man who has a large embolism that is occluding a middle branch of the right pulmonary artery. This patient presents with a history of advanced peripheral vascular disease involving the pelvic and leg veins bilaterally. In addition, this patient has hypertension and diabetes and is an alcoholic who smokes two packs of cigarettes daily.

Figure 7–47 A and B shows a pulmonary angiogram of a 27-year-old man who experienced severe dyspnea after long-term hospitalization and abdominal surgery. In these two images, the left pulmonary arteriogram and coned-down views reveal the presence of multiple pulmonary emboli in several of the lower arterial branches. Notice the dark areas (*arrows*) of embolic formation (see Fig. 7–47B).

Urokinase and streptokinase, which are two fibrinolytic agents, have proved useful in the treatment

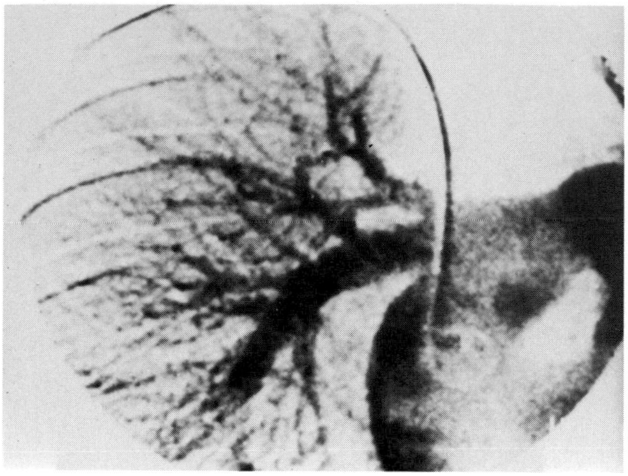

▶ Figure 7–45

A normal pulmonary angiogram.

of pulmonary embolism. However, fibrinolytic therapy is contraindicated when excessive bleeding is present.

As stated earlier, pulmonary embolectomy is the last resort for patients who suffer from a pulmonary embolism. Pulmonary embolectomy is the surgical removal of blood clots from the pulmonary circulation. This procedure has a high mortality rate.

Another alternative in the management of pulmonary emboli is the vena caval filter (or what we commonly refer to as the ''umbrella'').

Vena caval filters are used in patients who are at high risk for pulmonary emboli. High-risk patients can be identified as those in whom adequate anticoagulation fails to prevent a recurrent embolism. Patients may have pulmonary hypertension and cor pulmonale

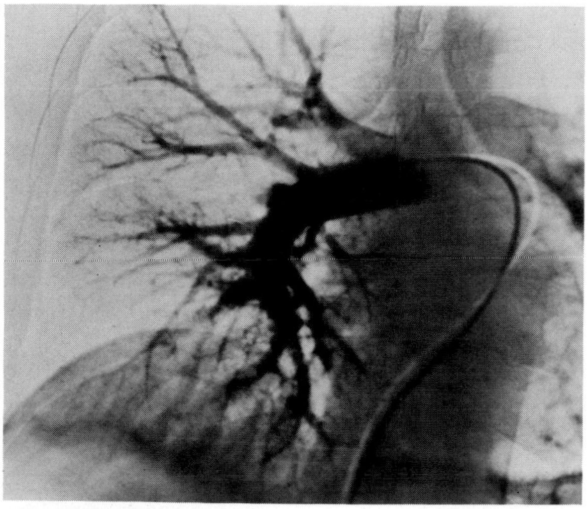

▶ Figure 7–46

A right pulmonary angiogram in a 77-year-old man who has a large embolism occluding a middle branch of the right pulmonary artery.

following an episode of massive pulmonary embolism. Under these circumstances, anticoagulant therapy may be discontinued.

There are some contraindications regarding caval filters. Patients suffering from congestive heart failure may have a vena cava that exceeds 28 mm. Proper function of the caval filter may be compromised when the caval diameter exceeds 28 mm. Thrombus formation at the puncture site may pose the risk of detachment of a thrombus during manipulation of the catheter. This is especially the case during the femoral vein approach.

One popular caval filter is the titanium Greenfield vena caval filter with a No. 12 French introducer system. This device is permanently implanted in the IVC and is designed to protect against pulmonary embolism while providing for continued patency of the vena cava. The titanium alloy used in the manufacture of the Greenfield vena caval filter allows for magnetic resonance imaging.

The titanium Greenfield vena caval filter comes preloaded with a jugular or femoral introducing catheter (Fig. 7–48). The femoral approach is advantageous because it eliminates the potential for anomalous puncture of the carotid artery and pneumothorax. It also reduces the risk of air embolism and cardiac arrhythmias. The femoral approach is difficult when vessel tortuosity is present, especially in the right iliac vein. In the femoral approach, there is always the danger of dislodging thrombi that may be adhering to the vessel wall.

It is essential that a routine cavagram first be performed. This is to determine whether the vein is free of thrombi (Fig. 7–49A and B). Once the preloaded introducer is in proper position, the release mechanism is activated to disengage the filter from the introducer (Fig. 7–50). The filter has specialized hooks that instantly secure the filter to the caval wall (Fig. 7–51A and B).

Arteriovenous Malformation

A pulmonary arteriovenous malformation (AVM), sometimes termed a fistula or aneurysm, is a congenital vascular anomaly through which a relatively large amount of nonoxygenated blood flows. The lesion, therefore, represents a right-to-left shunt and is associated with varying degrees of unsaturation of the arterial blood. The malformations are usually multiple and occur more frequently in the lower lobes than elsewhere. Because the caliber of vessels within the mass varies, there is no quantitative correlation between the size of the anomaly and the amount of shunt. The pulmonary lesions may be accompanied by hemangiomas or telangiectases elsewhere and are then part of a generalized angiomatous process. Because these are right-to-left shunts that may be quite large, the filtering effect of the pulmonary capillary circulation is lost, and any embolic process arising in the systemic venous system may result in systemic

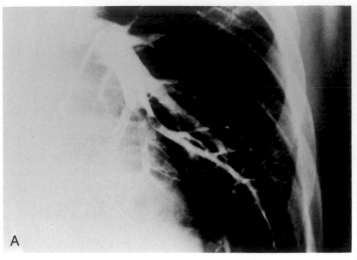

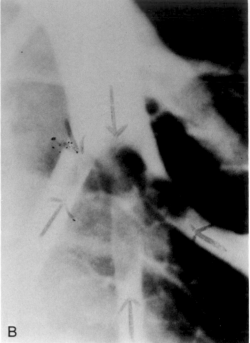

▶ **Figure 7–47**

A 27-year-old man who had complications after abdominal surgery. *A,* A coned-down pulmonary angiogram reveals the presence of multiple pulmonary emboli in several lower arterial branches. *B,* Notice the dark areas (*arrows*) of embolic formation.

embolization. A brain abscess, for example, is among the complications.

Radiographically, the malformation is represented by a round, oval, or lobulated mass or several masses, usually in the lower lobes. Linear tomograms and computed tomography scanning are useful in outlining the blood supply and in clearly defining the lesions. These lesions visually often seem to mimic metastatic lesions. Pulmonary arteriography is used to confirm the findings before surgical removal and also to determine the presence of smaller lesions that cannot be outlined on routine radiographs.

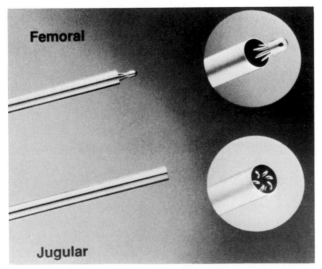

▶ **Figure 7–48**

Titanium Greenfield vena cava filter introducer. (Courtesy of Medi-tech/Boston Scientific Corporation, Watertown, MA.)

Figure 7–52 represents a PA chest, an AP right-sided chest tomogram, and a right selective pulmonary arteriogram of a 63-year-old man with a history of hemoptysis. The report identifies a lobulated density in the right upper lung, measuring 2 cm in diameter, with vascular densities, representing the feeding and draining vessels, extending to the right pulmonary artery and heart (left atrium). These abnormal structures are better outlined by the tomographic and angiographic examinations.

▶ THORACIC AORTA

Aneurysms

Aneurysms are localized dilatations of blood vessels (typically arteries) that are caused by an area of weakness in the vessel wall. Aneurysms can be classed into two primary groups: true and false. A *true aneurysm* structurally involves all three layers of the artery, namely the adventitia, media, and intima. Most true aneurysms affecting the thoracic aorta are atherosclerotic in origin. A *false* or *pseudoaneurysm* constitutes a destruction of the arterial wall. It may be limited to the intima, or it may involve all layers (Fig. 7–53).

Aortic Dissection

For the most part, dissecting aneurysms arise from a tear in the ascending aorta or arch. The length of dissection and the level of extension into vital structures determine the prognosis. The media and intima are usually involved, with an intimal flap presenting

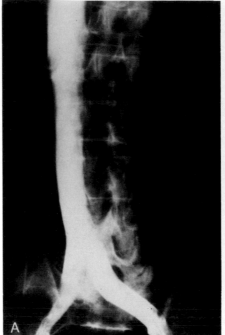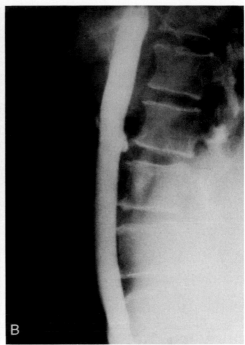

▶ **Figure 7–49**

A and *B,* Anteroposterior and lateral inferior vena cavagram; the result is normal.

entrance into a false lumen. Dissecting aneurysms are classed into two groups: (1) type A, which involves the ascending aorta or arch, and (2) type B, which involves the descending aorta only.

Hypertension is the single largest cause of aortic dissection. Patients younger than 40 years of age who have Marfan's syndrome, a collagen disorder, can be found to have a dissecting aneurysm. Pregnancy is also thought to be a precursor to aortic dissection. For the most part, middle-aged (older than 40 years of age), hypertensive men seem to suffer from aortic dissection more than any other age group.

Widening of the mediastinum appears to be the most common indication of aortic dissection on the routine PA chest film (Fig. 7–54).

If the dissection involves the aortic root, then echocardiography is preferred. Some studies indicate that computed tomography is more accurate than angiography in the diagnosis of aortic dissection; however, if the patient with dissection is a surgical candidate, then angiography should take precedence.

Angiography remains the best method of imaging for demonstrating occlusion of branch vessels and aortic regurgitation, both of which are important for planning surgery (Fig. 7–55).

Atherosclerotic Aneurysms

As stated previously, intrathoracic aneurysms are found most frequently in the descending thoracic aorta and have an atherosclerotic etiology.

Thoracic and thoracoabdominal aortic aneurysms are more difficult to treat and have a higher mortality rate than have those of the abdominal aorta. The most significant danger is rupture. The larger the aneurysm, the greater the risk of rupture. Studies indicate that more than 40% are over 10 cm in diameter.

Figure 7–56 is a PA chest radiograph of a 44-year-old woman who had an aortic arch aneurysm. Note the shifting of the trachea to the right. This patient's primary complaints were chest pain and dysphagia.

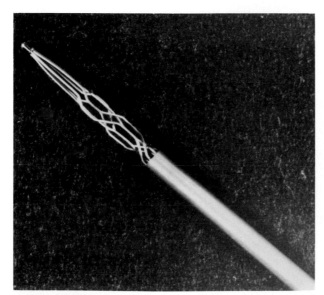

▶ **Figure 7–50**

Greenfield filter release mechanism. (Courtesy of Medi-tech/ Boston Scientific Corporation, Watertown, MA.)

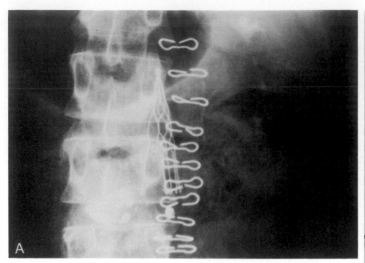

▸ **Figure 7–51**

A and B, Views of a Greenfield filter with specialized hooks affixed to the caval wall. (Courtesy of Medi-tech/Boston Scientific Corporation, Watertown, MA.)

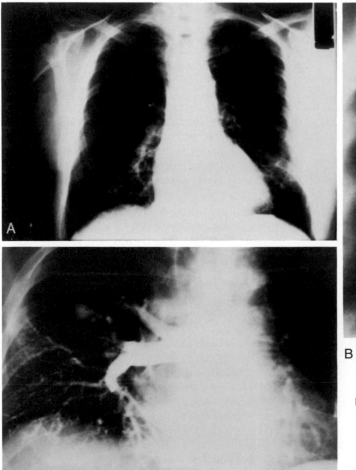

▸ **Figure 7–52**

A 63-year-old man with a history of hemoptysis.
A, Posteroanterior view of the chest.
B, Anteroposterior right chest tomogram.
C, A right selective pulmonary arteriogram. Lobulated densities (blood clot) measuring 2 cm in diameter are apparent in the right upper lung.

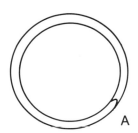
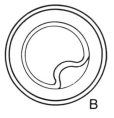
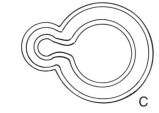

▶ **Figure 7–53**

Differentiation of a true aneurysm (A), a dissection (B), and a pseudoaneurysm (C). (Redrawn from an illustration by Martha J. Dane.)

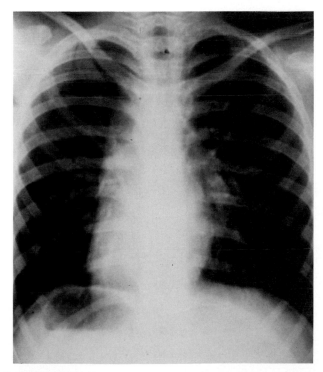

▶ **Figure 7–54**

Posteroanterior chest film demonstrating widening of the mediastinum.

Figure 7–57 shows a 55-year-old man who had chest pain and dyspnea. The PA chest radiograph revealed a huge thoracic aortic aneurysm that seemed to encompass the majority of the thoracic aorta. Unfortunately, it is difficult to determine the "exact" extent of this aneurysm owing to part rotation. The trachea is shifted to the right; however, owing to the rotation of the chest (noted by sternoclavicular asymmetry), it is not really possible to accurately determine the size of this aneurysm.

Figure 7–58 *A, B,* and *C* shows a PA view of the chest and two lateral views of the aorta (of the same image) with a conventional radiograph (see Fig. 7–58*B*) and a subtraction print (see Fig. 7–58*C*). Note the differences in the two radiographs. This patient is a 27-year-old man who was found to have this aneurysm during a pre-employment physical examination. He had no specific complaints or clinical history that would have indicated this lesion.

Figure 7–59 shows a patient who was asymptomatic but, upon direct questioning, recalled being involved in an automobile accident with injury to the thorax 15 years earlier. The plain x-ray film of the chest shows an enlargement that is associated with a calcific rim of the aortic knob. Thoracic aortography reveals a chronic saccular aneurysm of the descending thoracic aorta beyond the origin of the left subclavian artery. Aneurysms of the thoracic aorta after blunt trauma can be divided into the acute and chronic types. In the acute stage, multiple fractures, internal injuries, and shock may divert the attention from the thorax, so that rupture of the aorta is overlooked. The commonest site of rupture of the aorta is usually at the ligamentum arteriosum. This is explained by the fixation of the aorta by the brachiocephalic arteries and ligamentum arteriosum and by forces that result in deceleration. Very severe chest trauma causes complete rupture of the aorta and death. A linear tear may heal spontaneously or give rise to a dissecting aneurysm that progresses to form a false aneurysmal sac.

Syphilitic, arteriosclerotic, and congenital aneurysms found at the top of the descending aorta need to be differentiated, and the history of trauma is significant.

Figure 7–60 shows a patient with a large aneurysm at the top of the aortic arch, at a point where the aorta begins to course downward. The patient is a 55-year-old man who complained of chest discomfort. The cause of the aneurysm was unknown. The thoracic aorta and aneurysm are presented in the standard AP format (Fig. 7–60*A*) and with a subtracted image (Fig. 7–60*B*). Subtracted images are frequently included as an addition to the angiographic study.

Figure 7–61 is a lateral aortographic view of an adolescent with a subaortic stenosis (*arrow*) and a history of a VSD. Idiopathic hypertrophic subaortic stenosis is a special type of myocardial hypertrophy that involves the ventricular septum and encroaches on the left ventricular cavity. This condition usually manifests itself in late childhood or in early adult life.

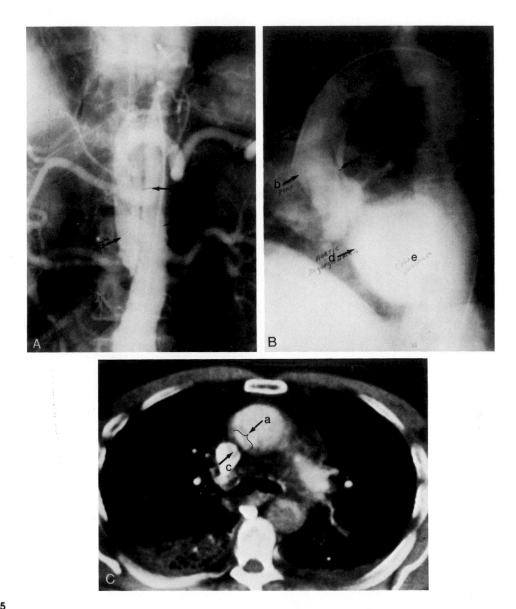

▶ **Figure 7–55**

Dissecting aneurysm. *A,* Anteroposterior aortogram. (a = false lumen; b = true lumen; c = intimal flap.) *B,* Lateral aortogram. (a = catheter; b = flap; c = flap; d = aortic regurgitation; e = left ventricle.) *C,* Computed tomography scan. (a = false lumen; b = aorta; c = superior vena cava.)

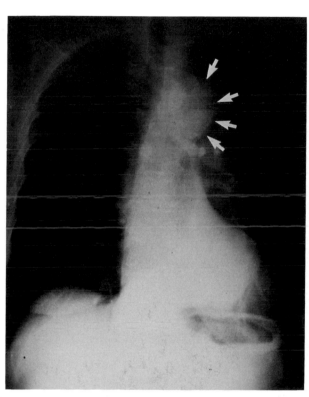

► **Figure 7–56**
Posteroanterior chest radiograph of a 44-year-old woman with an aneurysm of the aortic arch (*arrows*).

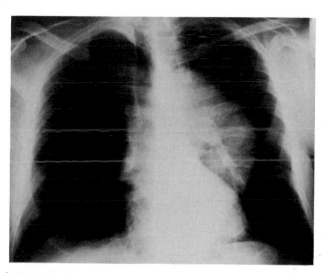

► **Figure 7–57**
Posteroanterior chest radiograph of a 55-year-old man with a huge aortic arch aneurysm.

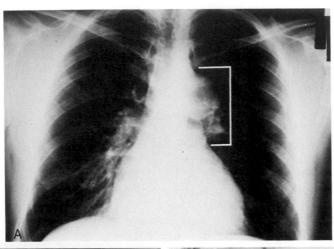

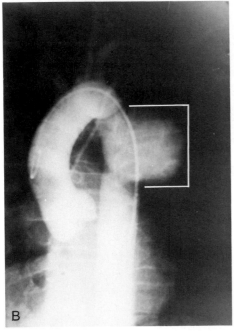

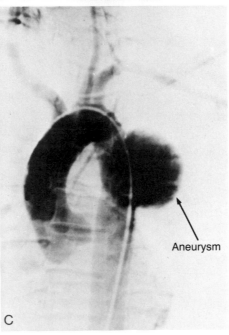

► **Figure 7–58**

A, Posteroanterior chest (bracket indicates aneurysm); *B,* Left posterior oblique chest (bracket indicates aneurysm); *C,* Left posterior oblique chest, subtraction image: thoracic aortic aneurysm.

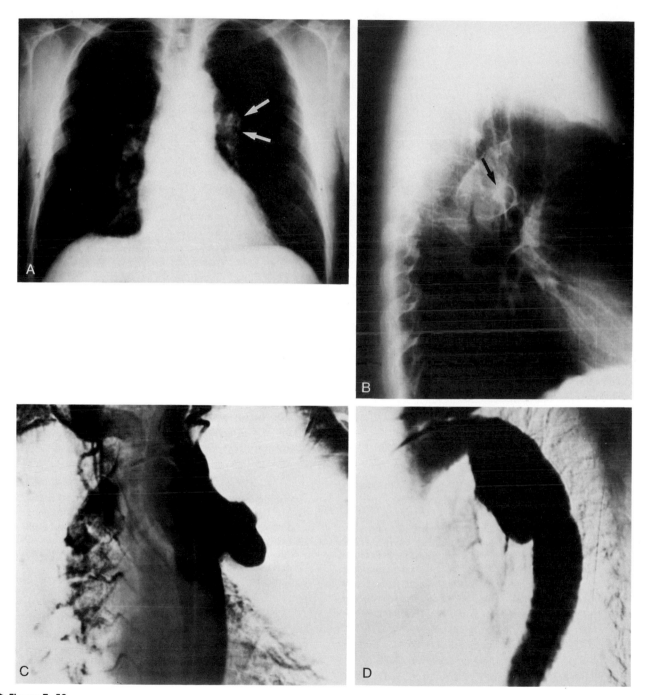

► Figure 7–59

A to *D,* A 15-year-old injury sustained in an automobile accident. A saccular aneurysm of the descending thoracic aorta is shown.

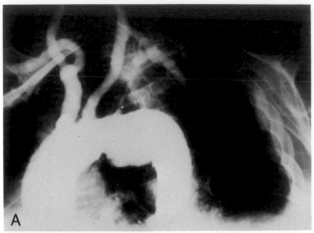

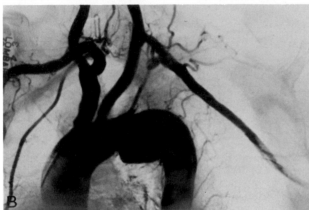

▶ **Figure 7–60**

A large aneurysm at the top of the aortic arch. *A,* Thoracic aortogram. *B,* Subtraction image of the same patient.

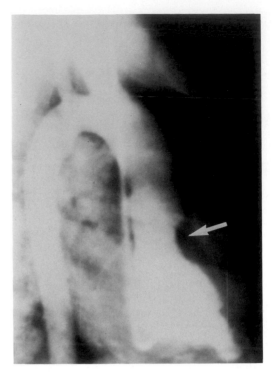

▶ **Figure 7–61**

Subaortic stenosis (*arrow*) in an adolescent patient who had a history of a ventricular septal defect.

▶ BIBLIOGRAPHY

Abrams HL: Abrams Angiography: Vascular and Interventional Radiology, Vol 1, 3rd ed. Boston, Little, Brown, 1983.

Benchimol A: Noninvasive Techniques in Cardiology for the Nurse and Technician. New York, John Wiley, 1978.

Carlton RR and Philpot D: Cardiovascular-Interventional Technology Exam Review. Philadelphia, JB Lippincott, 1991.

Cawson RA, McCracken AW, et al: Pathology: The Mechanisms of Disease. 2nd ed. St Louis, CV Mosby, 1989.

Des Jardins T: Clinical Manifestations of Respiratory Disease, 2nd ed. Chicago, Year Book Medical Publishers, 1990.

Gedgaudos E, Moller J, Castaneda-Zuniga W, and Amplatz K: Cardiovascular Radiology. Philadelphia, WB Saunders, 1985.

Greenfield LJ, Cho KJ, et al: Evolutions of hook design for fixation of the titanium Greenfield filter. J Vasc Surg 12:345, 1990.

Greenfield LJ, McCurdy JR, et al: A new intra caval filter permitting continued flow and resolution of emboli. Surgery 73(4):153, 1973.

Greenfield LJ and Michna BA: Twelve-year clinical experience with the Greenfield vena caval filter. Surgery 104:706, 1988.

Grossman W, et al: Cardiac Catheterization and Angiography, 3rd ed. Philadelphia, Lea & Febiger, 1986.

Judkins MP: Angiographic equipment: The cardiac catheterization laboratory. *In* Abrams HL (ed): Coronary Arteriography: A Practical Approach. Boston, Little, Brown, 1983.

Juhl JH and Crummy AB: Paul and Juhl's Essentials of Radiologic Imaging, 5th ed. Philadelphia, JB Lippincott, 1987.

Kandarpa K: Percutaneous transfemoral placement of Kimray-Greenfield inferior vena cava filters. *In* Handbook of Cardiovascular and Interventional Radiologic Procedures. Boston, Little, Brown, 1989.

Laudicina PF: Applied Pathology for Radiographers. Philadelphia, WB Saunders, 1989.

Meszaros WT: Cardiac Roentgenology. Springfield, IL, Charles C. Thomas, 1969.

Miller S (ed): Cardiopulmonary imaging. Radiol Clin North Am 27(6), 1989.

Miller S (ed): Advances in cardiac imaging. Radiol Clin North Am 23(4), 1985.

Robbins LL (ed): Golden's diagnostic radiology. *In* Davis LA and Shearer LT: Pediatric Radiology, 2nd ed. Baltimore, Williams & Wilkins, 1973.

Squire LF and Novelline RA: Fundamentals of Radiology, 4th ed. Cambridge, MA, Harvard Press, 1988.

Verel D and Grainger R: Cardiac Catheterization and Angiocardiography, 2nd ed. London, Churchill Livingstone, 1973.

Wojtowycz M: Interventional Radiology and Angiography. Chicago, Year Book Medical Publishers, 1990.

▶ SELF-ASSESSMENT QUIZ

1. Who first accomplished cardiac catheterization?
   a. Sones
   b. Bernard
   c. Forssmann
   d. Amplatz

2. Who was the first human to be catheterized?
   a. Sones
   b. Bernard
   c. Forssmann
   d. Amplatz

3. Who first described a technique for selective coronary arteriography using a brachial approach?
   a. Sones
   b. Bernard
   c. Forssmann
   d. Amplatz

4. Who first used the transfemoral route utilizing shaped selective catheters?
   a. Swan-Ganz
   b. Amplatz
   c. Forssmann
   d. Sones

5. Who first introduced a flow-guided balloon-tipped catheter that allowed for the introduction of a cardiac catheter at the patient's bedside?
   a. Swan-Ganz
   b. Sones
   c. Gruntzig
   d. Amplatz

6. Who is responsible for introducing a technique for coronary angioplasty in 1977?
   a. Sones
   b. Swan-Ganz
   c. Amplatz
   d. Gruntzig

7. Who are responsible for development of preformed catheters that resulted in lower mortality rates?
   a. Amplatz and Judkins
   b. Gruntzig and Amplatz
   c. Amplatz and Sones
   d. Gruntzig and Judkins

8. The outermost layer of the heart is the
   a. myocardium
   b. epicardium
   c. endocardium
   d. pleura

9. What is the name given to the largest branch of the RCA?
   a. circumflex
   b. diagonal
   c. acute marginal
   d. posterior descending

10. Venous blood returns to the right atrium by way of the
    a. coronary arteries
    b. venae cavae
    c. aorta
    d. pulmonary arteries

11. An instrument that is described as "a series of stopcocks" is called a (an)
    a. manometer
    b. adapter
    c. connector
    d. manifold

12. What type of catheters is often preferred for both right and left ventriculography?
    a. Sones
    b. Judkins
    c. pigtail
    d. sidewinder

13. What procedure is Moniz most noted for?
    a. coronary arteriography
    b. cardiac ventriculography
    c. cardiac catheterization
    d. pulmonary angiography

14. What is the preferred site of injection for pulmonary arteriography?
    a. right brachial vein
    b. aorta via translumbar puncture
    c. femoral vein
    d. femoral artery

15. The Grollman pigtail catheter and the NIH catheter are utilized with what procedure?
    a. pulmonary angiography
    b. coronary arteriography
    c. cardiac bypass surgery
    d. embolectomy

16. Which position best demonstrates the left pulmonary artery and its branches?
    a. RPO
    b. LPO
    c. RAO
    d. left lateral

17. The cardiac cycle occurs approximately how many times per minute?
    a. 17 to 20
    b. 50 to 70
    c. 75 to 80
    d. 80 to 100

18. _____ is the ventricular pressure measured just prior to contraction.
    a. systole
    b. mean pressure
    c. diastole
    d. end-diastole

19. What congenital cardiac disorder is the most common?
    a. tetralogy of Fallot
    b. atrial septal defect (ASD)
    c. aortic stenosis
    d. VSD

20. What are the two primary defects in tetralogy of Fallot?
    a. pulmonary stenosis and VSD
    b. VSD and ASD
    c. pulmonary stenosis and transposition of the aorta
    d. right ventricular hypertrophy and ASD

21. Infants born with transposition of the aorta exhibit severe cyanosis.
    a. true
    b. false

22. What congenital disorder results in differing arm and leg blood pressures?
    a. VSD

b. coarctation of the aorta
c. ASD
d. tetralogy of Fallot

23. An area of dead heart muscle is referred to as
a. fibrillation
b. fibrosis
c. infarct
d. thrombosis

24. Which of the following terms are examples of emboli?
1. disengaged thrombi
2. gas
3. fat particles
4. neoplastic particles
    a. 1 only
    b. 1 and 2
    c. 1, 2, and 3
    d. 1, 2, 3, and 4

25. Which procedures utilize radioactive material?
a. ventilation and perfusion scans
b. venograms
c. embolectomies
d. pulmonary arteriography

26. The titanium Greenfield vena caval filter is used to prevent
a. hemorrhage
b. spasm
c. pulmonary emboli from entering the lungs
d. claudication

27. The titanium Greenfield vena caval filter is often described by which term?
a. balloon
b. pigtail
c. umbrella
d. sidewinder

28. Most true aneurysms affecting the thoracic aorta are _____ in origin.
a. traumatic
b. mycotic

c. atherosclerotic
d. false

29. What is the most common indication of aortic dissection as seen on the PA chest radiograph?
a. elevation of the diaphragm
b. gross cardiomegaly
c. widening of the mediastinum

30. Which aneurysmal location is the most difficult to treat and has a higher mortality rate?
a. thoracic and thoracoabdominal aorta
b. aortic arch
c. abdominal aorta
d. at the level of the iliac bifurcation

► STUDY QUESTIONS

1. List the indications for cardiac catheterization.

2. Trace the path of pulmonary and systemic circulation.

3. List the branches of the RCA and LCA.

4. Describe the types and sizes of catheters used in selective coronary arteriography.

5. Why do cardiologists prefer pigtail catheters for both right and left ventriculography?

6. Describe the three primary approaches for pulmonary arteriography.

7. What are the purposes of pulmonary hemodynamic evaluation?

8. What is meant by the terms strain-gauge and Wheatstone bridge?

9. What is meant by the terms systolic pressure, diastolic pressure, and mean pressure?

10. List and describe three congenital disorders of the heart and aorta.

► CHAPTER EIGHT

► VISCERAL ANGIOGRAPHY

► CHAPTER OUTLINE

► CHAPTER OBJECTIVES

Upon completion of Chapter 8 the technologist will be able to:

1. List and explain at least three applications for visceral angiography
2. List and describe the equipment and accessories utilized in visceral angiography
3. List the vessels that are visualized in visceral angiography
4. List the contraindications and complications of visceral angiography
5. Describe the routine angiographic positioning for visceral angiography
6. Explain the differences between flush and selective visceral angiography
7. List the indications and contraindications for portal venography
8. List the indications and contraindications for splenic arteriography
9. List the indications and contraindications for pancreatic arteriography
10. List the indications and contraindications for renal arteriography
11. Describe how to select the appropriate injection rates for visceral angiography
12. Describe how to select the appropriate filming rates for visceral angiography
13. List the types of contrast media employed in visceral angiography
14. Describe the selection criteria for contrast media utilized in visceral angiography
15. Describe the catheter types and designs used for the various visceral angiograms

The primary use of angiography in the gastrointestinal (GI) system is to locate the source of GI bleeding. The positive diagnosis of a bleeding source provides for diagnostic determination of both surgical and nonsurgical choices of treatment or intervention.

The 1980s have seen the widespread use of both endoscopy and radionuclide scanning in conjunction with angiography for hemorrhage localization. Endoscopy often provides preliminary information as to which individual patient might benefit from selective angiography.

In upper GI bleeding, the regions of potential hemorrhage can be generally subdivided into the *esophagogastric* and *gastroduodenal* areas. The left gastric artery (LGA) is catheterized for gastric bleeding and the gastroduodenal artery (GDA) for pyloroduodenal hemorrhage.

In small and large intestinal bleeding, which is often referred to as a "lower GI bleed," the sources of blood supply are the superior and inferior mesenteric arteries. The superior mesenteric artery (SMA) is evaluated for small bowel bleeding and suspect areas of the proximal colon extending to the middle transverse colon. The remainder of the transverse colon, descending and sigmoid colon, and rectum are visualized by selective catheterization of the inferior mesenteric artery (IMA).

The two most frequent causes of UGI hemorrhage are *peptic ulcer disease* and *esophageal varices*. Other causes include gastritis, neoplasms, arteriovenous fistula, pancreatitis, hemobilia, aneurysms, and arteriovenous malformations (AVMs).

In an acute lower GI bleed, *diverticula* have been found responsible in approximately one half of all cases. This is followed by *angiodysplasia* (small vascular abnormalities), commonly found in the intestine in patients older than 60 years of age. Angiodysplasia tends to originate in the cecum and ascending colon.

The angiographic confirmation of GI bleeding, the extravasation of the contrast medium, is noted in the capillary and venous phases of circulation. If extravasation is to be observed, bleeding must generally exceed 0.5 ml/min.

▶ ANATOMY

The *celiac axis* is a short, thick trunk artery that arises from the anterior surface of the abdominal aorta just below the aortic hiatus of the diaphragm between T-12 and L-1. In most patients, the celiac trunk presents a trifurcation of the left gastric, hepatic, and splenic arteries (Fig. 8–1*A* and *B*).

The *left gastric* artery is the smallest of the three branches and passes upward and to the left of the aorta toward the gastric cardia. This artery provides blood flow to the distal end of the esophagus and passes along the lesser curvature toward the pylorus, giving off branches to the adjacent anterior and posterior walls of the body of the stomach and anastomosing (usually) with the right gastric artery.

The *common hepatic* artery is directed to the right and anteriorly, giving off the GDA. Beyond the origin of the GDA, the common hepatic artery is called the *proper hepatic* artery. The proper hepatic artery travels inferiorly to the area of the porta hepatis where it divides into the *right* and *left hepatic* arteries that supply the corresponding lobes of the liver. In approximately 10% of the population, there is a *middle hepatic* artery arising from either the right or left hepatic artery. The middle hepatic artery supplies blood to the caudate lobe of the liver.

The GDA is a major branch arising from the common hepatic artery. The GDA descends toward the stomach and provides blood flow to the anterior and pyloric areas of the stomach. The GDA divides at the lower border of the duodenum and produces two important branches, the *pancreatoduodenal* and the *gastroepiploic* (gastro-omental) arteries.

The *splenic* artery is the longest branch of the celiac axis and is often noted for its tortuousity. The splenic artery passes horizontally and to the left behind the stomach. It passes along the dorsal margin of the body and tail of the pancreas, and as it approaches the splenic hilum it divides into two or three branches that enter the spleen.

The splenic artery gives off several branches to the pancreas and stomach. These branches are the pancreatic arteries and the right and left gastroepiploic arteries. The splenic is often the first visceral artery to show evidence of atherosclerosis.

The SMA, the second unpaired visceral branch of the abdominal aorta, arises from the anterior or ventral surface of the aorta near the first lumbar body (L-1), approximately 2 cm below the celiac trunk. The SMA passes downward and supplies the small intestine, the cecum, the ascending portion of the colon, and approximately one half of the transverse portion of the colon.

The SMA in its caudal course gives off several major branches: the *inferior pancreatoduodenal, jejunal, ileal, ileocolic, right colic,* and *mid-colic* arteries (Fig. 8–2*A, B,* and *C*).

The IMA is smaller than the SMA and arises 3 to 4 cm above the bifurcation on the anterior or ventral surface of the aorta at the level of the third lumbar vertebra (L-3). The IMA passes caudal to the left side of the aorta and provides blood flow to the distal half of the transverse colon, the descending and sigmoid colon, and the rectum (Fig. 8–3*A* and *B*).

The major branches of the IMA are the *left colic, sigmoid,* and *superior hemorrhoidal* or *rectal* arteries.

▶ PROCEDURAL ANGIOGRAPHY

Percutaneous Puncture Procedure

In earlier chapters, it was stated that abdominal aortography can be performed by the femoral, translumbar, and axillary approaches. In renal angiography, "*flush*" aortography is often utilized for the evalu-

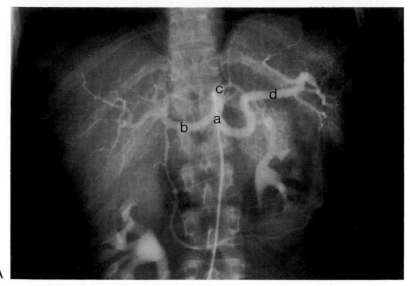

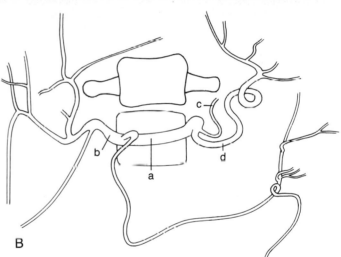

► **Figure 8–1**

A, Normal celiac
arteriogram. (a = celiac
trunk/axis; b = hepatic
artery; c = gastric artery;
d = splenic artery.)
B, Diagram of the celiac
arterial anatomy.
(a = celiac trunk/axis;
b = hepatic artery;
c = gastric artery;
d = splenic artery.) (*B,*
Redrawn from an
illustration by Martha J.
Dane).

ation of large tumors and hypertension and to investigate the origins of the renal arteries. *Selective* catheterization is essential for the evaluation of intrarenal disease.

Arterial puncture is the method utilizing the *Seldinger* technique. The vessel most preferred for access is the *common femoral* artery. The pulse is palpated just below the inguinal ligament, and an 18-gauge arterial needle is introduced at an angle of 45 degrees (see Fig. 10–35). If the tip of the needle is in the artery lumen, bright red pulsating streams of blood will exit the needle hub. When the presence of arterial blood is confirmed, a "*floppy*" guidewire is introduced through the needle and into the lumen of the common femoral artery. The guidewire should progress without difficulty. If difficulty is encountered, the guidewire should be removed and needle placement should be checked.

The guidewire for renal flush aortography should be placed near the level of the origins of the renal artery. This will place the guidewire in the vicinity of L1–L2. Many radiologists prefer to perform an aortic flush

when only the renal system is under evaluation. Placing the catheter at the level of the diaphragm will fill the celiac and SMA systems and can obscure renal vasculature.

Following placement of the guidewire on or near the renal origins, the arterial needle is removed and a catheter is placed over the guidewire.

Many radiologists prefer a flush *pigtail* catheter for abdominal aortography. The pigtail contains multiple side holes for optimum dispersion of the contrast medium. The pigtail end reduces lateral *whipping* or *recoil* often present in straight-end flush catheters.

The flush aortogram will outline or delineate the renal artery for the radiologist and provide him or her with information suggesting the size of the renal arteries, the number of renal arteries, and perhaps the type of catheter that might be used for selective catheterization.

The flush injection often presents immediate evidence of an abnormality. Aortic aneurysms are frequently found just below the renal arteries and above the distal aortic bifurcation (common iliac arteries).

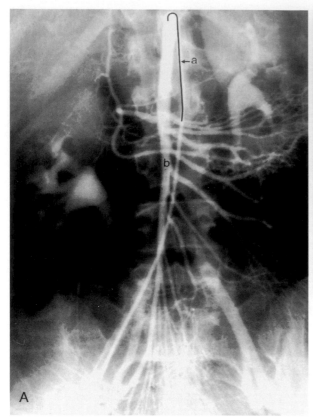

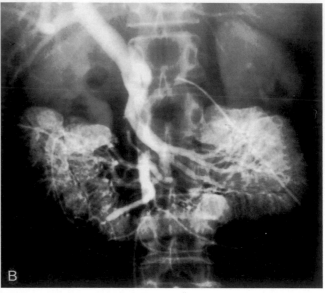

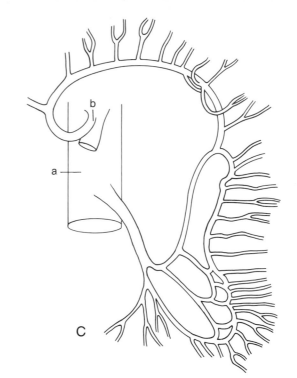

▶ **Figure 8–2**

A, Normal superior mesenteric arteriogram. (a = catheter selectively placed into superior mesenteric artery; b = superior mesenteric artery.) *B,* A percutaneous puncture of the superior mesenteric artery and demonstration of arterial branches and the small intestine and proximal colon. *C,* Diagram of the superior mesenteric artery. (a = abdominal aorta; b = entrance into superior mesenteric artery.) (*B,* Redrawn from an illustration by Martha J. Dane.)

An abdominal aortic aneurysm is a very common finding in the older adult patient (Fig. 8–4).

Atherosclerotic changes in the older adult often lead to complete occlusion of the abdominal aorta. Biplane filming is routine in abdominal aortography (Fig. 8–5).

Although coarctation of the aorta is not as common as some of the other congenital malformations, this abnormality can be seen on the abdominal flush arteriogram. This condition varies from stenosis to atresia and develops early in intrauterine life, resulting in stimulus to the formation of collateral circulation to the lower body (Fig. 8–6).

▶ **CATHETERS**

Selective renal catheterization requires the use of a special catheter with a shaped tip to enter a specific selected artery.

The most commonly used catheters for selective visceral angiography are termed *multiple-curve* catheters. Popular names used to describe these selective visceral catheters include *headhunter, cobra,* and *sidewinder.* Each of these special catheters is available in a "series," which offer a variety of sizes of outer catheter diameter (French number), number and spacing of side holes, and angle of the shaped tip.

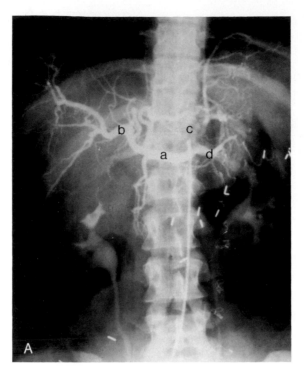
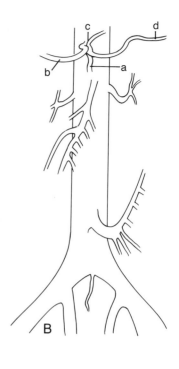

▶ **Figure 8–3**

A, A normal celiac arteriogram. (a = celiac trunk/axis; b = common hepatic artery; c = left gastric artery; d = splenic artery.) B, Diagram of the inferior mesenteric artery. (a = celiac trunk/axis; b = common hepatic artery; c = left gastric artery; d = splenic artery.) (B, Redrawn from an illustration by Martha J. Dane.)

It is important to understand that the selection of one of these catheters depends on the diameter of the aorta. For example, a cobra C-1 or a sidewinder S-1 curve is used in an aorta with a lumen that is anatomically narrow or pathologically stenotic. The cobra C-2 or sidewinder S-1 is used for an average-sized aorta, and a cobra C-3 or a sidewinder S-2 catheter is used for a wide- or large-diameter aorta. The diameter of the aorta will generally parallel body habitus. Hypersthenic persons usually have a wide aorta; asthenic, hyposthenic, and pediatric patients usually have an aorta that is smaller and narrow. The aorta in a young person usually runs a straight course, whereas in an older individual, the aorta runs a tortuous course.

Once the selective catheter has been chosen, the procedure requires a catheter exchange. The guide-

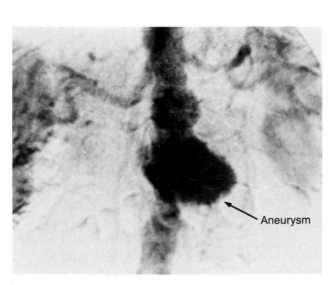

▶ **Figure 8–4**

A subtraction film of an abdominal aortic flush showing an aortic aneurysm in a 68-year-old man with a history of hypertension.

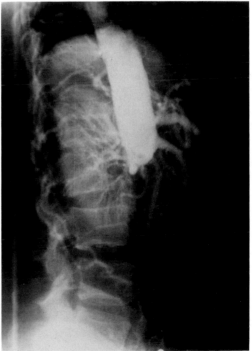

▶ **Figure 8–5**

Lateral view of a completely obstructed abdominal aorta just below the level of the superior mesenteric artery.

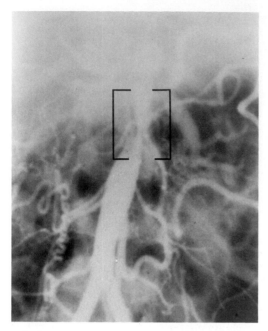

▶ **Figure 8–6**

Abdominal flush aortogram reveals coarctation of the aorta (*brackets*) in a 6-year-old boy.

wire is reinserted, and the flush catheter is removed. The selective catheter is passed over the guidewire and placed in the mid-abdominal aorta.

Curved catheters straightened out by the guidewire are often taken to the area of the aortic arch or ascending aorta in order to reconstruct their original shape. This is often required using a *Simmons* or sidewinder catheter. Catheters with good *memory* are preferred for selective catheterization.

The use of a selective catheter requires that the catheter tip be placed in a plane that coincides with the origin of the artery. When the catheter appears to enter a vessel origin, a hand injection of contrast medium can be made to identify the vessel and its location. The injection rate and volume depend on the size of the renal artery as observed fluoroscopically during the test injection.

▶ INJECTION VOLUME AND FILM SEQUENCING

Table 8–1 lists the contrast medium injection volume and film sequencing for abdominal aortic flush aortography and selective renal arteriography.

Radiographic Projections

The projections used in abdominal aortography and selective renal arteriography are most likely determined by the pathologic process being examined. Some radiologists prefer abdominal flush aortography prior to selective catheter placement.

The anteroposterior (AP) projection is generally performed first. Variations in patient anatomy, disease process, or vessel tortuosity may require left and right posterior oblique views (LPO/RPO) to clearly delineate the vessel origins or small neoplastic lesions. Two projections, AP and lateral, are required to correctly evaluate aneurysms and arterial trauma.

Following selective catheter placement, the superior and inferior levels of the kidney or the position of the hilum can be marked under fluoroscopic guidance to assist in proper patient positioning. The central ray will enter at the level of the hilum in the expiratory phase of respiration. Collimation is essential to enhance contrast by reducing scatter radiation.

Catheters

For visceral angiography, a visceral hook catheter can be utilized, as can the cobra (C-2) and sidewinder catheter series. Sizes of catheters are usually within the No. 5 to No. 7 French size range. Many radiologists prefer No. 5 French catheters because they are often easier to advance over the guidewire into selected mesenteric branches.

The flow rates for a given patient vary. Certain pathologic conditions (e.g., portal hypertension and cirrhosis) increase arterial flow and require increased injection rates. The increased flow rate is often necessary due to vascular stenosis. In the elderly, children, and patients with atherosclerosis, the volumes are decreased. A test injection of contrast medium indicates vessel condition, which then determines the injection flow rate. Table 8–2 presents injection rate examples for four different vessels. A 60 or 76% contrast medium is being used for each study.

Technical Considerations

In an acute (GI) bleed, the suspected vessel is injected first. Once the test injection is complete, mesenteric angiography proceeds. Mesenteric angiography re-

▶ **Table 8–1**

ABDOMINAL AORTIC FLUSH AND SELECTIVE RENAL
INJECTION/FILMING RATES

Contrast Medium	60% or 70% Diatrizoate meglumine
Injection Rate/Volume	Small arteries—2–4 ml/sec, total: 10 ml
	Average to large—5–6 ml/sec, total: 10–15 ml
Film Rate	2/sec × 4 sec
	1/sec × 6 sec

► **Table 8–2**

CONTRAST MEDIUM/INJECTION RATES FOR VISCERAL ANGIOGRAPHY

Contrast Medium (usually nonionic)	60 or 70% Diatrizoate meglumine
Injection Rate/Volume	
Celiac/superior mesenteric artery	8–10 ml/sec; total: 45–60-ml volume
Inferior mesenteric	3–5 ml/sec; total: 20–30-ml volume
Left gastric	3–5 ml/sec; total: 10–15-ml volume
Gastroduodenal	3–8 ml/sec; total: 12–15-ml volume

quires several individual injections of contrast medium. When lower GI hemorrhage is being investigated, angiography of the pelvic region should be completed first. This decreases the chances of a contrast-filled bladder overlying and decreasing image detail.

The filming sequence depends on the arterial flow to the selected vessel and the diagnostic information that is required. Filming should be rapid during the arterial flow. A suggested filming sequence may be two films per second for a total of 4 seconds, next one exposure per second for 4 seconds, followed by one film every 3 seconds for 15 seconds. This long sequence allows for the contrast medium to pass completely through the arterial, capillary, and venous phases of circulation and is necessary to assess contrast extravasation in GI bleeding.

Conventional cut-film serial changers are generally preferred for mesenteric angiography. Digital subtraction angiography (DSA) tends to be difficult in patients who are severely ill or uncooperative. DSA requires that the patient is still for longer periods. From our experience, the long duration of an exposure run of 25 to 30 seconds, combined with the addition of moving bowel gas, can yield a less than optimum digital angiographic study.

When the source of hemorrhage is identified during the course of mesenteric angiography, transcatheter-interarterial injection of vasopressin or therapeutic embolization can be performed while the patient is still on the table. Therapeutic embolization is one of the many vascular interventional procedures that are discussed in Chapter 11. Figure 8–7 represents a selective celiac arteriogram that reveals active hemorrhage involving the LGA in a 57-year-old male patient. Figure 8–8 shows a selective study of the SMA. A postoperative bleed is noted in the middle colic artery.

Equipment

The equipment criteria for visceral angiography varies somewhat from those required for neuroradiology and cardiac imaging.

Generally, biplane filming capabilities are not required for visceral angiography. However, consideration must be given to a lateral projection (view) when pathology such as abdominal angina or mesenteric ischemia is suspected.

The abdomen is the thickest body part imaged in visceral angiography/aortography. Optimum kilovoltage (70 kVp) is necessary to obtain a study that can differentiate between the contrast-filled vessels and the surrounding tissues. Thus, 70 to 75 kVp is recommended for visceral angiography. One may be tempted to use higher kilovoltage levels in a larger patient. However, higher levels of kilovoltage only serve to produce additional secondary radiation and subsequent fog that decreases the desired subject contrast. In order to avoid motion unsharpness, the longest exposure time recommended for visceral angiography is 100 msec.

The two requirements of 70 kVp and 100 ms seem to push one toward the selection of high-speed film-screen combinations and generators with a three-phase output in the area of 800 to 1000 mA. This high x-ray generation output allows for rapid serial filming at reasonably short exposure times while maintaining an acceptable heat load in the range of 50 to 95%.

Angiography in the 1990s has been enhanced due to innovative technical advancements such as high-resolution/high-speed screens and the continued development of rare-earth phosphors. Image sharpness is reduced as screen speed increases. However, in visceral angiography, sharpness of the image is not as

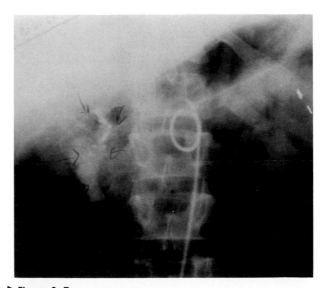

► **Figure 8–7**

Active hemorrhage (*arrows*) of the left gastric artery as seen on this selective celiac arteriogram.

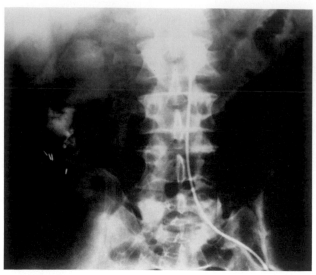

▶ **Figure 8–8**
Selective injection of the superior mesenteric arteriogram indicates a pooling of contrast in the area of the middle colic artery.

critical as it is in neuroangiography and peripheral angiography. Care must be taken to choose a system that allows enough exposure latitude yet avoids too much speed and radiographic mottle.

Two techniques that can be used to improve studies in obese patients are a faster film/screen combination and a reduction of the source-image-receptor distance (SID/FFD).

The preliminary or scout film is extremely important in visceral angiography. Felt-tipped markers can be used to identify the entrance site of the x-ray beam (central ray). One can mark this site in the desired phase of respiration. This allows for fine tuning (placement) of the site of interest prior to the injection of the contrast agent.

In many visceral procedures additional subtraction angiography may be required following the examination. This requires informing the patient how important cessation of breathing is through the entire series run, which may last for 25 to 30 seconds. Respiratory motion and peristalsis become a problem in evaluating the abdominal viscera.

If subtraction technique is a consideration, the injector should be delayed 0.1 to 0.2 second in order to ensure a scout film for subtraction masking. Subtraction is always an integral requirement in suspected GI bleeds.

DSA is often utilized in visceral angiography. Digital venous imaging (DVI), as it was called in its formative period, was heralded as the procedure that would greatly reduce the risk as well as the cost of angiography. Many physicians believed that DVI would replace arterial injections with a less invasive peripheral-venous injection.

Problems encountered with DVI included motion, peristalsis, cardiac output, and the volume of contrast needed. Because of these problems, the radiologist

tended to shy away from a procedure that would tend to render poor images.

The value of DSA is with intra-arterial injections. Intra-arterial injections can be made using smaller volumes of a contrast medium and often with a diluted contrast medium that reduces the burning sensation.

Timing is the same as conventional filming runs, so motion becomes less of a factor. The trade-off tends to be in the size of the image-intensifier used. The large field intensifiers cover larger field sizes but will have less mottle (spotted resolution) than a smaller field.

▶ ANGIOGRAPHY OF THE LIVER, SPLEEN, AND PANCREAS

Angiographic studies of the liver, spleen, and pancreas are invasive procedures that are being replaced with lower-risk, noninvasive imaging procedures. Computed tomography (CT), ultrasound (US), and magnetic resonance imaging (MRI) are capable of demonstrating solid and cystic lesions with a high degree of accuracy while substantially lowering the procedural risks. However, angiography of the liver is still essential for the evaluation of certain pathologic conditions (Table 8–3).

Although its use has diminished, hepatic angiography remains an important imaging tool in prediagnostic procedural assessment of interventional treatment and management.

Hepatic Angiography

The liver differs from the other visceral organs in that it has a dual blood supply; the *hepatic arteries* and the *portal venous system*. Venous drainage takes place through the *hepatic veins* and into the *inferior vena cava (IVC)*.

In the normal patient, approximately 20 to 30% of hepatic blood comes from the hepatic arteries. The remainder or majority of blood flow comes from the portal venous system. If either of these systems is reduced, the other flow system will generally increase to compensate. This compensation or dilatation becomes an important angiographic presentation to the radiologist, especially in patients with advanced cirrhosis (Figs. 8–9 and 8–10).

▶ **Table 8–3**
INDICATIONS FOR HEPATIC ANGIOGRAPHY

Portal hypertension
Hepatic neoplasms
Differentiating hepatic and extrahepatic masses
Hepatic trauma
Hemobilia
Pre-liver transplantation
Vascular malformations
Budd-Chiari syndrome

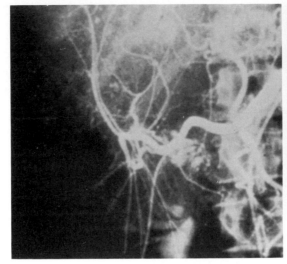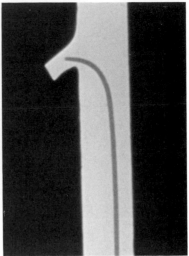

▶ **Figure 8–9**

Normal selective hepatic arteriogram. The adjacent diagram shows the entry of a selective catheter into the celiac axis.

Selective hepatic angiography is used to demonstrate numerous pathologies including hepatic metastases (Fig. 8–11), cavernous hemangioma (Fig. 8–12*A* and *B*), and hepatic stenosis (Fig. 8–13).

Catheters

Catheters commonly used in hepatic arteriography are the types with reverse curves, such as the sidewinder, cobra, or MK-2 series. Many radiologists prefer smaller, high-torque catheters for their ability to pass deeper and more distal in the hepatic and branch arteries. Side-hole placement near the catheter tip is often used in the belief that it reduces the "jet-whip" effect during pressurized injections. A contraindication for side-hole catheters would be selective catheterization for embolization. End-hole

catheters would be recommended in order to decrease the chance of the embolic material's becoming obstructed in the catheter lumen and side holes.

Contrast Medium/Flow Rates

A test injection under fluoroscopic control will give the angiographer an idea of the flow rate within the artery as well as the stability of the catheter within the arterial lumen.

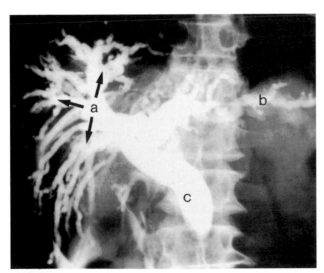

▶ **Figure 8–10**

Percutaneous transhepatic cholangiogram. Hepatic (*a*) and pancreatic (*b*) fibrosis with fibrosis of the distal common bile duct (*c*).

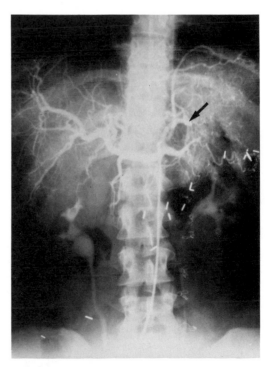

▶ **Figure 8–11**

A celiac arteriogram with hepatic metastases. Note the presence of hepatomegaly in the right upper quadrant. The tumor, which is seeding via the bloodstream, resulted in an obstruction of the splenic artery (*arrow*).

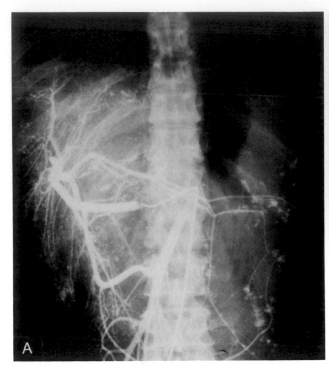

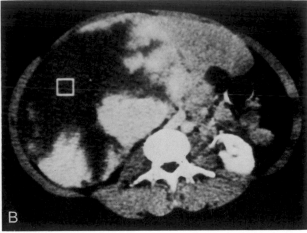

▶ Figure 8–12

A, A selective hepatic arteriogram demonstrating a huge cavernous hemangioma with slow blood flow, encompassing the entire liver in this 66-year-old man. *B,* A computed tomography image of a cavernous hemangioma (same patient as in *A*).

A 76% solution of diatrizoate meglumine is often used to improve the contrast opacity in both the parenchymal and venous phases of circulation.

Arteriographic detail is much better if selective angiography of the common hepatic artery is performed instead of a celiac axis flush angiogram. The suggested flow rate for hepatic angiography is 5 to 10 ml/sec with a 30- to 40-ml volume.

▶ Figure 8–13

A selective hepatic arteriogram revealing stenosis (*arrows*) of the proximal portion of the hepatic artery in this 65-year-old man.

Film Rate

Filming should be rapid, suggesting two films per second for 4 or 5 seconds. The second phase may vary depending on the need to visualize the later venous phase and require filming up to 25 seconds. This is often a consideration in a history of portal hypertension. The suggested filming rate is 2/sec × 4 or 5 seconds, then 1/sec for 5 seconds, then 0.5/sec for 4 seconds.

Radiographic Projections/Positioning

Selective celiac angiography can be utilized to provide a "roadmap" for visceral artery anatomy. If celiac occlusion is a clinical possibility, a serial lateral view may be a necessity.

From our experiences, selective common hepatic injection is usually performed in the AP position. The central ray will bisect a line between the xiphoid process and the right iliac crest, and it will also bisect the midsagittal plane and the right lateral margin of the body. Reduced collimation or the addition of a cone is suggested to reduce scatter radiation and enhance subject and film contrast.

Arterial Computed Tomography/Angiography

Following conventional hepatic angiography and with the catheter tip securely in place in the common hepatic artery, CT angiography has been and can be used in certain clinical situations. This procedure has been especially effective in diagnosing *hepatoma/ hepatocellular carcinoma* (primary liver cell cancer) and suspected hypovascular lesions (Fig. 8–14*A*, *B*, *C*, and *D*).

With the catheter left in place, the patient is transported to the CT suite. Progressively, 8-mm scans of the selected liver areas are obtained following an additional infusion of 8 to 10 ml of 30% contrast medium injected at a rate of 3 ml/sec. (The contrast medium [ionic versus nonionic] is selected in accordance with radiologist's preference.) The scan is started approximately 10 seconds post injection.

Portal Venography

The portal venous system drains the small bowel, colon, stomach, spleen, and pancreas. The indications for portal venography are listed in Table 8–4.

Several techniques are currently being utilized to evaluate the portal venous system. They include arterial portography, percutaneous transhepatic catheterization, and percutaneous splenoportography.

Arterial portography relies on selective catheterization of either the SMA or splenic artery. Opacification is dependent on high-volume contrast injection with relevant serial filming taking place in the later phases of venous circulation. The primary problem associated with this procedure is the resultant contrast dilution that occurs and significantly reduces the diagnostic appearance of the angiogram. *Percutaneous transhepatic catheterization* and *percutaneous splenoportography* are alternatives for visualizing the portal venous system.

Both procedures require a percutaneous needle puncture utilizing a 6″, 20-gauge portal vein polyethylene sheath needle system.

Transhepatic catheterization is attempted in the right mid-axillary plane with needle placement in the area of the porta hepatis below the right hemidiaphragm.

Percutaneous *splenoportography* is a direct needle

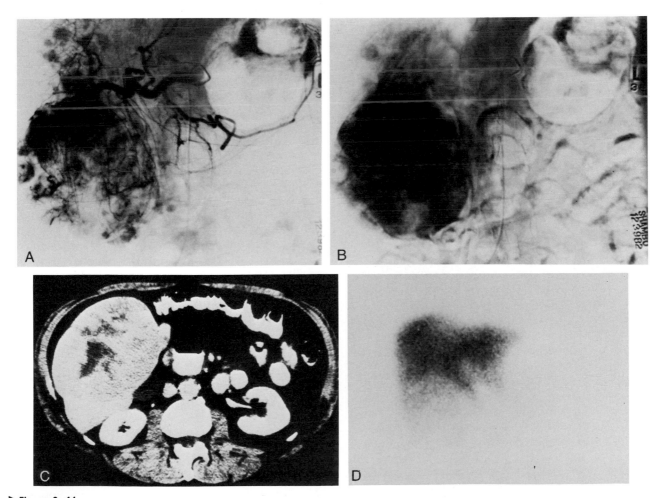

▶ **Figure 8–14**

A, A selective hepatic arteriogram of the early arterial phase demonstrates hepatocellular carcinoma in this 64-year-old man. *B*, Venous phase in the same patient. *C*, A computed tomography image of the same patient. *D*, A nuclear medicine image revealing an area of decreased uptake in the right lower lobe of the liver in the same patient.

INDICATIONS FOR PORTAL VENOGRAPHY

Portal hypertension
Evaluation of mesenteric, splenic and portal veins prior to shunt
    placement
Suspected thrombosis
Prehepatic transplantation
Laennec's cirrhosis
Colon or small bowel varices
Measurement of portal wedge pressures

▶ **Table 8–5**
COMPLICATIONS OF PERCUTANEOUS
TRANSHEPATIC ARTERIOGRAPHY AND
PERCUTANEOUS SPLENOPORTOGRAPHY

Percutaneous Transhepatic Arteriography	Percutaneous Splenoportography
Hemorrhage	Hemorrhage
Traumatic aneurysm and fistula	Splenic rupture
Pneumothorax	Splenic aneurysm and fistula
Portal vein thrombosis	Puncture of other organs
Puncture of the intestine	

puncture of the splenic capsule, in the posterior axillary line at the point of maximal splenic dullness and under fluoroscopic guidance. The usual site of puncture is generally in the area of the eighth and ninth ribs (Fig. 8–15).

Both of the aforementioned procedures are indicated when portal arteriography has not provided diagnostic information as to the patency of the portal vein. The incidence of complications tends to be higher for both procedures than arterial portography (Table 8–5).

Splenic Angiography

The primary indications for splenic angiography are listed in Table 8–6.

From the femoral approach, the splenic artery can be selectively catheterized using a sidewinder or cobra series catheter. If the axillary approach is used, a headhunter catheter may be a better choice. Table 8–7 lists an example of an injection rate of contrast medium and film rate for a splenic arteriogram.

Radiographic Positioning/Projections

An AP, single-plane, serial arteriogram generally provides adequate information. Many radiologists may request a right posterior oblique (RPO) view if the splenic artery appears tortuous on the test injection.

Splenic arteriography usually reveals a wide spectrum of pathology. Elderly patients with advanced arteriosclerosis often present arterial calcification such as is demonstrated in Figure 8–16.

The spleen is the abdominal organ that is most frequently damaged in automobile accidents. Blunt abdominal trauma often results when the left quadrant abruptly comes in contact with the steering wheel of a vehicle (Figs. 8–17 A and B and 8–18 A, B, and C).

Pancreatic Angiography

Pancreatic angiography has decreased considerably with the arrival of noninvasive diagnostic CT and US.

As a diagnostic tool, CT has a high level of accuracy in diagnosis of pancreatic carcinomas. Arteriography remains valuable in diagnosing small tumors and in examining specific clinical situations in which noninvasive diagnostic tests have been inconclusive. The primary indications for pancreatic angiography are listed in Table 8–8. Table 8–9 presents sample injection/film rates for the pancreatic artery and its branches.

Catheters

The catheters utilized will depend upon the specific area of pancreas being examined and the curve desired. The cobra and sidewinder series are commonly

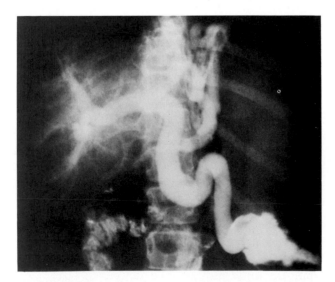

▶ **Figure 8–15**
A splenoportogram with a negative result on examination.

▶ **Table 8–6**
INDICATIONS FOR SPLENIC ANGIOGRAPHY

Portal hypertension
Aneurysms/atherosclerotic disease
Differentiation of accessory spleens
Therapeutic embolization
Trauma

▶ **Table 8–7**

INJECTION/FILM RATES FOR SPLENIC ANGIOGRAPHY

Contrast Medium	60% Diatrizoate meglumine
Injection Rate/Volume	5 ml/sec for a total of 30–45 ml
Film Rate	2 films/sec × 4 sec; then 1
	film/sec × 6 sec*

*Note: In patients with portal hypertension, the duration of filming should be prolonged to cover 25 to 30 seconds.

used to selectively evaluate both the pancreatic head and body.

The arterial supply to the pancreas can be quite variable. Complete examination will often call for subselective catheterization of the gastroduodenal and occasionally the dorsal pancreatic and superior mesenteric arteries in order to project a complete study of the pancreatic circulation (Fig. 8–19).

▶ RENAL ANGIOGRAPHY

Today, selective renal arteriography is most commonly used for the evaluation of renovascular hypertension, for the "roadmapping" and diagnosis of renal tumors, and for the preoperative assessment of donor kidneys in renal transplant. The effects of renal trauma, especially suspected arterial injury, are also a clinical indication (Fig. 8–20A and B).

The indications for renal venography includes a laboratory assay of renin levels, a diagnosis of renal vein thrombosis, and the evaluation of tumor invasion of the renal vein and IVC. Table 8–10 lists the indications for renal arteriography.

Anatomy

The kidneys are usually supplied by a single artery originating from the lateral aspect of the abdominal aorta at the level of the first or second lumbar vertebral body (L1–L2). Multiple renal arteries to one or both kidneys occur in approximately 33% of individuals.

Arterial System

The kidneys are located in the posterior part of the abdomen, behind the peritoneum on either side of the vertebral column. The right kidney is usually located slightly lower than the left kidney due to the presence of the right lobe of the liver. The renal arteries lie behind the renal veins, and the origin of the left renal artery is usually somewhat higher than that of the right.

The medial border of the kidney is concave in the center and contains an indented fissure that is referred to as the hilum. The hilum allows for entry or exit of the arteries, veins, ureter, and nerves into the kidney.

When the main renal artery enters the hilum, there is a division into five branches or segments. These vascular segments are the *apical, upper, middle, lower,* and *posterior* branches.

These *segmental* branches extend into the kidney, run between the pyramids, and become the *interlobar* arteries. At the juncture between the cortex and medulla they become the multiple *arcuate* arteries and eventually give off the *interlobular* arteries that course perpendicular to the arcuate arteries into the cortex. The interlobular arteries continue as the *afferent arterioles* and feed into the renal glomeruli.

Venous System

The venous return of blood through the renal system uses much the same terminology as its counterpart in the arterial system.

The *efferent glomerular* vessel forms a plexus in the area of Henle's loop. This plexus or network carries blood into the *interlobular* veins, then into the *arcuate* veins, on to the *interlobar* veins, and finally into the *renal* vein with discharge back into the IVC.

Renal Angiography Phases

Renal arteriography phases can generally be divided into three phases of circulation: arterial, capillary (nephrogram) and venous. Following injection, the arterial phase is seen during the first 1 to 3 seconds depending upon the injection rate. The capillary phase follows and is visible at 3 to 8 seconds following injection. The nephrogram visualizes the contrast medium in the

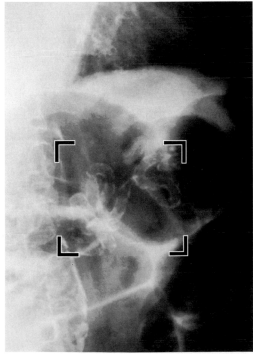

▶ **Figure 8–16**

Splenic artery calcification (*brackets*) in an 88-year-old woman.

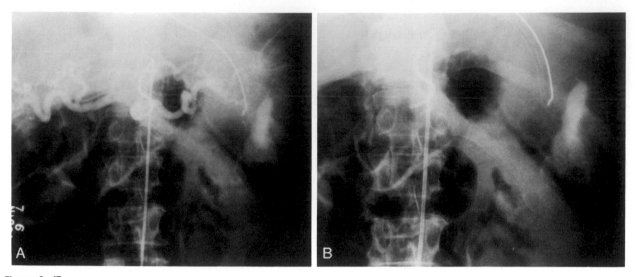

▶ **Figure 8–17**

A and *B*, A selective splenic arteriogram revealing a splenic hematoma. The injury was sustained as a result of blunt abdominal trauma from an automobile accident.

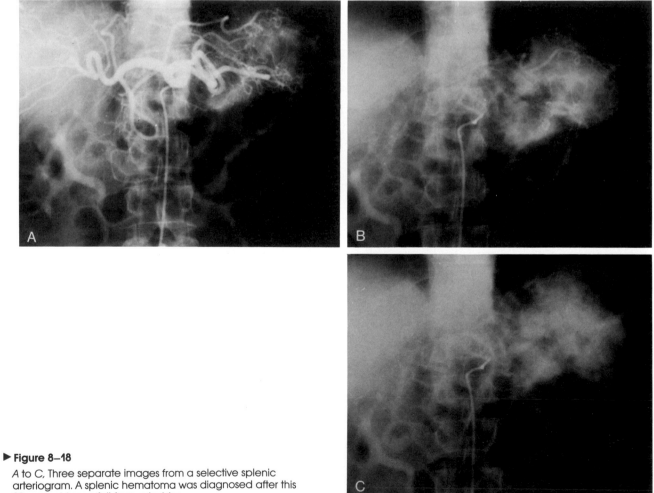

▶ **Figure 8–18**

A to *C*, Three separate images from a selective splenic arteriogram. A splenic hematoma was diagnosed after this 33-year-old man fell from a ladder.

▶ **Table 8–8**

INDICATIONS FOR PANCREATIC ANGIOGRAPHY

Localization of endocrine tumors
Hemorrhage
Vascular mapping for resection
Vascular tumors
Atherosclerotic disease

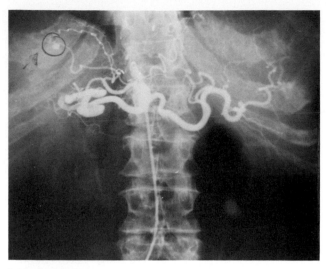

▶ **Figure 8–19**

Subselective catheterization of the gastroduodenal artery with identification of a small aneurysm of the artery (circle) in a 58-year-old man.

renal capillaries and passing through the excretory tubular systems. The venous phase can be variable. It may be seen as soon as 4 seconds or as late as 10 to 12 seconds following injection. A correctly sequenced diagnostic renal angiogram will show all three phases of circulation. The radiologist will make several test injections before establishing the injection and filming sequences (Fig. 8–21 *A, B,* and *C*).

Contrast Media

In selecting a contrast medium, the radiologist will take into consideration its viscosity, osmolality, toxicity, and mode of excretion.

Contrast agents with sodium have a greater toxicity than do contrast agents with methylglucamine. Thus, the radiologist must weigh toxicity versus viscosity in his or her choice of a contrast medium. This is especially important with patients who present a higher risk for renal arteriography. Many institutions are converting from an ionic to a nonionic contrast medium for all venography and arteriographic studies.

▶ VENOUS SAMPLING

The primary indications for renal vein catheterization are venous sampling for renin determination, diagnosis of renal vein thrombosis, and evaluation of neoplasms.

The renal vein can be catheterized selectively via the femoral vein approach. Catheter selection varies, yet many radiologists prefer catheters with side holes placed near the tip of the catheter. The cobra (C-2), Simmons, and multipurpose catheters are widely utilized. The Simmons and multipurpose catheters often require the use of a deflecting guidewire. Deflecting wires are very useful in bending straight catheters, recurving C-shaped or sidewinder catheters, advanc-

ing catheters selectively, and retrieving intravascular foreign bodies.

The contrast medium is injected to check the catheter's position in the renal vein. Following correct placement, 2 to 5 mm of blood are removed to cleanse the catheter of any flush solution and contrast material. Next, 10 to 15 ml of blood is withdrawn and injected into an appropriate laboratory test tube containing edetate calcium disodium (ECD) (material found inside a lavender-top blood collection tube). The collected venous blood is mixed with ECD to prevent blood clotting. The sample test tube should be marked as to location of the sample and patient identification and should be placed in an ice bath until the samples reach the laboratory. After centrifugation, the plasma is separated, frozen immediately to preserve renin activity, and sent to a special laboratory. Each blood sample requires the use of a separate sterile syringe and separate test tube containing ECD.

Samples are drawn from each renal vein and from the IVC above the renal veins and below the renal veins.

Several maneuvers can be used to stimulate renin secretion from the kidneys. Captopril and Lasix can be injected intravenously beforehand, or the patient

▶ **Table 8–9**

INJECTION/FILMING RATES FOR PANCREATIC ANGIOGRAPHY

Contrast Medium	76% Diatrizoate meglumine
Injection Rates/Volume	Dorsal pancreatic: 3 ml/sec for 10–12 ml total
	Gastroduodenal: 4 ml/sec for 10–15 ml total
	Superior mesenteric: 6–8 ml/sec for 50–60 ml total
Film Rate	Dorsal pancreatic: 1/sec for 6 seconds; then 1 every other second × 6 sec
	Gastroduodenal: 2/sec for 3 sec; then 1 every other second × 6 sec

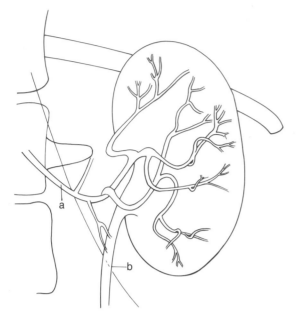

▶ **Figure 8–20**

Diagram of the renal artery in a left selective renal
arteriogram. (a = left renal artery; b = proximal left ureter.)
(Redrawn from an illustration by Martha J. Dane.)

may be elevated to a semi-upright or sitting position
for about 20 minutes (before sampling) to encourage
renin secretion.

Other laboratory studies that may be performed in
conjunction with venous sampling include split renal
function studies to determine volume, sodium, and
creatinine levels and osmolality. Further explanation
of these laboratory studies is beyond the scope of this
text.

▶ COMMON PATHOLOGY

Congenital

Both the flush and selective methods reveal a wide
variety of congenital variation and diseases of the
kidney. Talk to any vascular surgeon, and he or she
will recall a situation in which several renal vessels
were present. Renal arteriography plays an important
role in detailing congenital anomalies and normal
variants involving the renal vasculature (Fig. 8–22). A
horseshoe kidney is another common normal variant
seen on flush angiography (Fig. 8–23).

▶ **Table 8–10**
INDICATIONS FOR RENAL ANGIOGRAPHY

Arterial Disease/Disorders	Atherosclerotic stenosis
	Aneurysms
	Arteriovenous malformation
	Arteriovenous fistula
	Aortic dissection
	Fibromuscular dysplasia
	Neurofibromatosis
	Congenital stenosis
	Vasculitis
Inflammatory/Parenchymal Disease	Chronic glomerulonephritis
	Chronic pyelonephritis
	Acute tubular disease
	Cyst
	Hydronephrosis
Renal/Adrenal Tumors	Benign tumors
	Hypernephroma/adenocarcinoma
	Renal cell carcinoma (metastatic)
	Wilms' tumor (nephroblastoma)
Venous Diseases/Disorders	Renal vein thrombosis
	Testicular varicocele
	Ovarian vein syndrome
	Renal vein varices
	Agenesis
	Dysgenesis
	Hypoplasia
	Renin assay
Trauma	Aneurysm
	Parenchymal/arterial laceration
	Intimal flap
	Perirenal
	Retroperitoneal hematoma
	Renal vein thrombosis
	Iatrogenic/postprocedural trauma
Renal Transplant	Stenosis
	Occlusion/thrombosis
	Infarct
	Arteriovenous fistula
	Chronic rejection

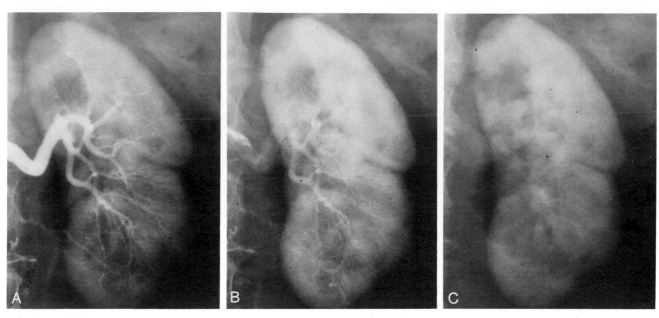

► **Figure 8–21**

A, Arterial phase of a selective renal arteriogram. *B,* Capillary phase of the same patient. *C,* Venous phase of the same patient.

Atherosclerosis

Atherosclerotic plaque-type lesions are the most dominant in causing renal artery stenosis (Fig. 8–24).

Fibromuscular Hyperplasia

Also common, but usually in younger females, is fibromuscular hyperplasia (Fig. 8–25). Both atherosclerosis and fibromuscular hyperplasia can cause renovascular hypertension. Once these lesions are identified, it must be determined if the lesions are hemodynamically significant.

Renal Artery Aneurysms

Although renal artery aneurysms are not common, they are usually apparent to the radiologist because 25 to 30% of these aneurysms contain sufficient calcium to be radiographically identifiable. They may be congenital, atherosclerotic, or post-traumatic (false aneurysms) (Fig. 8–26).

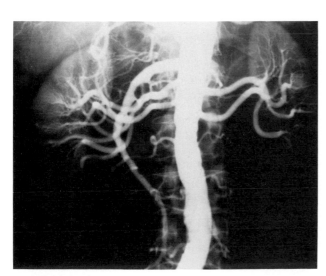

► **Figure 8–22**

An abdominal aortic flush study of a 67-year-old man with a history of diffuse peripheral vascular disease. The presence of an extra pair of renal arteries is noted. This is a normal variant but could be significant if the patient ever requires kidney surgery.

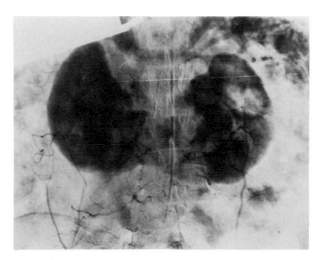

► **Figure 8–23**

A venous phase subtraction study of the kidneys reveals a common normal variant—horseshoe kidneys. The lower poles of the kidneys are joined across the midline.

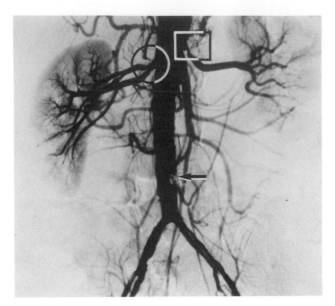

▶ **Figure 8–24**

An aortic flush arteriogram that demonstrates an atherosclerotic plaque (*arrow*) in the distal aorta; two renal arteries to the right kidney (*circle*); and left renal artery stenosis (*box*).

Renal Artery Thrombosis

Renal artery thrombosis is another consequence of atherosclerosis. Thrombolytic therapy is an effective method of dissolving a thrombus in the renal artery (Fig. 8–27*A*, *B*, and *C*).

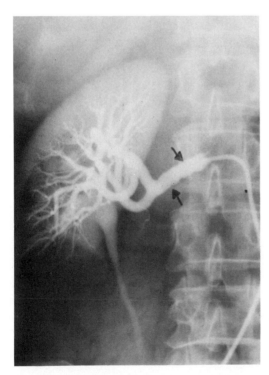

▶ **Figure 8–25**

Fibromuscular hyperplasia of the left renal artery (*arrows*) in this selective renal arteriogram.

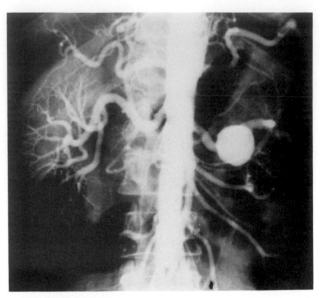

▶ **Figure 8–26**

A large aneurysm of the left renal artery is shown.

Renal Cyst

Renal cysts currently are well demonstrated on CT and MRI, which are adjuncts to renal arteriography. These two modalities are best in differentiating solid tumors from cysts. Figures 8–28, 8–29, and 8–30 are three examples of renal cysts.

Renal Tumors

Although malignant tumors of the kidney can be divided into six different types, the overwhelming majority of primary renal tumors are renal cell carcinoma, also referred to as adenocarcinoma or hypernephroma. These malignant tumors can occur almost anywhere in the kidney and usually predominate in men between 40 and 60 years of age. The tumor is usually quite large and highly vascular. Five separate case studies involving this tumor follow (Figs. 8–31, 8–32*A* and *B*, 8–33*A* and *B*, 8–34*A* and *B*, and 8–35).

Tuberculosis

Tuberculosis is not limited to the chest but can be found in any organ, including the kidney. Because the spread of tuberculosis is hematogenous, the abnormalities may be seen on flush and selective renal angiography (Fig. 8–36*A*, *B*, and *C*).

Renal Trauma

Two common ways in which the kidneys are traumatized are automobile accidents and penetrating high-velocity missile (gunshot) wounds to the abdomen. CT and angiography are utilized in studying these types of injury to the kidney (Figs. 8–37 and 8–38).

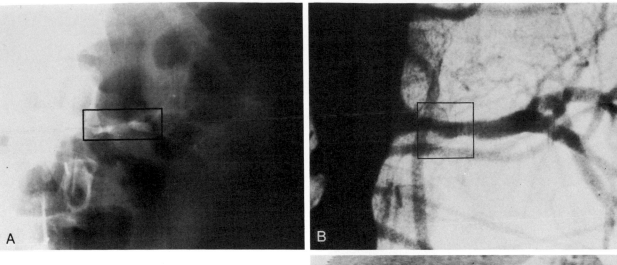

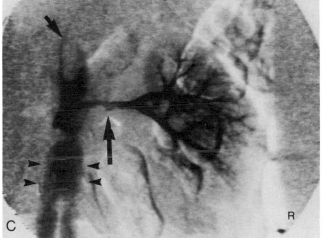

▶ **Figure 8–27**

A, A demonstration of a thrombus in the left renal artery (*box*). B, The thrombus (*box*) as seen on a subtracted abdominal flush arteriogram. C, On this digital subtraction study, the thrombus is once again identified (*long arrow*). Note the presence of the catheter (*short arrow*), which was passed via the axillary artery because of the history of synthetic graft replacement of the distal aorta (*arrowheads*).

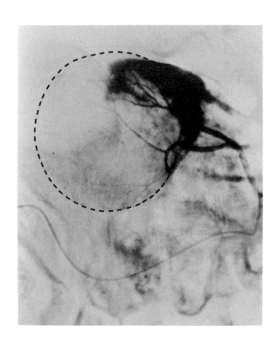

▶ **Figure 8–28**

This selective, subtraction right renal arteriogram reveals the presence of a huge renal cyst (*dotted line*) occupying the lower two thirds of the kidney.

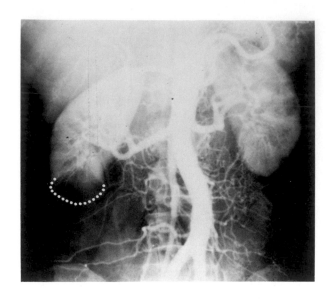

▶ **Figure 8–29**

This aortic flush arteriogram reveals a simple cyst of the lower pole of the right kidney (*dotted line*).

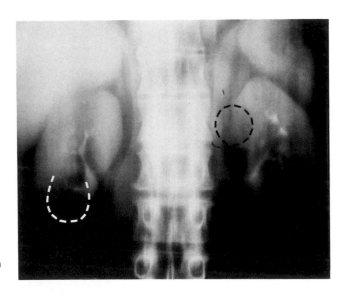

▶ **Figure 8–30**

A nephrotomogram revealing a right lower pole renal cyst (*dotted line*) and a left upper pole renal cyst (*dotted line*) in this 75-year-old man.

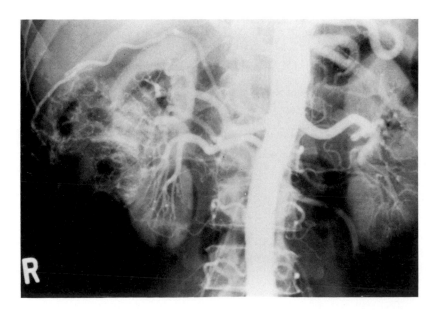

▶ **Figure 8–31**

This aortic flush arteriogram demonstrates a large hypernephroma originating in the mid-portion of the right kidney and extending completely outside of the kidney in this 56-year-old man.

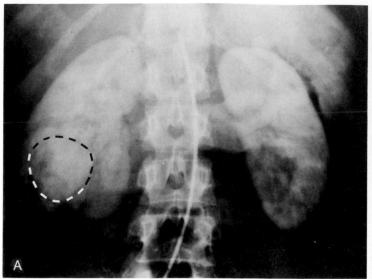

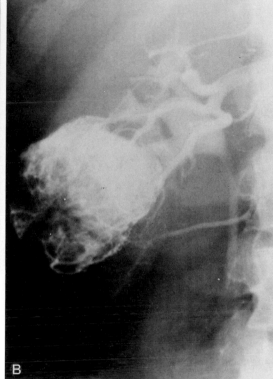

▶ **Figure 8–32**

A, This is a nephrogram/capillary phase of the kidneys in an arteriogram of a 55-year-old man with a right lower pole hypernephroma (*dotted line*). *B,* The same patient is shown. A selective injection is given into vessels that indicate the right lower pole hypernephroma.

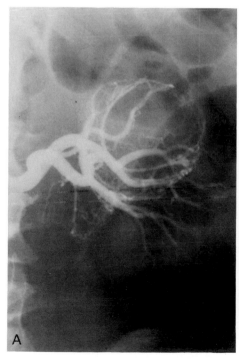

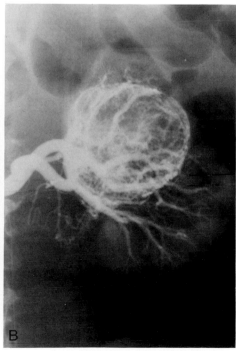

▶ **Figure 8–33**

Early (*A*) and (*B*) arterial phases in this left selective renal arteriogram that demonstrates an upper pole hypernephroma.

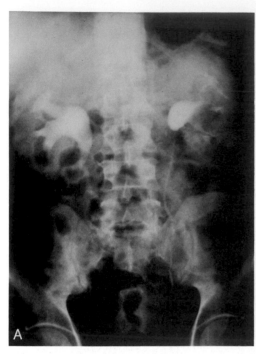
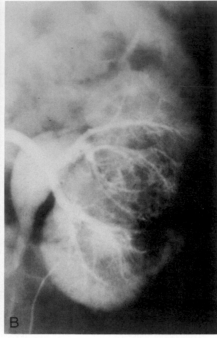

▶ **Figure 8–34**

A left middle hypernephroma comparatively observed on an IVP (*A*) and left selective renal arteriogram (*B*).

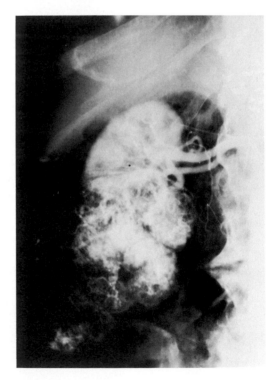

▶ **Figure 8–35**

This selective right renal arteriogram demonstrates an extensive metastatic (renal cell) carcinoma in this 77-year-old woman.

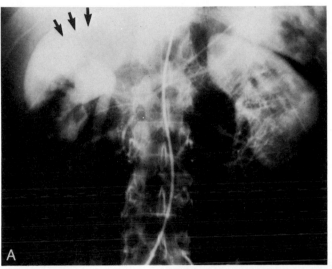

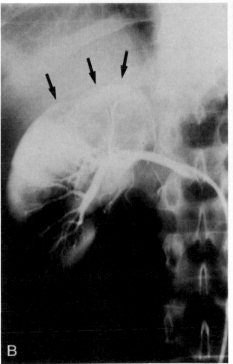

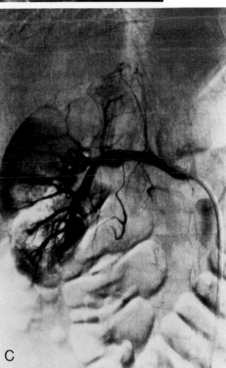

▶ **Figure 8–36**

This aortic flush (*A*) and selective right renal arteriogram (*B*) demonstrate nonfilling of the upper-pole vasculature (*arrows*), indicating an obstructive infundibulum due to tuberculosis in this 44-year-old man. *C*, A digital subtraction image of an upper pole defect in the same patient.

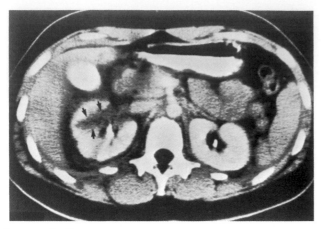

▶ **Figure 8-37**

This computed tomography scan shows a simple corticomedullary laceration (*arrows*) of the anterior portion of the right kidney without extravasation of perirenal fluid. This is considered a minor renal injury and was thus treated nonoperatively. (From Gay SB, Sistrom CL: Computed tomographic evaluation of blunt abdominal trauma. Radiol Clin North Am 30(2): 383, 1992.)

▶ **BIBLIOGRAPHY**

Abrams HL: Abrams Angiography: Vascular and Interventional Radiology, 3rd ed. Boston, Little, Brown, 1983.

Beckmann CF and Abrams HL: Renal venography anatomy: Technique and applications. Cardiovasc Intervent Radiol 3:45–70, 1980.

Kadir S: Diagnostic Angiography. Philadelphia, WB Saunders, 1986.

Kandarpa K: Handbook of Cardiovascular and Interventional Radiographic Procedures. Boston, Little, Brown, 1989.

Reuter S, Redman H, Cho K: Gastrointestinal Angiography. Philadelphia, WB Saunders, 1986.

Swamy S, Segal L, Mouli S: Percutaneous Angiography. Springfield, IL, Charles C. Thomas, 1977.

Williams, PL: Gray's Anatomy, 37th ed. New York, Churchill-Livingstone, 1993.

Wojtowycz M: Interventional Radiology and Angiography. Chicago, Year Book Medical Publishers, 1990.

▶ **SELF-ASSESSMENT QUIZ**

1. The primary indication for visceral angiography is for
   a. trauma
   b. tumors
   c. vascular malformations
   d. GI bleeding

2. What are the two most common causes of GI hemorrhage?
   1. trauma
   2. peptic ulcer
   3. vascular malformations
   4. esophageal varices
      a. 1 and 2
      b. 2 and 3

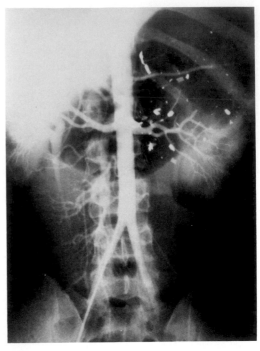

▶ **Figure 8-38**

A gunshot wound of the left kidney. This aortic flush arteriogram reveals the complete loss of the upper pole with evidence of multiple metallic remnants of a bullet that fragmented on contact. A massive peritoneal hemorrhage was present. The patient had an immediate left total nephrectomy.

   c. 3 and 4
   d. 1 and 3
   e. 2 and 4

3. What kind of film changer is preferred for visceral angiography?
   a. roll film
   b. cut film
   c. cassette

4. Visceral angiography always requires biplane filming.
   a. true
   b. false

5. What kilovoltage range is preferred for visceral angiography?
   a. 70 to 75 kVp
   b. 80 to 85 kVp
   c. 90 to 95 kVp
   d. over 100 kVp

6. In order to avoid motion unsharpness, the longest exposure recommended for visceral angiography is
   a. 25 msec
   b. 50 msec
   c. 75 msec
   d. 100 msec

7. Subtraction technique is always an integral requirement in suspected GI bleeds.
   a. true
   b. false

8. Which of the following produces the greatest vessel opacification?
   a. digital venous imaging
   b. digital subtraction angiography (intra-arterial)

9. What is the name of the vessel that is described as a short, thick trunk artery that arises from the anterior surface of the abdominal aorta?
   a. superior mesenteric
   b. right or left renal
   c. inferior mesenteric
   d. celiac axis/trunk

10. The celiac trunk has _____ branches.
    a. one
    b. two
    c. three
    d. four

11. What is the smallest branch of the celiac trunk?
    a. common hepatic
    b. left gastric
    c. splenic

12. What is a primary advantage of catheters that have side holes?
    a. decreases jet-whip
    b. prolongs the life of the catheter
    c. injection time is faster
    d. injection is made easier

13. The portal-venous system drains what organs?
    1. small bowel
    2. colon
    3. stomach
    4. spleen
    5. pancreas
       a. 1 only
       b. 1 and 2
       c. 1, 2, and 3
       d. 1, 2, 3, and 4
       e. 1, 2, 3, 4, and 5

14. Hemorrhage and pneumothorax are complications of what procedure?
    a. renal angiography
    b. femoral angiography
    c. percutaneous transhepatic cholangiography
    d. gastric embolization

15. Which procedure has almost been entirely replaced by computed tomography and ultrasound?
    a. hepatic angiography
    b. splenic angiography
    c. pancreatic arteriography
    d. renal angiography

16. Which catheters are commonly employed in selective pancreatic arteriography?
    a. straight and pigtail
    b. pigtail and headhunter
    c. cobra and sidewinder
    d. sidewinder and pigtail

17. Renal arteriography is most commonly used for the evaluation of
    a. renovascular malformation
    b. tumors
    c. renovascular hypertension
    d. trauma

18. What percentage of individuals will have more than one artery serving each kidney?
    a. 10%
    b. 22%
    c. 33%
    d. 50%

19. The right kidney is usually lower than the left kidney.
    a. true
    b. false

20. The "nephrogram" represents which phase of renal circulation?
    a. arterial
    b. capillary
    c. venous
    d. collateral

21. Flush aortography is often utilized for the evaluation of
    1. large renal tumors
    2. hypertension
    3. the origins of the renal arteries
       a. 1 only
       b. 1 and 2
       c. 1, 2, and 3

22. What is the name of the injection technique preferred for arterial puncture?
    a. flush technique
    b. common femoral technique
    c. selective technique
    d. Seldinger technique

23. What catheters are commonly used for selective visceral angiography?
    a. straight-end
    b. single-curve
    c. double-curve
    d. multiple-curve

24. What projections are usually required to correctly evaluate aneurysms and arterial trauma?
    1. AP
    2. lateral
    3. decubitus
    4. oblique
       a. 1 only
       b. 1 and 2
       c. 1, 2, and 3
       d. 1, 2, 3, and 4

25. What is the purpose of a deflecting guidewire?
    a. it helps the examination go faster
    b. it is easier on the patient's arterial system
    c. it is thrombogenic
    d. it is useful for bending straight catheters

▶ STUDY QUESTIONS

1. List five frequent causes of upper GI hemorrhage.

2. List the major vessels of the abdominal aorta.

3. Describe the location of the major vessels of the abdominal aorta.

4. List and describe five types of catheters used to perform visceral arteriography.

5. Describe the imaging equipment used to perform visceral arteriography.

6. Explain the differences between a flush, selective, and subselective catheterization.

7. List the imaging modalities (other than angiography) that are used to demonstrate vascular abnormalities of the abdomen.

8. What are the purposes of portal venography?

9. List and describe three important abnormalities found in the kidney.

10. What are the purposes of venous sampling?

► CHAPTER NINE

► PERIPHERAL ANGIOGRAPHY

► CHAPTER OUTLINE

Risk Factors
Anatomy
    Aorta and Its Branches
    Venous System
Injection Methods For Peripheral Angiography
    Femoral
    Axillary
    Translumbar Aortography
    Cubital Vein Puncture
Equipment
    Catheters
    Guidewires
    Contrast Material
Radiographic Technique
    Milliampere-Seconds
    Kilovoltage
    Film-Screen Combinations
Imaging Protocol
    Abdominal Aorta and Pelvis

Pelvic Angiography
    Injection Volumes and Filming Sequences
    Lower Extremity Arteriography Via a
        Programmed Stepping-Table
    Determination of Flow Rate
    Program for Table-Stepping
    Long-Film Cassette Changers
    Digital Subtraction Angiography
Pharmaceutical Enhancement of Arterial
  Opacification
Venography
    Lower Extremities
    Patient Preparation
    Techniques
    Venipuncture Injection Protocol
    Contrast Media
    Imaging Protocol
    Systemic Heparinization—Postprocedural Care
Pathology

► CHAPTER OBJECTIVES

Upon completion of Chapter 9 the technologist will be able to:

1. List the risk factors associated with peripheral angiography
2. List the primary vessels arising off the abdominal aorta
3. Identify the primary opacified abdominal arteries on an aortographic flush study
4. List the major arteries of the pelvis, thigh, leg, and foot
5. Identify the primary opacified arteries of the pelvis, thigh, leg, and foot on an arteriographic study
6. List the major veins of the deep and superficial venous system
7. Identify the veins of the deep and superficial venous system on a venogram study
8. Describe the primary injection methods for aortography
9. Describe the criteria for technique selection for angiography of pelvic vessels and its peripheral flow
10. Explain the principle of the "stepping-table"
11. Explain the principles of flow rate

Despite the technologic advancements in the non-invasive evaluation of peripheral vascular disease (PVD), contrast angiography remains the most widely utilized and reliable procedure for outlining and diagnosing aortic and lower and upper extremity disease.

PVD is a common health problem in the United States. The most common disease of the arterial system is *atherosclerosis*. Intimal atherosclerosis is seen primarily in men older than 50 years of age, and statistics reveal that 3% of men and 1% of women older than 60 years of age are affected. This disease is frequently present in patients who are hypertensive, who smoke, and who have diabetes.

Atherosclerosis is characterized by the formation of elevated *plaques* called *atheromas* on the intima. The word atherosclerosis comes from the Greek, athere, meaning "soft, fatty, gruel-like" and from scler, which means "hard." In the earliest stage of atherosclerosis, fatty streaks form along the intima. The lesions are widely scattered at first, but as the disease progresses they become more numerous and can eventually cover the entire intimal surface of an artery.[1] Later, atheromas or plaques of newly formed muscle cells filled with cholesterol build up and protrude into the lumen of the vessel. These deposits cause the inner wall to become roughened and also cause the muscle wall to be rigid and inelastic.

Atheromas narrow arterial channels, damage the underlying tunica media, and may progress to calcification, ulceration with thrombosis, and intraplaque hemorrhage. Vascular narrowing or stenosis may lead to *ischemia* of the areas served by the vessel and to the development of clots within the vessel itself. The process also damages and deforms the muscle wall to the extent that it becomes weakened and may develop into an aneurysm (Fig. 9–1 *A* and *B*).

▶ RISK FACTORS

The process of atherosclerosis is accelerated by hypertension. This is due to the additional stress placed on the lining of large blood vessels. Persons who have diabetes are especially susceptible and tend to develop atherosclerosis earlier in life than do persons who do not have diabetes and hypertension. Patients with hyperlipidemia, particularly high serum cholesterol, are also at higher risk. High serum cholesterol is thought to be closely associated with the development of coronary artery disease. Cigarette smoking, obesity, and genetic predisposition are other factors that are associated with the development of atherosclerosis.

The presence of atherosclerotic plaque provides an additional complication because of its embolic potential. Fragments of plaque may be dislodged by turbulent blood flow, in the presence of pelvic and extremity trauma, and as the result of penetrating injury from projectiles.

Atherosclerosis is an unwanted complication when associated with tumors, arteriovenous malformations, Buerger's disease, frostbite, popliteal disease, and cystic adventitial disease.

Direct injury to a vessel is associated most with catheterization. Bleeding at the puncture site may produce a *hematoma*. Most hematomas occur in patients who are hypertensive. Injury can also result from vascular occlusion from the subintimal passage of a catheter or guidewire.

▶ ANATOMY

Demonstration of the peripheral vascular system often takes place in conjunction with abdominal aortography. This study is referred to as an aortogram with a distal runoff. This means that the abdominal

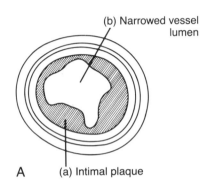

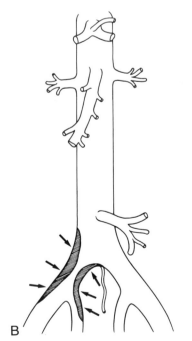

▶ **Figure 9–1**

A, Cross-sectional diagram of an artery. The shaded region (a) shows the accumulation of lipid-rich plaque that has accumulated on the vessel intima. The clear region in the center of the vessel (b) shows the remaining vessel lumen. *B,* A frontal diagram of the aorta and iliac bifurcation. Note the plaque (*arrows*) in the proximal right iliac artery. The arterial lumen has been significantly narrowed. (Redrawn from illustrations by Martha J. Dane.)

aorta and its branches will be imaged first, then, sequentially, the arteries of the pelvis, thighs, legs, and feet. Because atherosclerosis is often a widespread disease, it is often necessary to visualize both visceral and peripheral vascular systems. This information is critical to the surgeon and the surgical approach that may be employed. The abdominal aortogram visualizes these vessels by way of flush injections. Each anatomic area is flushed with a contrast medium while being sequentially imaged with an angiographic stepping-table. A stepping-table is a device that permits a sequential series of "steps" or shifting of the angiographic table to different stations or locations that result in multiple images of the vasculature. This table may step during an abdominoaortic run to obtain views of the vasculature of the pelvis, thigh, leg, and foot. Digital subtraction angiography also may be considered for complete lower extremity arteriography.[2]

In this chapter, it is necessary to discuss in anatomic terms the primary visceral branches as they relate to the peripheral vessels, although the procedural and pathologic focus is on the peripheral vascular system (Figs. 9–2 *A* to *D* and 9–3 *A* to *E*).

Aorta and Its Branches

At the level of the diaphragmatic hiatus, the descending (thoracic) aorta descends into the abdominal cavity. Inside the abdomen, this blood vessel is known as the abdominal aorta. It usually lies slightly to the left of the midline and parallel to the anterior surface of the vertebral column.

The first major visceral branch of the abdominal aorta is the *celiac axis,* which originates from the anterior (ventral) surface of the aorta at the approximate level of the superior surface of the T12–L1 intervertebral disk space (Fig. 9–4 *A* and *B*).

The *superior mesenteric* artery (SMA) arises 1 or 2 cm below the celiac axis and emerges from the anterior surface of the abdominal aorta near the inferior border/surface of the first lumbar vertebral body (Fig. 9–5 *A* to *C*).

The paired *renal* arteries originate opposite each other about 2 cm below the SMA anterior to the level of the second lumbar vertebra (L2). The origin of the renal arteries is at the lateral aspect of and is almost at right angles to the abdominal aorta (Fig. 9–6).

The smaller *inferior mesenteric* artery exits the anterior surface at the level of the L2–L3 intervertebral disk space (Fig. 9–7 *A* and *B*).

The *terminal aorta* is the portion of the abdominal aorta that is situated between the renal arteries and iliac bifurcation. The abdominal aorta usually terminates at the inferior surface of the fourth lumbar vertebra (L4), bifurcating at that point into the *right* and *left common iliac* arteries. The common iliac arteries are the primary arteries of the pelvis and lie adjacent to the common iliac veins.

At the level of the second sacral vertebra (S2), approximately in the middle of each sacroiliac joint, the common iliac artery bifurcates into the *internal* and *external iliac* arteries.

The *internal iliac* or *hypogastric* artery can be divided into anterior and posterior branches. The posterior branch furnishes blood flow to the superior gluteal, iliolumbar, and sacral arteries. The anterior branch supplies blood to the pelvic organs, including the bladder, rectosigmoid colon, and uterus.

The *external iliac* artery becomes the arterial trunk to the lower limb and has no major branches until it reaches the area where the inguinal ligament and the inferior epigastric and deep circumflex iliac arteries arise. As it passes under the inguinal ligament, the external iliac arterial conducting trunk to the lower limb is renamed the *femoral* artery.

The preferred approach for abdominal aortography is percutaneous catheterization of the *common femoral* artery. Arterial puncture is accomplished over the femoral head below the inguinal ligament.

The origin of the *deep femoral* artery (profunda femoris) marks the end of the common femoral artery. The deep femoral artery provides the major branches in the area of the femoral neck and also blood flow to the large muscular branches of the upper and midthigh. At its beginning, it lies at first lateral to the femoral artery and then runs behind it to traverse distally along the medial plane of the femur.

The *superficial femoral* artery (SFA) is a continuation of the common femoral artery. The bifurcation of the common femoral artery into the deep and superficial femoral branches takes place near the inferior border of the femoral head. The SFA extends distally, medial to the femur to the level of the adductor canal (Hunter's canal) in the distal third of the femur.

The *popliteal* artery is the continuation of the SFA and travels through the popliteal fossa (posterior to the intercondyloid fossa) of the femur to the lower border of the popliteus muscle, near the head of the fibula.

The *anterior tibial* artery commences at the bifurcation of the popliteal artery near the head of the fibula. The anterior tibial artery is the smaller of the terminal divisions of the popliteal and is the most lateral of the tibial bifurcation that originates from the popliteal artery. Near the ankle, the artery continues into the foot as the dorsalis pedis artery.

The *posterior tibial* artery is also a continuation of the popliteal artery. The tibioperoneal trunk originates from the popliteal artery and bifurcates into the posterior tibial and peroneal arteries and several small branches. The posterior tibial artery courses distally toward the foot, where it passes between the medial malleolus and over the calcaneus and terminates at the plantar arch of the foot.

The *peroneal* artery is located deeply on the back of the fibular (lateral) side of the leg. The peroneal artery does not connect with any major pedal vessels. It primarily supplies the lateral and medial malleolar arteries, which are often important collateral vessels

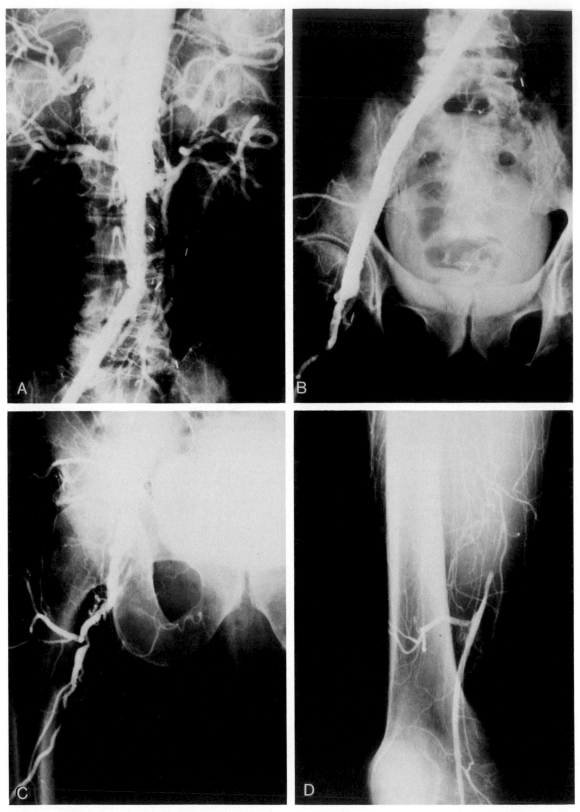

▶ Figure 9–2

A–D, Aortic flush and distal runoff procedure. This 54-year-old man has diffuse peripheral vascular disease. There is an aortofemoral graft and total blockage of the iliac artery at the bifurcation. *A,* The aortic flush injection. *B,* The second step in the injection and imaging sequence with visualization of the right iliac graft and continuation of the arterial blockage on the left side. *C,* Atherosclerotic disease of the right iliofemoral arterial system in the third step of the filming sequence. *D,* This shows a complete blockage of the midportion of the right superficial femoral artery, collateralization, and reconstitution of flow as the vessel passes down behind the knee in the fourth image of this sequence. Imaging of the lower leg and foot may also be desirable.

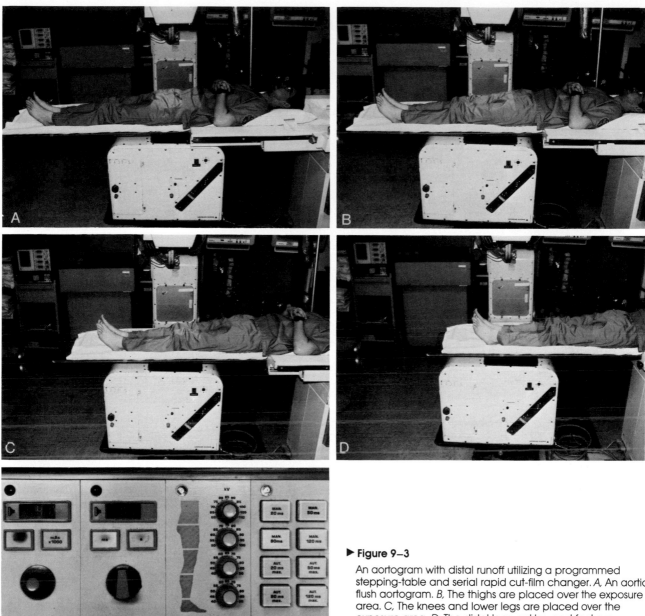

▶ **Figure 9–3**

An aortogram with distal runoff utilizing a programmed stepping-table and serial rapid cut-film changer. *A*, An aortic flush aortogram. *B*, The thighs are placed over the exposure area. *C*, The knees and lower legs are placed over the exposure area. *D*, The distal legs, ankles, and feet are placed over the exposure area. *E*, An example of a fixed mA, variable-kVp step control unit.

in occlusive disease of the lower leg vasculature (Fig. 9–8).

In the upper extremity, the *innominate-brachiocephalic* artery, which is the first branch of the aortic arch, gives rise to the *right subclavian* artery. The *left subclavian* artery is the third branch of the aortic arch. The subclavian arteries, after giving off their neck branches, continue as the great arterial system of the upper limb.

At the outer border of the first rib, the subclavian artery becomes the *axillary* artery. The distal boundary of both the axilla and its artery is formed by the lower border of the teres major muscle as it approaches the upper shaft of the humerus for insertion. From this point to the elbow, the arterial stem to the upper limb takes the name *brachial* artery. The brachial artery usually divides into two terminal branches, the ulnar and radial arteries, in the depths of the antecubital fossa. The *ulnar* artery courses with the ulnar nerve toward the wrist and gives off to smaller branches. The *radial* artery is a direct continuation of the brachial artery. The radial artery is quite superficial along its course and proceeds distally along the lateral side of the anterior compartment of the forearm. The superficial location permits easy compression of the artery against the radius and allows for the pulse to be taken. The blood supply to the wrist and hand comes from interconnecting networks of the ulnar and radial arteries (Fig. 9–9).

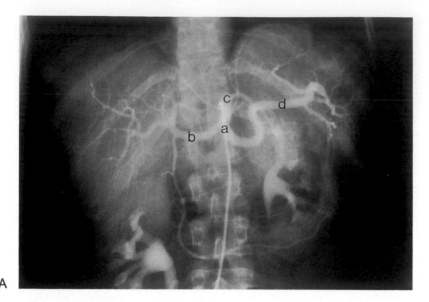

A

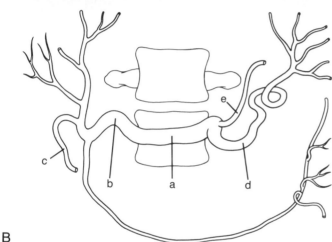

B

▶ **Figure 9–4**

A, A normal anteroposterior celiac arteriogram. (a = celiac trunk/axis; b = hepatic artery; c = gastric artery; d = splenic artery.)
B, Diagram of a celiac arteriogram. (a = celiac trunk/axis; b = common hepatic artery; c = right gastric artery; d = splenic artery; e = left gastric artery.) (*B,* Redrawn from an illustration by Martha J. Dane.)

Venous System

The veins of the pelvis and legs are drained by *deep* and *superficial* venous systems. The deep veins of the pelvis and legs provide the majority of venous return to the heart. The deep veins travel parallel to the course of the arterial flow but drain in the opposite direction. The primary communication between the deep and superficial venous systems is via the perforating veins located in the lower legs and distal thighs.

Blood normally flows from the *superficial system* into the deep system by way of perforating veins. The valves in the perforating veins are unidirectional, thus preventing back-flow. The primary veins of the superficial venous system include the *greater saphenous* vein, which is the longest vein in the body. The greater saphenous vein originates in the medial foot (medial marginal vein near the great toe) and terminates at the *common femoral* vein. The *lesser saphenous* vein arises posteriorly from the lateral foot (lateral marginal vein near the 5th toe) and goes to the

knee joint, where it joins the popliteal and greater saphenous veins.

The *deep venous system* runs parallel to the distal arterial system (superficial femoral artery system) and often assumes the same names; the popliteal vein, superficial femoral vein, deep femoral vein, external iliac vein, and common iliac veins are examples.

The common iliac veins join together anterior to the fifth lumbar vertebra (L5) to form the *inferior vena cava* (IVC). The IVC is located to the right of the abdominal aorta and just anterior to the lumbar vertebral bodies (Fig. 9–10).

The venous system of the upper extremity is similar to that of its arterial counterpart. The *superior vena cava* (SVC) forms into the innominate/ brachycephalic veins, subclavian veins, and axillary veins. On the lateral aspect, the axillary vein forms into the cephalic vein, which winds around onto the anterior aspect of the forearm and in front of the elbow joint communicates with the basilic vein through the median cubital vein, which is often se-

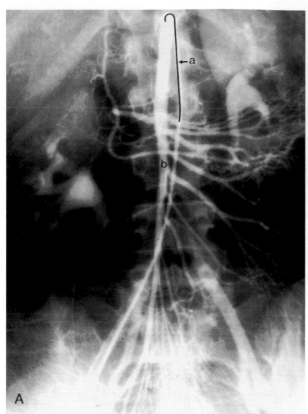

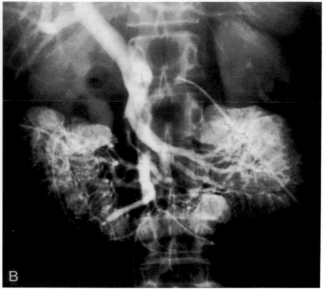

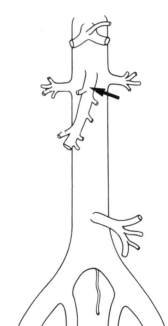

▶ **Figure 9–5**

A, A normal superior mesenteric arteriogram. (a = a catheter selectively placed into the superior mesenteric artery; b = superior mesenteric artery.) *B,* Percutaneous puncture of a superior mesenteric artery and a demonstration of arterial branches and the small intestine and proximal colon. *C,* Diagram of normal superior mesenteric artery anatomy demonstrated on frontal view (*arrow*). (C, Redrawn from an illustration by Martha J. Dane.)

lected for venipuncture. A median vein of the forearm is also often prominent. This vein drains the central portion of the palm and joins the median cubital vein (Fig. 9–11).

▶ INJECTION METHODS FOR PERIPHERAL ANGIOGRAPHY

Femoral

Abdominal aortography and lower extremity angiography can be performed via the femoral, axillary, brachial, and translumbar approaches. The artery of

choice is generally the common femoral. The femoral access is preferred because site compression is much safer and effective over the femoral head. The radiologist selects the femoral artery that has the strongest palpable pulse (Fig. 9–12*A* and *B*).

Axillary

The axillary artery is used routinely for arterial puncture in the absence of competent femoral blood flow, which can result from obstructive disease of the bilateral common femoral or the iliac arteries. In our experience, many radiologists prefer axillary

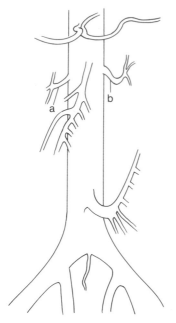

▶ **Figure 9–6**

Diagram of the renal arteries as they arise off the abdominal aorta. (a = right renal artery; b = left renal artery.)

puncture when synthetic graft material is in place. Axillary puncture is preferred from the left upper extremity to decrease the chance of embolization. The risks of axillary puncture are cerebral stroke, vessel spasm, patient discomfort, and resultant site hematoma. The complication rate of axillary puncture is twice that of femoral catheterization (Fig. 9–13).

Translumbar Aortography

If the femoral, axillary, and brachial routes are unacceptable, translumbar aortography (TLA) is an option. The translumbar approach requires the patient to be in a prone position on the angiographic table. The percutaneous puncture (18-gauge needle with a No. 6 French sheath) is made in an area below the 12th rib to the left of the midline, approximately 3 to 4″ to the left of the 12th thoracic spinous process. TLA is contraindicated in patients with coagulation disorders and in those with hypertensive states due to bleeding. The problem of hemorrhage, especially following multiple needle sticks, places patients at increased risk. Another disadvantage is that with most needle systems, only a flush injection is possible. Selective catheterization of target vessels is difficult with the translumbar approach (Fig. 9–14).

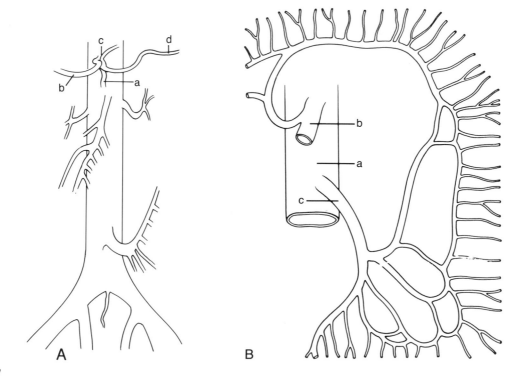

▶ **Figure 9–7**

A, Diagram of a normal abdominal aorta. (a = celiac trunk/axis; b = hepatic artery; c = gastric artery; d = splenic artery.) B, Diagram of the anatomy of a normal inferior mesenteric artery and its relationship to the aorta and superior mesenteric artery. (a = aorta; b = superior mesenteric artery; c = inferior mesenteric artery.) (Redrawn from illustrations by Martha J. Dane.)

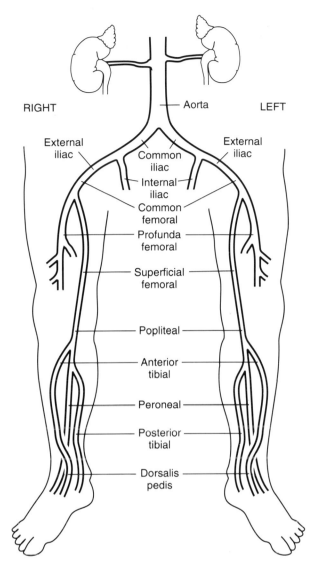

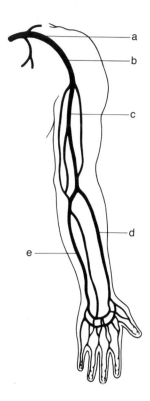

▶ **Figure 9–8**
Diagram of the arterial anatomy of the pelvis, thigh, and leg.

▶ **Figure 9–9**
Diagram of the arterial anatomy of the upper extremity. (a = subclavian artery; b = axillary artery; c = brachial artery; d = radial artery; e = ulnar artery.) (Redrawn from an illustration by Martha J. Dane.)

Cubital Vein Puncture

For this puncture, the arm is abducted 45 degrees. The antecubital fossa is prepared and draped. A tourniquet is affixed over the upper arm, and the median cubital vein is pierced with a 16-gauge angiocatheter or 19-gauge butterfly needle. Two techniques are frequently employed for cubital vein puncture: the angiocath technique and the butterfly technique.

▶ EQUIPMENT

Catheters

Abdominal aortography via the transfemoral approach can be accomplished by utilizing a 60-cm, No. 5 or 6 French (5F or 6F) multiple-hole "flush" pigtail

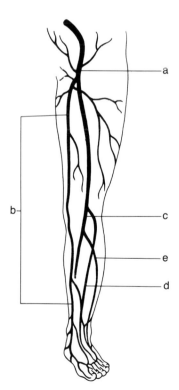

▶ **Figure 9–10**
Diagram of the lower extremity venous system, anterior aspect. (a = femoral vein; b = long saphenous vein; c = popliteal vein; d = anterior tibial vein; e = peroneal vein.) (Redrawn from an illustration by Martha J. Dane.)

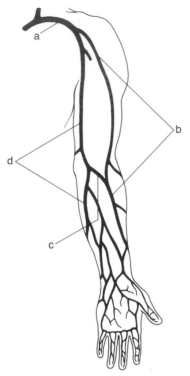

▶ **Figure 9–11**

Diagram of the upper extremity venous system, palmar aspect. (a = subclavian vein; b = cephalic vein; c = median cubital vein; d = basilic vein.) (Redrawn from an illustration by Martha J. Dane.)

or straight catheter. The catheter is placed at the approximate level of the renal arteries, thus decreasing the chance of filling of the celiac trunk and superior mesenteric arteries. An alternative is to place the catheter above the celiac axis in order to better opacify the visceral arteries. This is especially relevant if an abdominal aortic aneurysm is suspected.

An axillary approach requires a longer catheter, usually an 80- or 100-cm, No. 5 or 6 French (5F or 6F) flush pigtail. Catheter placement is in the approximate area of T12 to L2.

The translumbar approach utilizes an 18-gauge, translumbar needle with an attached No. 6 French (6F) sheath. Sheaths can be used with an end hole, or flush sheaths can be used with side holes.

Selective examination of the lower extremities is done using the retrograde femoral, translumbar, and axillary approach. For better lower extremity contrast filling, the catheter is placed approximately 5 cm above the aortic bifurcation.

One of the important considerations for the radiologist is the size of the catheter compared with the inner diameter of the vessel that is being examined. The narrower the catheter, the greater the potential for thrombus production.

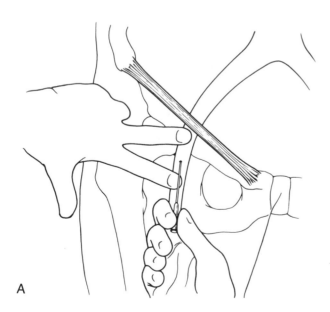

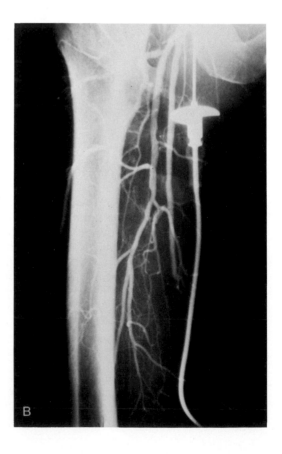

▶ **Figure 9–12**

A, Diagram of an arterial puncture below the inguinal ligament. (Redrawn from an illustration by Martha J. Dane.) B, Percutaneous right transfemoral arterial puncture technique.

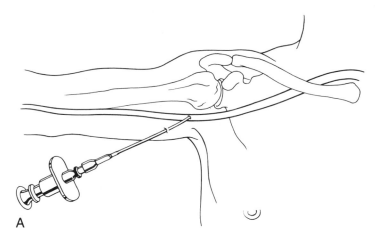

A

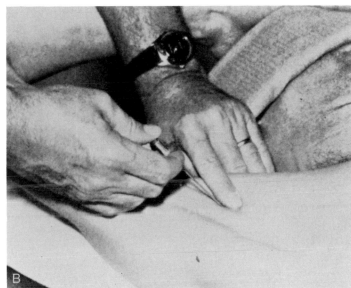

B

▶ **Figure 9–13**

A, Diagram showing the technique for retrograde axillary artery puncture. (Redrawn from an illustration by Martha J. Dane.) *B,* Retrograde puncture of the right axillary artery is shown. The patient had a suspected occlusion in a vascular graft located in the distal aorta and common iliac arteries.

Guidewires

Standard stainless-steel guidewires for adult use are 145 cm long. These wires are consistently used with catheters up to 100 cm in length. In selective arteriography, longer exchange guidewires 260 to 300 cm in length are used for catheter exchange without losing position in a selected vessel.

The radiologist today has many different types of guidewires to choose from. Major considerations include J tip configuration: straight, 1.5 mm, 3 mm, 7.5 mm, and 15 mm in diameter. The J tip wires are required in the presence of severe stenotic arteries and in the presence of severe plaque.

The newer guidewires are coated in Teflon and impregnated with heparin. Teflon coating of the wire results in a lower coefficient of friction, thus reducing the chance of catheter "sloughing" (scraping of the inner catheter wall) when the wire is being advanced or retracted. Heparin reduces the thrombogenicity of the guidewire. The latest technology employs hydrophilic guidewires with polymer coatings that further reduce the coefficient of friction. The coefficient of friction refers to the friction created when a guidewire is passed inside a catheter. Guidewires awaiting use during a given procedure should be immersed in a heparinized bath consisting of 3000 IU of heparin per 500 ml of normal saline (Fig. 9–15).

Contrast Material

The contrast medium is selected by the radiologist. The choice depends on the preangiographic history of the patient, a physical examination, and a laboratory assessment. Optimal angiographic image quality must be weighed against the potential morbidity caused by contrast overload. Injection of a contrast medium produces an initial vasodilatation that is followed by reactive vasoconstriction in the renal circulation, an effect implicated in renal toxicity.

For healthy patients, the type of contrast agent used has very little influence on morbidity. The newer low osmolar or nonionic contrast materials are be-

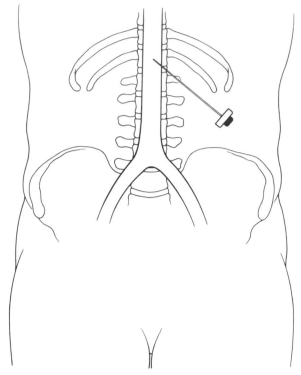

▶ **Figure 9–14**

In percutaneous translumbar aortography, a special 18-gauge needle is placed directly into the abdominal aorta from a left flank approach.

lieved to cause fewer adverse reactions, produce less pain, and reduce renal toxicity.

▶ RADIOGRAPHIC TECHNIQUE

Angiographic imaging equipment varies considerably depending on generators, film-screen combinations, and radiographic tube and heat unit ratings.

Milliampere-Seconds

Milliampere-seconds (mAs) provide for the overall density of the image. In serial contrast imaging, the highest mAs and shortest possible exposure time is required. The exposure time in abdominal aortography should not exceed 100 msec in order to eliminate motion artifacts and vessel spasm.

Kilovoltage

Kilovoltage (kVp) dictates the radiographic contrast of the image. Contrast in the abdominal aortogram (arteriogram) should have sufficient penetration to optimize contrast opacification in comparison with surrounding abdominal structures. Depending on the film-screen combination, 65 to 75 kVp is the ideal range for anteroposterior (AP) abdominal arteriography. Lateral abdominal projections usually require 80 to 85 kVp in order to adequately penetrate and demonstrate the abdominal structures of interest.

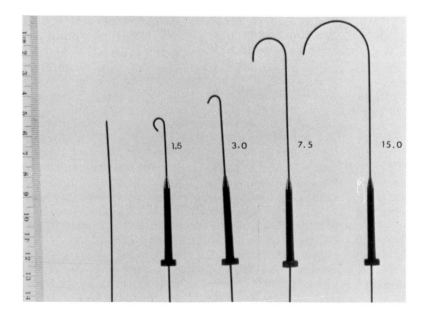

▶ **Figure 9–15**

Basic guidewire shapes. The numbers represent the sizes of the J tip in millimeters (manufacturer's specifications). (From Kadir S: Diagnostic Angiography. Philadelphia, WB Saunders, 1986, p 12.)

Film-Screen Combinations

Film-screen technology has improved greatly during the last decade. Slower systems will always provide better resolution; however, in angiography, radiographic contrast is most important, in addition to a motion-free image. These needs have been addressed by rare earth phosphor film-screen systems. The rare earth systems and advanced "grain" technology have allowed for much better detail requiring less kilovoltage and reduced exposure times, resulting in high-quality angiograms. A film-screen speed combination of 750 to 900 is most satisfactory for aortography and extremity runoff. The film-screen system speed becomes an important factor in delivering both desirable contrast and density in serial angiography.

If patient obesity or musculature results in a radiographic technique that exceeds manufacturer or equipment safety limits, we utilize the inverse square law rather than increase the exposure time. Reduction of the source-image distance (SID) in either filming plane (AP and lateral) often keeps the exposure time at 100 msec or less and still minimizes motion artifacts.

▶ IMAGING PROTOCOL

Abdominal Aorta and Pelvis

It is recommended that biplane filming be utilized for abdominal aortography. Two views, placed at right angles to each other, provide for a more complete diagnostic presentation.

The lateral projection provides valuable information in assessing disease processes of the posterior aortic wall, in evaluating the size of an abdominal aortic aneurysm, and in visualizing those arteries arising from the anterior surface of the aorta, such as the celiac and the superior and inferior mesenteric arteries. Biplane aortography allows for better angiographic presentation of irregular and ulcerated plaques and embolized clots.

Scout radiographs should be taken to ensure that the bowel is clean of opaque contrast material and to enable the technologist to adjust technique factors for optimal image enhancement. The positioning for the AP or frontal abdominal projection includes a radiograph from the level of the diaphragm at the superior level of the film taken on full expiration. We have found that "marking" the scout film position with a felt-tip marking pen allows for fine adjustment in positioning prior to the injection of the contrast medium. The central ray for both AP and lateral projections should be directed to the plane of the lumbar spine, approximately at the level of L1 (Fig. 9–16).

Pelvic Angiography

Pelvic angiography also requires AP and lateral biplane filming, especially in the presence of significant

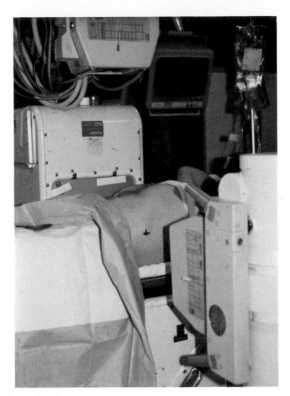

▶ Figure 9–16

An example of a biplane filming protocol for an abdominal flush aortogram. A mark on the left side of the patient's abdomen indicates the centering point for the lateral projection.

atherosclerotic occlusive disease. These projections allow the radiologist to better evaluate the severity of the stenotic areas and also provide an oblique view of the aortic bifurcation, the posterior origins of the internal iliac arteries, and an oblique view separating the superficial and deep femoral systems in most views.

The oblique view for pelvic angiography is accomplished by using an angle sponge to raise the pelvis to a 45-degree elevation. The right posterior oblique (RPO) position shows the origin of the right internal iliac artery and the left deep femoral artery. The left posterior oblique (LPO) position presents the left internal iliac artery and the right deep femoral artery. Dual C-arm devices can be used to accomplish these oblique images while the patient remains supine on the table.

Anatomic positioning can be more accurately determined by observing the area of aortic bifurcation on the television monitor while the radiologist injects the test dose to relocate the catheter in the distal aorta. The level of aortic bifurcation varies from one patient to another. The top of the film should be placed above the aortic bifurcation (Fig. 9–17).

Following abdominal aortography and prior to injecting the pelvic angiogram, it is recommended that the patient be asked to urinate in order to decrease the amount of residual contrast in the bladder. This is also recommended prior to stepping-table angiography of

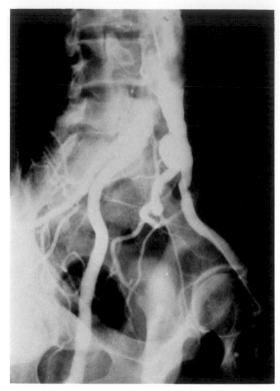

▶ **Figure 9–17**
A small iliac pseudoaneurysm, distal aortic atherosclerosis, and an aneurysm at the aortoiliac graft site in a 67-year-old man. Notice how the oblique view of the pelvis demonstrates the iliac bifurcation.

the lower extremity vasculature. The patient is given a bed pan, or the urinary bladder is drained by way of a Foley catheter that is inserted as part of the pre-procedural work-up.

Injection Volumes and Filming Sequences

The radiologist evaluates blood flow with a test injection following placement of the catheter. The patient's age and physiology vary the speed of blood flow. In older patients, blood flow is slower, especially in those with atherosclerotic occlusive disease. In younger adults and pediatric patients, the blood flow is fast and may require a more rapid filming rate. The filming rates should allow for arterial opacification and the contrast flow through the capillary to the venous system. Table 9–1 lists the injection and filming rates for abdominal and pelvic angiography when utilizing a 76% diatrizoate meglumine contrast medium.

Lower Extremity Arteriography Via a Programmed Stepping-Table

With a programmed stepping-table top, the peripheral arteries from the lower pelvis to the pedal arches

can be visualized utilizing a single injection. The runoff vessels can be filmed using four or five overlapping radiographs on a standard 14 × 14″ serial film changer.

Scout films are taken during the initial prepuncture period. Once again, patient centering is marked on the patient in the event that adjustments are required before the contrast injection is given.

The radiographic technique is adjusted according to the type of generator selection equipment used. Some types of equipment use a fixed kVp (70 to 75 kVp) to penetrate all steps and allow for a variable mA rate to be adjusted for each body part or position. Conversely, some control units accomplish this change of technique by using a fixed mA density level with variable kVp stations adjusted for each body part.

The stepping-table is first engaged and locked over the first position, usually in the lower pelvic area. The patient is then moved and positioned under the field light by sliding him or her into place on the table mattress. Prior to scout exposure, the table is manually stepped through the overlapping program to visually ensure that both adequate proximal and distal coverage is attained. The scout films allow for adjustments in both technique and positioning prior to contrast injection. The scout filming process also allows the technologist to give the patient a preview of the process and table movement that will take place during the contrast injection.

Determination of Flow Rate

The programming of the angiographic "run" depends on the *flow rate* of the patient's blood. A minimum program run of 25 seconds is utilized for patients with a rapid flow. Patients presenting with a slower flow need a program run of at least 30 seconds to visualize distal vessels.

Following abdominal aortic injection, the catheter is relocated to just above the aortic bifurcation. Under fluoroscopy, the patient and the table are moved to place the popliteal area of the symptomatic leg in the center of the fluoroscopy (C-arm) unit. A rapid bolus of 10 ml of contrast medium is injected, and, using a watch, the time of transit is monitored and computed until the contrast medium reaches the popliteal artery. This time value is used in selecting the injection flow rate and gives an indication of how long it will take the contrast medium to arrive at the "third step," which is adjacent to the popliteal area. If the flow rate is quick (between 6 and 8 seconds), an injector flow rate of between 10 and 12 ml/sec for a total volume of 70 ml can be used. If the flow rate to the popliteal area is slow (between 10 and 13 seconds), the injector flow rate is adjusted to ensure a longer injection time. This can be accomplished with an injection rate from 6 to 8 ml/sec for a total of 70 ml.

▶ **Table 9-1**

INJECTION VOLUMES AND FILMING SEQUENCES

	Contrast Medium	Injection Rate/Volume	Film Rate
Abdominal Angiography	76% Diatrizoate meglumine	20 ml/sec (total of 45 ml)	2/sec × 4 sec; followed by 1/sec × 4 sec
Pelvic Angiography	76% Diatrizoate meglumine	10 ml/sec (total of 30 ml)	2/sec × 3 sec; followed by 1/sec × 4 sec

Program for Table-Stepping

The timed delay between contrast medium injection and the first film exposure varies. The correct sequencing of the table shift is crucial in obtaining a diagnostically acceptable study. When computing the program, it must be kept in mind that each table shift takes 1 second.

If the patient's blood flow to the popliteal area is quick (6 to 8 seconds), a film delay of 2 to 3 seconds is recommended. If the blood flow on the symptomatic side is slow (10 to 13 seconds), a film delay of 3 to 5 seconds is recommended. Table 9-2 lists an example of a program for lower extremity runoff when using a stepping-table.

Long-Film Cassette Changers

Long-film cassette changers are still used in some institutions. These systems use a 72 to 90″ SIRD, which is a graduated filter in an extension cone that covers the length of the cassette. The cassette contains three different screen speeds, which are used to obtain an even density along the entire length of the leg. These systems employ a special table that holds long-field cassettes (14 × 36″ with a single screen or 14 × 51″ with three screens). The field size varies with individual units, as does the cassette capacity (four to six cassettes). The basis of this system is to present the entire distal extremity arterial flow from the aortic bifurcation to beyond the popliteal arteries on a single film.

Filming time is computed according to its arrival in the popliteal flow of the symptomatic extremity. A 5- to 7-second delay is normally seen. Since the contrast medium is injected over 8 to 10 seconds, the filming is adjusted to permit maximum arterial filling. If an injection rate of 6 ml/sec for a total volume of 60 ml is used, filming should begin approximately 2 seconds prior to completion of the injection phase. This allows for opacification of the iliac arteries and for maximum opacification distally.

The large-cassette programmer allows for selection of a time delay before changing the cassette. This allows delays of between 1 and 8 seconds between each film cassette.

Digital Subtraction Angiography

The vascular radiologist may utilize digital subtraction angiography (DSA) in combination with routine film arteriography. One of the advantages of this system is that it provides a method to visualize and evaluate the small vessel disease processes that are distal to the popliteal system. DSA uses a computer to enhance the diagnostic information by electronically removing undesirable bone and soft tissue that may hide these small collateral systems. The distal collateral flow is important in order to allow the vascular surgeon to assess and plan distal graft procedures and is also important in confirming the possible utilization of vascular interventional procedures (e.g., transluminal angioplasty).

▶ PHARMACEUTICAL ENHANCEMENT OF ARTERIAL OPACIFICATION

Intra-arterial injection of vasodilators can be used to enhance optimal visualization of distal vessels. The most well known are as follows:

1. *Tolazoline (Priscoline)*—an arterial vasodilator. The angiogram should be performed in 1 to 3 minutes following injection. The preparation would consist of 25 mg of tolazoline in 10 to 15 ml of 5% glucose solution.

2. *Papaverine*—a myovascular relaxant, useful in

▶ **Table 9-2**

PROGRAM FOR LOWER EXTREMITY RUNOFF WITH A STEPPING-TABLE

Injector Flow Rate	Total Volume	Film Delay
6–12 ml/sec*	70 ml	2–5 sec*

Film Program
Step 1. Pelvis: 3-sec delay; then 1/sec for 3 sec > shift
Step 2. Thighs: 1/sec for 3 sec > shift
Step 3. Knees: 1/sec for 4 sec > shift
Step 4. Feet:† 1/sec for 4 sec; then 1/sec every other sec for 3 sec

* Injector flow rate and film delay are dependent on the rapidity of the patient's arterial vascular flow.
† If the patient is tall, a fifth step can be added.

treatment of arterial spasm. A suitable amount of 20 to 30 mg is injected for 60 to 65 seconds.

3. *Lidocaine*—a systemic analgesic. A quantity of 50 mg of 2% lidocaine (Xylocaine) is diluted in 10 to 15 ml of 5% glucose solution. Lidocaine produces vasodilatation, and its effects last from 30 minutes to 1 hour.

4. *Reserpine*—an adrenergic, reduces peripheral vasospasm. A quantity of 0.5 to 1.5 mg of reserpine is injected into the arterial system by way of a catheter.

▶ VENOGRAPHY

Lower Extremities

The most common reason for lower limb venography is to rule out suspected deep venous thrombosis. It is often impossible to clinically distinguish between deep vein thrombosis and thrombophlebitis; however, in most patients, inflammation is present and the patient is symptomatic (Fig. 9–18).

Lower limb venography is also used when evaluating varicose veins and also when assessing the state of venous stasis.

Patient Preparation

Patients with deep vein thrombosis often exhibit a swollen edematous lower extremity. Pre-examination

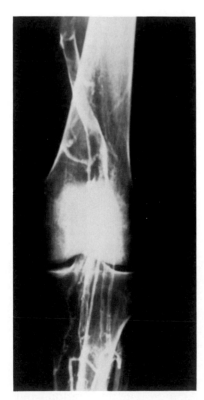

▶ **Figure 9–18**

A 56-year-old man with deep vein thrombosis.

preparation orders often include elevation of the symptomatic extremity, and occasionally an order is placed for an elastic wrap, which is designed to decrease edema. If extensive varicosities (varicose veins) are apparent, the entire calf can be wrapped with the elastic bandage. This provides for better contrast filling of the deep veins and can decrease the amount of contrast material needed to opacify these enlarged, tortuous veins.

Techniques

There are many techniques in use for lower leg venography. Venography can be performed in the supine or semiupright (Fowler's) position and with many types of imaging equipment. Venography can utilize fluoroscopy and spot filming and may be accomplished using conventional 14 ×17″ cassettes. The advantage of fluoroscopy is that it allows for the radiologist to assess the contrast flow in "real time."

Supine or semiupright venography is often preferred by the radiologist. The semiupright, angled-table technique is preferred because the contrast material is held in the extremity by gravity. This allows for more time to complete the filming process, and the delayed passage of contrast allows for less contrast material to be injected (Fig. 9–19*A* and *B*).

The patient is placed on the fluoroscopic tilt table, and the patient's head is elevated 35 to 45 degrees. The patient's weight is borne on the opposite foot, and a wooden box is used to elevate the patient over the table filming area. This box also allows for the "hanging" leg to be completely relaxed, thus preventing muscle contraction in the affected leg (which can affect contrast opacification) (Fig. 9–20). Patients who are unable to stand or who are weak can be assisted with the use of restraint bands. The bands can be placed over the chest and under the affected leg and over the knee of the weight-bearing leg. This allows for at least some elevation of the table in all examinations, including in debilitated and seriously ill patients, and assists in providing maximum opacification. Even if the patient can tolerate only a 25-degree elevation, we have found that this assists in delaying contrast passage.

Venipuncture Injection Protocol

With the patient in a semiupright position, tourniquets are placed above the ankle and above the knee. These tourniquets provide for obstruction of the superficial veins and furnish better opacification of the deep venous system, without the "spaghetti-like" filling of the superficial system that overlies the deep veins (Fig. 9–21).

The venipuncture is accomplished over the instep of the foot. A 19- to 21-gauge butterfly needle is inserted, preferably in a direction toward the toes. This downward insertion provides for better opacification

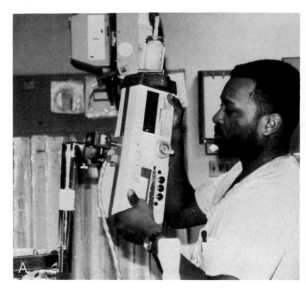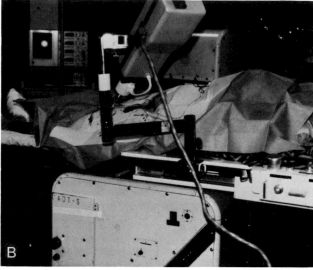

▶ **Figure 9–19**

A, The technologist prepares to attach the injector arm swivel to the angio table. *B,* The injector arm swivel is attached to the stepping-table.

of the deep veins of the calf. The butterfly needle is taped into position after a test injection is given to rule out extravasation.

The injection of contrast may be by hand, by slow-delayed power injection, or by drip infusion. From our experience, hand injection allows for more constant control of contrast, especially when fluoroscopy is used. Fluoroscopy is often indicated even when

14 × 17″ plain filming is employed in order to evaluate and decrease the chance of extravasation.

Contrast Media

Many radiologists advocate the use of a 60% contrast medium. Nonionic (low osmolar) contrast media have been proved to reduce a patient's discomfort during

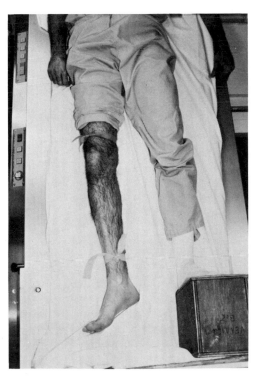

▶ **Figure 9–20**

The patient's opposite leg is placed with the foot in contact with the wooden box.

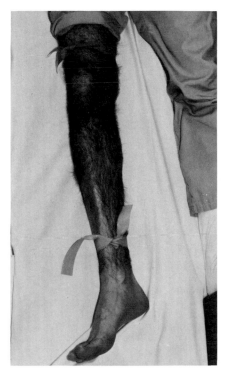

▶ **Figure 9–21**

Tourniquets are placed above the knee and ankle.

injection and to further reduce the possibility of postvenogram thrombosis. A total of 80 to 100 ml of contrast medium is injected over 1 to 3 minutes.

Imaging Protocol

If fluoroscopy is used, the flow of contrast is followed up the leg. Filming begins when the contrast bolus fills and reaches the proximal popliteal vein. If fluoroscopy is not being used, radiography should begin after an injection of 30 to 40 ml of contrast medium. Table 9–3 lists a suggested filming sequence for a lower extremity venogram.

Prior to radiographing the pelvic veins and IVC, the patient is brought back to the supine position. Many radiologists prefer to apply manual compression to the femoral area while the table is leveled and the technologist is preparing for the next exposure. Once the filming routine is established, the radiologist releases compression, elevates the extremity, and asks the patient to take a deep breath and strain down (Valsalva maneuver) during the exposure. These methods are used to enhance contrast filling of the pelvic and caval vessels.

Systemic Heparinization— Postprocedural Care

When filming is completed, many radiologists prefer to infuse heparinized solution (heparin and normal saline or dextrose and water) into the veins of the leg to reduce the chance of postprocedural thrombophlebitis and to flush the contrast medium out of the leg veins. The leg can also be elevated on pillows or given suitable support to encourage drainage.

▶ PATHOLOGY

Many diseases and conditions are diagnosed and treated by way of peripheral angiography. Several examples are presented in the succeeding paragraphs.

Leg pain is a common complaint of older individuals and is apparent after weight bearing and excessive exercise. The pain is often relieved by simply

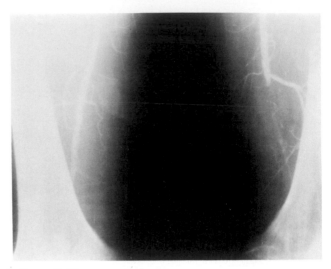

▶ **Figure 9–22**

An occlusion of the distal portion of the left superficial femoral artery.

resting. Upon resumption of exercise, pain is again experienced. This is referred to as *intermittent claudication*. Atherosclerosis is often the cause of this condition (Fig. 9–22).

Buerger's disease affects medium-sized blood vessels (particularly the arteries of the legs). This disease can cause severe pain and, in severe cases, can lead to gangrene. *Thromboangiitis obliterans* (another term

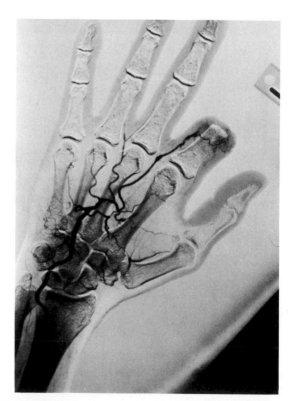

▶ **Figure 9–23**

Subtraction film describing a postsurgical demonstration of the left hand.

▶ **Table 9–3**

LOWER EXTREMITY VENOGRAM

Suggested Filming Sequence

1. AP* and external rotation of the calf (2 films)
2. AP and external rotation of the knee (2 films)
3. Removal of the tourniquets; repeat steps 1 and 2 (1 film for each step)
4. AP distal thigh (1 film)
5. AP pelvis-proximal thigh (1 film)

* AP = anteroposterior.

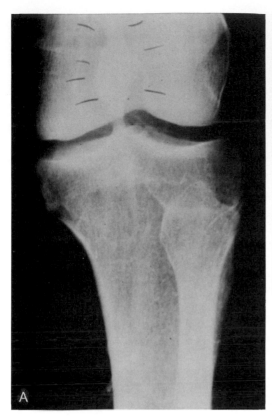

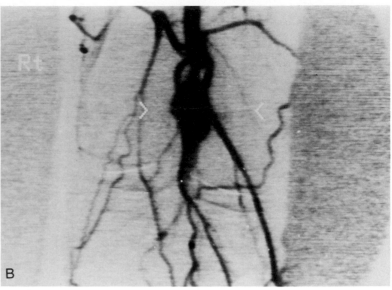

▶ **Figure 9-24**

A, An angiographic demonstration of a popliteal aneurysm of the left knee.
B, A digital subtraction angiography study of the left popliteal aneurysm.

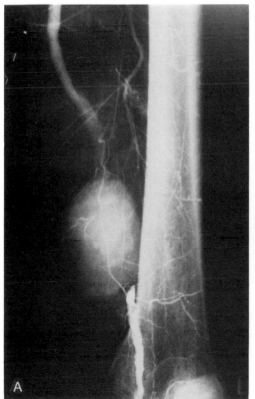

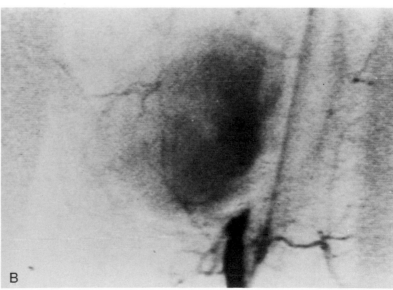

▶ **Figure 9-25**

A, Mycotic aneurysm of the left thigh. *B,* A digital subtraction angiography
demonstration of a mycotic aneurysm.

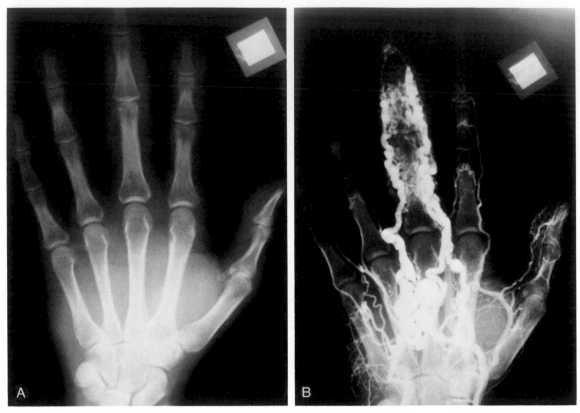

▶ Figure 9–26

A, A scout film of the left hand. *B,* An arteriovenous malformation of the left hand and middle finger.

for Buerger's disease) refers to the clotting, pain, and inflammation that occur in this disease and to the fact that it can obliterate, or destroy, blood vessels. Figure 9–23 is an angiographic study of a 59-year-old man who had a partial surgical amputation of the left index finger. The patient had a long history of alcohol abuse and had smoked for 40 years. The patient's finger became gangrenous and had to be amputated.

Aneurysms can be found almost anywhere in the vascular system. Aneurysms are saccular lesions formed by the localized dilatation of the wall of an artery, vein, or the heart. Aneurysms can develop from many sources; for example, as a result of a congenital vessel weakness, as a complication of atherosclerosis, from an infection, and as a late effect of trauma. Figure 9–24 *A* and *B* is an angiographic study

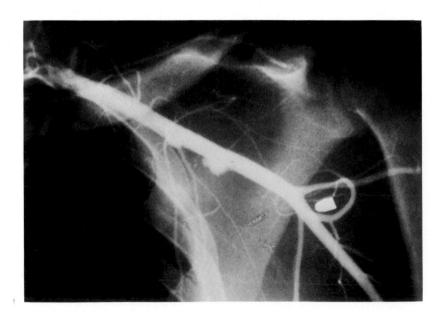

▶ Figure 9–27

A gunshot wound with a bullet lodged in the left axillary region.

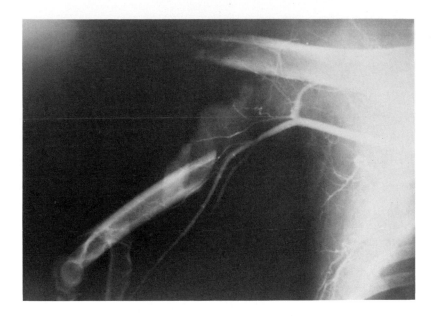

▶ **Figure 9–28**

A compound fracture of the right humerus with no evidence of vascular injury.

of a patient's lower leg that was injured during a football game. The angiogram demonstrates a popliteal aneurysm.

Aneurysms often develop as a post-traumatic complication. The individual in Figure 9–25A and B was

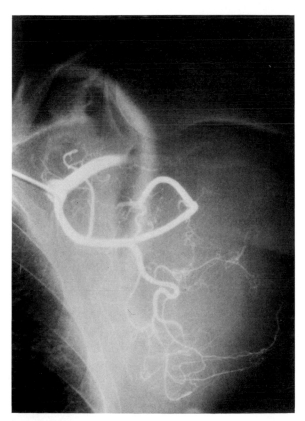

▶ **Figure 9–29**

A hemangiosarcoma of the left axillary region and artery.

stabbed in the thigh during a domestic dispute. Following initial emergency treatment, the patient's leg became painful and swollen. An infection was suspected, and the patient was hospitalized. A femoral arteriogram revealed a mycotic aneurysm at the wound site. Reconstitution of the superficial femoral artery is seen distal to the aneurysm.

Figure 9–26A and B involves a 25-year-old man whose left hand was stepped on during a football game. The hand was significantly bruised, but the initial radiographs demonstrated no bone abnormality, only some soft tissue swelling. After about 3 weeks, the patient's index finger became swollen and almost doubled in size. The patient complained of severe pain. A brachial arteriogram revealed an arteriovenous malformation of the hand and middle finger.

In Figure 9–27, a 27-year-old man was shot in the left upper torso in a drive-by shooting. A subclavian arteriogram revealed that the vasculature was not damaged by the missile. Arteriography of the limbs and abdomen is frequently performed to rule out vascular injury.

Industrial accidents frequently result in major injury involving bone, soft tissue, and the adjacent vascular supply. Figure 9–28 shows an injury caused when a 27-year-old laborer was shoveling a mixture of sand and gravel into a cement mixer. The shovel flew out of his hand and into the cement mixer. While attempting to retrieve his shovel, his arm somehow got caught inside the mixer, resulting in a compound, badly displaced fracture of the right humerus. Amazingly, the arteriography of the upper limb revealed that the subclavian and brachial arteries remained intact.

Vascular tumors that are situated adjacent to a vascular supply or that develop within a vessel are frequently identified via peripheral arteriography. Fig-

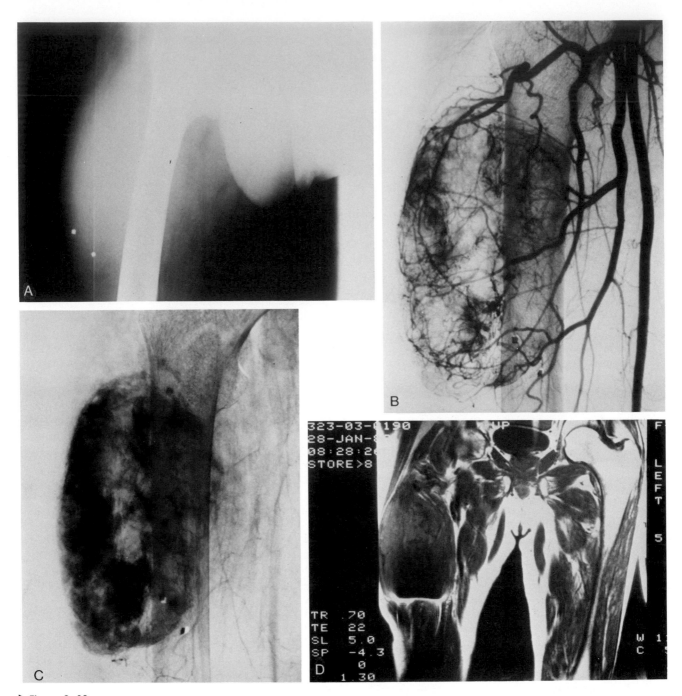

► **Figure 9–30**

A, A scout film of the right thigh revealing swelling. *B,* Histocytoma: late arterial phase. *C,* Histocytoma: venous phase. *D,* Histocytoma as seen on magnetic resonance imaging.

ure 9–29 reveals a hemangiosarcoma of the right axillary region and artery in a 44-year-old man.

Figure 9–30*A* to *D* demonstrates a malignant histoma of the right anterolateral aspect of the right thigh in a patient who reported significant swelling and pain. This tumor was demonstrated on plain films of the thigh, on femoral arteriography, and on a magnetic resonance imaging scan.

► **REFERENCES**

1. O'Toole M (ed): Miller-Keane Encyclopedia and Dictionary of Medicine, Nursing, and Allied Health, 5th ed. Philadelphia, WB Saunders, 1992.
2. Wojtowycz M: Interventional Radiology and Angiography. Chicago, Year Book Medical Publishers, 1990.

► BIBLIOGRAPHY

Abrams HL: Abrams Angiography: Vascular and Interventional Radiology, 3rd ed. Boston, Little, Brown, 1983.

Gaspar M and Barker W: Peripheral Arterial Disease, 3rd ed. Philadelphia, WB Saunders, 1981.

Golman K and Almen T: Contrast media-induced nephrotoxicity: Survey and present state. Invest Radiol 27:92, 1985.

Hessel SJ and Adams DF: Complications of angiography. Radiology 138:273, 1981.

Huff JA, Kasemeyer B, and Lutjen G: Bilateral femoral angiography: A step-by-step approach. Radiol Technol 16(1):35, 1989.

Johnsrude IS, Jackson DC, and Dunnick NR: A Practical Approach to Angiography, 2nd ed. Boston, Little, Brown, 1987.

Kadir S: Diagnostic Angiography. Philadelphia, WB Saunders, 1986.

Kandarpa K: Handbook of Cardiovascular and Interventional Radiologic Procedures. Boston, Little, Brown, 1989.

► SELF-ASSESSMENT QUIZ

1. Which of the following best describes an atheroma?
   a. a ballooning out of an artery
   b. a lesion produced as the result of vessel dissection
   c. plaque-like lesions of the arterial intima
   d. a type of arteriovenous malformation

2. Which of the following are considered to be risk factors for atherosclerosis?
   1. obesity
   2. cigarette smoking
   3. diabetes mellitus
   4. hypertension
      a. 1 only
      b. 1 and 2
      c. 1, 2, and 3
      d. 1, 2, 3, and 4

3. The first major branch of the abdominal aorta is the
   a. celiac axis/trunk
   b. superior mesenteric
   c. renal artery
   d. inferior mesenteric

4. Which artery supplies blood to the distal colon?
   a. celiac axis/trunk
   b. superior mesenteric
   c. deep femoral
   d. inferior mesenteric

5. The longest vein in the body is the
   a. popliteal
   b. great saphenous
   c. femoral
   d. lesser saphenous

6. Which artery is the artery of choice for percutaneous needle puncture when performing abdominal aortography?
   a. axillary
   b. brachial
   c. common femoral
   d. abdominal aorta

7. Which artery is the artery of choice when synthetic graft material is in place?
   a. common femoral
   b. axillary
   c. abdominal aorta
   d. external iliac

8. Translumbar aortography is usually accomplished with the patient in the _____ position?
   a. supine
   b. LPO
   c. prone
   d. lateral

9. Which of the following catheters can be used selectively as well as for flush injections?
   1. pigtail
   2. straight end
   3. headhunter
   4. sidewinder
   5. cobra
      a. 1 only
      b. 1 and 2
      c. 1, 2, and 3
      d. 1, 2, 3, and 4
      e. 1, 2, 3, 4, and 5

10. Which of the following injection approaches is actually a "retrograde" injection?
    a. axillary
    b. brachial
    c. translumbar
    d. common femoral

11. Standard guidewires for adult use are approximately how long?
    a. 50 cm
    b. 100 cm
    c. 145 cm
    d. 175 cm

12. Which guidewire configuration is the most common?
    a. J
    b. C
    c. L
    d. I

13. In order to reduce the coefficient of friction
    a. guidewires are impregnated with heparin
    b. guidewires contain a wetting agent
    c. the guidewire is twice as long as the catheter
    d. guidewires are coated in Teflon

14. Which of the following reduces the thrombogenicity of the guidewire?
    a. heparin
    b. Teflon
    c. wetting agents
    d. the stainless-steel quality of the wire

15. Exposure factors in abdominal aortography should not exceed _____ milliseconds in order to eliminate motion artifacts and vessel spasms.
    a. 50
    b. 75
    c. 100
    d. 200

16. What is the ideal kVp range of AP abdominal arteriography?
    a. 65 to 75

    b. 75 to 80
    c. 85 to 90
    d. over 90

17. Lateral abdominal arteriography usually requires what kVp range to adequately penetrate and demonstrate abdominal arterial anatomy?
    a. 65 to 75
    b. 75 to 80
    c. 80 to 85
    d. over 90

18. What film-screen speed combination is recommended for aortography and extremity runoff?
    a. 500 to 600
    b. 600 to 700
    c. 700 to 750
    d. 750 to 900

19. Which position reveals the left internal iliac and right deep femoral arteries?
    a. RAO
    b. RPO
    c. LAO
    d. LPO

20. Approximately how long does it take to completely demonstrate the blood vessels from the pelvis to the foot, utilizing a stepping-table?
    a. 10 to 15 seconds
    b. 15 to 20 seconds
    c. 25 to 30 seconds
    d. 30 seconds to 1 minute

21. A long-film cassette changer utilizes what size of cassettes?
    a. 14 × 14″
    b. 14 × 17″
    c. 7 × 17″
    d. 14 × 36″

22. Tolazoline hydrochloride (Priscoline) acts as a/an
    a. arterial vasodilator
    b. myovascular relaxant
    c. arterial vasoconstrictor
    d. analgesic

23. Which drug is used to treat an arterial spasm?
    a. papaverine
    b. lidocaine
    c. tolazoline hydrochloride (Priscoline)
    d. epinephrine

24. A wooden box is used for what special procedure?
    a. translumbar aortography
    b. peripheral angiography
    c. venography
    d. aortogram with distal runoff

25. Which type of injection allows for more constant control of contrast media administration for venography?
    a. hand injection
    b. drip infusion
    c. slow, delayed power injection
    d. rapid power injection

▶ STUDY QUESTIONS

1. List and describe three indications for visceral angiography.

2. List and describe three contraindications for visceral angiography.

3. List all the trunk vessels and major branches of the arteries and veins of the peripheral vascular system.

4. Describe the structure and function of a peripheral stepping-table.

5. List and describe three types of catheters used in selective peripheral angiography.

6. List and describe three guidewire configurations used in peripheral angiography.

7. Describe two ways to enhance radiographic technique when performing peripheral angiography.

8. List and describe three pharmaceutical agents that are used to enhance arterial opacification.

► CHAPTER TEN

► NEUROANGIOGRAPHY

► CHAPTER OUTLINE

► CHAPTER OBJECTIVES

Upon completion of Chapter 10 the technologist will be able to:

1. Define (a) carotid arteriography; (b) vertebral arteriography; and (c) cerebral angiography
2. List the indications and contraindications for (a) carotid arteriography; (b) vertebral arteriography; and (c) cerebral angiography
3. List the primary types of equipment employed in neuroangiography
4. List the names or types of needles, guidewires, and catheters utilized in neuroangiography
5. List the major arteries of cerebral circulation
6. Describe the patient care/nursing management procedures that are unique to neuroangiography
7. Describe the procedural considerations for neuroangiography
8. Explain the criteria of contrast medium selection
9. Describe the rationale for subtraction enhancement film technique
10. Explain the positioning and filming protocol for neuroangiography
11. List the most common neoplasms of the brain and spinal cord that are demonstrated with angiography
12. List the most common diseases and conditions affecting the brain and spinal cord that are demonstrated with angiography

The techniques of cerebral angiography have progressed greatly since the Portuguese neuroradiologist Moniz performed the first carotid angiogram on a patient in 1927. Moniz performed a surgical cut-down of the carotid artery and introduced a needle under visual guidance.

Historically, the progression of neuroangiography, from the 1930s to the present, was dependent on technologic advancements in radiology. A few of these advancements include the percutaneous injection technique that was developed by Seldinger in 1953; the increased capabilities of rapid film changers and contrast medium injectors; the development of smaller x-ray tube focal spots; the improvement of intensifying screens and radiographic film; the addition of computer applications to angiography; the development of water-soluble and nonionic contrast material; and further development of needle, guidewire, and catheter science.

▶ INDICATIONS

The indications for cerebral angiography and the appropriateness of any percutaneous contrast procedure is a shared medical decision between the patient's physician and the vascular radiologist or neuroradiologist. It depends on the patient's clinical history, physical examination, and expectant diagnostic results. In many pathologic protocols, computed tomography (CT) has become the imaging procedure of choice. Magnetic resonance (MR) imaging of vascular anatomy and pathology is only beginning to develop. MR angiography is now a reality and is becoming a valuable addition to the field of neuroimaging. This concept is discussed later in the chapter.

Cerebral angiography is an important procedure in the diagnostic evaluation of atherosclerotic occlusive disease, aneurysms, arteriovenous malformations (AVMs), and thrombotic/embolic pathology. Cerebral angiography is designed to locate vascular abnormalities and to provide the surgeon with a preoperative display of the vascular anatomy and pathologic lesion. It is also useful in the diagnosis of vascular complications following surgery or other invasive studies such as angioplasty, embolization, and therapeutic drug infusion. In cerebral trauma, CT scanning is often the definitive imaging modality, yet angiography is still one of the primary methods of specifically demonstrating abnormal vascular details following trauma (e.g., intracerebral, subdural, or epidural hematomas and the anatomic displacement of the cerebral vessels). Table 10–1 lists the indications and contraindications for cerebral angiography.

▶ CONTRAINDICATIONS

Contraindications for cerebral angiography must be evaluated with the patient's overall condition in mind. Clinical studies and observations indicate that major procedural complications are related directly to the severity of the patient's illness. Thus, patients with multisystem abnormalities (e.g., cardiac, renal, and pulmonary) are often considered to be too unstable to have angiography. Prior history of adverse reactions to intravascular contrast media, recent myocardial infarction, unstable angina, congestive heart failure, and severe hypertension can increase the probability of major complications. Cerebral angiography can be hazardous in elderly patients with advanced arteriosclerosis, in pregnant women, and in patients with active intracerebral hemorrhage. These patients are more likely to experience sudden changes in their cardiac status following injection of a contrast medium. They are also likely to suffer ischemic injury and possibly show symptoms and signs of a cerebrovascular accident (CVA) or stroke.

▶ VASCULAR ANATOMY

Aortic Arch

The blood supply that feeds the cerebral vascular system originates from the superior surface of the

▶ **Table 10–1**

INDICATIONS AND CONTRAINDICATIONS
FOR CEREBRAL ANGIOGRAPHY

Indications	Contraindications
Cerebrovascular disease	Contrast media sensitivity
Carotid artery disease	Advanced arteriosclerosis
Cerebral thrombosis	Severe illness
Cerebral embolism	Comatose patients
Cerebral hemorrhage	Severe hypertension
Aneurysm	Severe subarachnoid hemorrhage
Arteriovenous fistula/malformation	Severe intracerebral hemorrhage
Congenital malformation	Advanced age
Primary neoplasm	
Trauma	
Presurgical evaluation	
Postsurgical evaluation	

aortic arch, which is located behind the sternum (manubrium portion). There are variations in their origins, yet most individuals have three major branches that arise directly off the aortic arch. The *brachiocephalic* artery (BCA), also known as the *innominate* artery, which is the first branch of the aortic arch, emanates behind the manubrium of the sternum and is usually 3 to 4 cm in length and courses superiorly (cranially) along the right side of the trachea. It bifurcates into the right common carotid and right subclavian arteries at the level of the right sternoclavicular joint. The *left common carotid* artery (LCCA) is the second branch of the aortic arch. The LCCA is longer than the *right common carotid* artery (RCCA) because its origin is directly from the aortic arch. The *left subclavian* artery (LSA) is the third and final major branch of the aortic arch. The LSA courses cranially and provides an origin for the left vertebral artery (Figs. 10–1 and 10–2).

Common Carotid Arteries

The *common carotid* arteries (CCAs) are enclosed within their individual carotid sheaths; run parallel to the jugular vein system; and are located lateral to the thyroid cartilage. The common carotids usually bifurcate at the level of the superior lateral borders of the thyroid cartilage. The bifurcation level often varies according to body habitus—for example, it is higher in short-necked (hypersthenic) patients and lower in long-necked (hyposthenic and asthenic) patients and children (C3 to C5) (Figs. 10–3 and 10–4). The two main branches of the CCAs are the internal and external carotid.

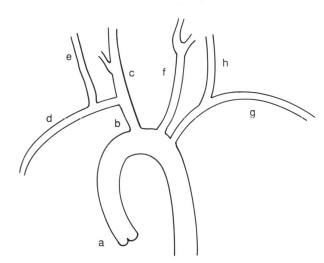

▶ Figure 10–2

A diagram of the aortic arch. (a = ascending aorta; b = innominate or brachiocephalic artery; c = right common carotid artery; d = right-subclavian artery; e = right vertebral artery; f = left common carotid artery; g = left subclavian artery; h = left vertebral artery.) (Redrawn from an illustration by Martha J. Dane.)

External Carotid Arteries

The *external carotid* arteries exit medial and anterior to the internal carotid arteries. Branches can be divided into the *anterior* segment, which is directed toward the facial and mandibular regions, and the

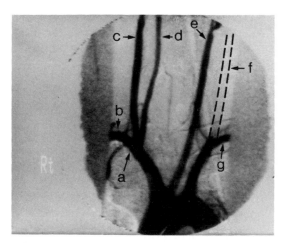

▶ Figure 10–1

Digital subtraction angiography of a normal aortic arch. (a = innominate artery; b = right subclavian artery; c = right common carotid artery; d = left vertebral artery; e = left common carotid artery; f = left vertebral artery; g = left subclavian artery.)

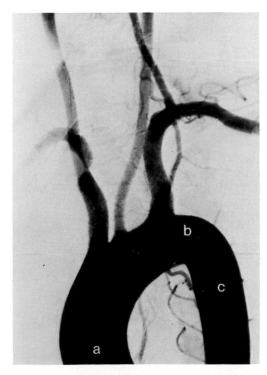

▶ Figure 10–3

The bilateral common carotid arteries (a = ascending artery; b = arch; c = descending artery.)

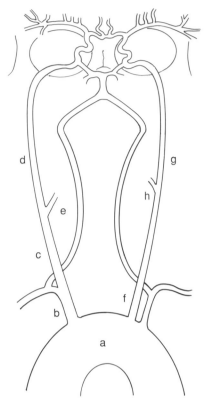

▶ **Figure 10–4**

Frontal view of the carotid arteries. (a = aortic arch;
b = innominate or brachiocephalic artery; c = right common
carotid artery; d = right internal carotid artery; e = right
external carotid artery; f = left common carotid artery; g = left
internal carotid artery; h = left external carotid artery.)
(Redrawn from an illustration by Martha J. Dane.)

posterior segment, which courses toward the neck and occipital region. Table 10–2 lists the branches of the external carotid artery.

Internal Carotid Arteries

The *internal carotid* arteries originate at the carotid bifurcation (C3–C4). There is a dilatation at the terminal portion of the CCA, and its evolution into the internal carotid artery is called the *carotid sinus*. This area contains special sensory cells (pressure receptors) that play a specific role in the regulation of blood pressure in the brain. The carotid body monitors the oxygen partial pressure (Po_2). Special radiographic

▶ **Table 10–2**
BRANCHES OF THE EXTERNAL CAROTID ARTERY

Anterior Branches	Posterior Branches
Superior thyroid	Pharyngeal
Lingual	Auricular
Facial	Occipital
Internal maxillary	

views (i.e., half-axial obliques) are often required in angiography of this area, because the carotid bifurcation is often a repository for intimal atherosclerotic plaque build-up.

The *cervical portion* of each internal carotid artery runs perpendicularly (superiorly) upward through the foramen lacerum and becomes the *petrous portion* at the level of the temporal bone. It curves forward and medially and ascends through the sphenoid region of the petrous bone. The *cavernous* segment (also known as the carotid siphon) begins at the apex of the petrous bone and exits from the carotid canal, courses upward, and passes forward along the lower border of the sella turcica. The cavernous segment of the internal carotid artery is easily noted on the lateral angiogram by its S shape. The posterior curve of the S is located adjacent to the dorsum sellae, and the anterior portion of the S passes adjacent to the medial side of the anterior clinoid process. (The cavernous segment or sella turcica can be located at a point ¾″ anterior and ¾″ superior to the external auditory meatus.) Several branches originate from the cavernous segment. The *ophthalmic* artery accompanies the optic nerve, gives off the central retinal artery, which enters the optic nerve, and courses anteriorly through the optic foramen. Its branches supply the eye, ocular muscles, ethmoid, and nasal mucosa. The *posterior communicating* artery passes posteriorly above the oculomotor nerve and connects the internal carotid system and the posterior cerebral artery. The third branch is the *anterior choroidal* artery. This artery arises at a point that coincides with a bifurcation, which becomes the anterior and middle cerebral arteries. Displacement of these branches is often seen with intracranial masses, and the posterior communicating artery can often play an important role in collateral circulation (through the circle of Willis) in certain occlusive pathologic conditions (Figs. 10–5 and 10–6).

The two terminal branches of the internal carotid arteries are the *anterior cerebral* artery (ACA) and *middle cerebral* artery (MCA). The ACA arises from the bifurcation of the terminal internal carotid artery and courses medially and horizontally to the longitudinal fissure separating the hemispheres of the brain. The ACAs are located very near the median sagittal plane and are connected across the midline by the *anterior communicating* artery, which completes the anterior connection in the circle of Willis. The anterior communicating arteries supply the medial surface of the frontal and parietal cerebral cortices. Very often, in order to visualize the anterior communicating artery angiographically, special patient positioning and auxiliary techniques must be used. Anterioposterior (AP) obliques and submentovertical (SMV) positions can frequently be used to demonstrate this tiny artery angiographically by eliminating overlap of the artery upon itself. The degree of central ray angulation varies according to the body habitus. Cross-compression of the contralateral (opposite) in-

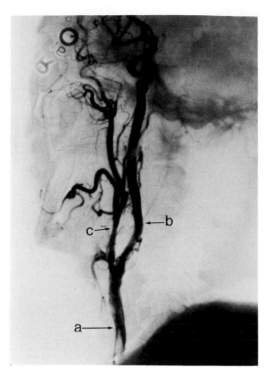

▶ **Figure 10–5**

Lateral cerebral arteriogram showing the internal and external carotid arteries. (a = right common carotid artery; b = right internal carotid artery; c = right external carotid artery.)

ternal carotid cervical branch can sometimes improve opacification.

The MCA also begins at the terminal portion of the internal carotid bifurcation. It extends laterally and terminates upon entering the *sylvian fissure*. It divides into a number of branches that are distributed to the lateral surface of the cerebral hemisphere. It supplies most of the lateral surface of the cerebral cortex.

The *lenticulostriate* arterial branches supply the basal ganglia, the thalamus, and the internal capsule. These arterial branches are commonly the site of hemorrhage or thrombus, which causes the familiar pattern of contralateral paralysis called a *stroke*.

The MCA is the largest branch of the internal carotid artery. The sylvian portion of the MCA provides an important baseline used by radiologists or neuroradiologists in assessing neurovascular disease. The *sylvian triangle* is an important anatomic landmark that sometimes indicates an abnormal position of certain arteries of the brain. It is very important with regard to the presence of mass lesions and their ability to push the intracranial vessels out of normal position. Anterior masses push the triangle posteriorly; posterior masses push the triangle anteriorly; superior masses push the triangle inferiorly; and inferior masses push the triangle superiorly. This landmark is bordered superiorly, anteriorly, and inferiorly by levels of the branches of the sylvian portion of the MCA (Figs. 10–7 to 10–11). Table 10–3 lists the important structures of the internal carotid artery.

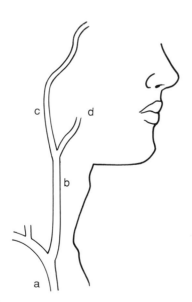

▶ **Figure 10–6**

Lateral view of the carotid arteries. (a = innominate or brachiocephalic artery; b = right common carotid artery; c = right internal carotid artery; d = right external carotid artery.) (Redrawn from an illustration by Martha J. Dane.)

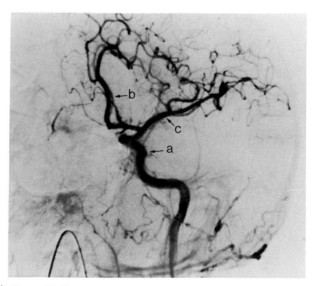

▶ **Figure 10–7**

Lateral cerebral arteriogram showing the internal carotid artery, anterior cerebral artery, and middle cerebral artery and their branches. (a = internal carotid artery; b = anterior cerebral artery; c = middle cerebral artery.)

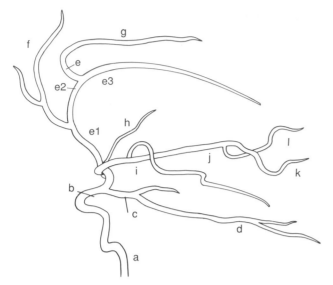

▶ **Figure 10–8**

A diagram of a lateral cerebral arteriogram demonstrating the internal carotid artery and its branches. (a = internal carotid [extradural] artery; b = internal carotid [intradural] artery; c = posterior communicating artery; d = posterior cerebral artery; e = anterior cerebral artery; e1 = pericallosal-inferior artery; e2 = pericallosal-anterior artery; e3 = pericallosal superior artery; f = frontopolar artery; g = callosomarginal artery; h = frontal ascending artery; i = middle cerebral artery; j = posterior temporal artery; k = angular artery; and l = posterior parietal artery.) (Redrawn from an illustration by Martha J. Dane.)

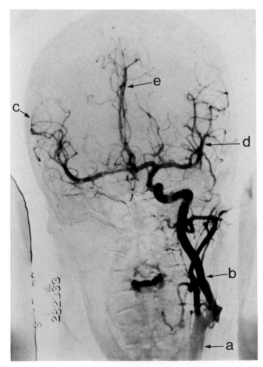

▶ **Figure 10–9**

Anteroposterior cerebral showing the anterior and middle cerebral arteries. (a = left common carotid artery; b = left internal carotid artery; c = right middle cerebral artery; d = left middle cerebral artery; e = anterior cerebral artery.)

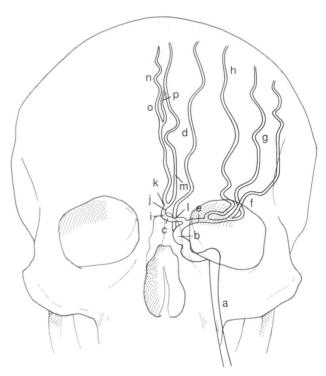

▶ **Figure 10–10**

Frontal diagram of the anterior cerebral circulation. (a = internal carotid [extradural] artery; b = internal carotid [intradural] artery; c = posterior communicating artery; d = posterior cerebral artery; e = middle cerebral artery; f = posterior temporal artery; g = angular artery; h = posterior parietal artery; i = anterior communicating artery; j = pericallosal inferior artery; k = pericallosal anterior artery; l = anterior cerebral artery; m = frontopolar artery; n = anterior cerebral artery; o = pericallosal superior artery; p = callosomarginal artery.) (Redrawn from an illustration by Martha J. Dane.)

Vertebrobasilar System

The arterial flow to the posterior portion of the brain and brain stem is supplied by the *vertebrobasilar system* (VBS). The origin of vertebral arteries bilaterally is the subclavian arteries. The vertebrals ascend through the cervical transverse foramina of C1 to C6. The vertebral arteries enter the skull through the foramen magnum, and at the lower level of the pons, the contralateral vessels unite, forming the *basilar* artery. The basilar artery ends by dividing and forming the *posterior cerebral* arteries (PCAs). The PCA links the internal carotid artery through the posterior communicating artery and forms the lateral borders of the circle of Willis. The PCAs supply areas important to eye function and to the production of cerebrospinal fluid (Figs. 10–12 to 10–15). Table 10–4 lists the arteries and branches of the vertebrobasilar system.

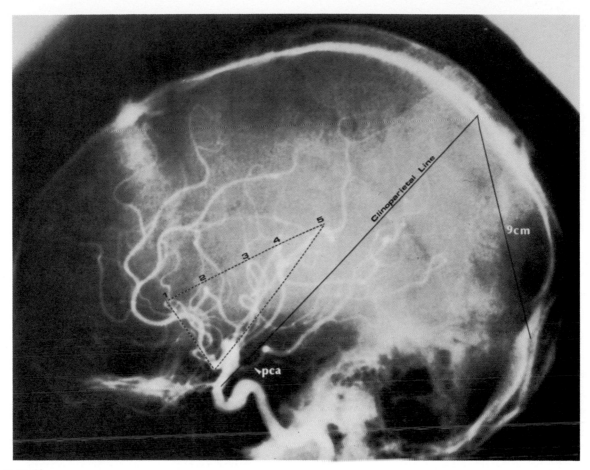

▶ Figure 10–11

Lateral projection of the skull showing the middle cerebral artery and its branches. The triangular-shaped dotted line illustrates the sylvian triangle. The upper border or roof can be formed by drawing a line across the loops of the branches of the middle cerebral artery (numbered from 1 to 5 as they rise to the top of the sylvian fissure). Number 5 denotes the angular branch and the sylvian point. The floor of the sylvian triangle is shown by a dotted line drawn from the sylvian point to the genu (the area in which the middle cerebral artery bifurcates at its most lateral point.) The anterior part of the sylvian triangle is demonstrated by connecting the anterior loop of the middle cerebral artery with the genu. (From Ramsey RG: Neuroradiology with Computed Tomography, Philadelphia, WB Saunders, 1982.)

Arterial Collateral Circulation

It is important to note that the internal carotid artery system provides branches that supply blood flow to

▶ Table 10–3

STRUCTURES OF THE INTERNAL CAROTID ARTERY

Cervical Portion	Petrous Portion
Carotid bifurcation	Carotid siphon
Carotid sinus	Ophthalmic
Carotid body	Posterior communicating
	Anterior cerebral
	Anterior communicating
	Middle cerebral
	Lenticulostriate

the frontal portion of the brain, and the vertebrobasilar artery has branches that supply blood flow to the posterior portion of the brain. By the anastomosis or joining of several arterial branches, a collateral circulation system is formed in the cerebral arterial system of the brain. It is called the *circle of Willis*. When a cerebral vessel is occluded, collateral blood flow may occur between the external and internal carotid arterial system and between the basilar and carotid systems. The circle of Willis consists anteriorly of an anastomosis between the anterior cerebral arteries in the midline, joining both hemispheres via the small anterior communicating artery. Laterally, the posterior communicating artery joins the posterior cerebral arteries, thus creating a circle. When one of the major arterial routes in this circle is occluded, blood flows from a normal pressure area to the lower or

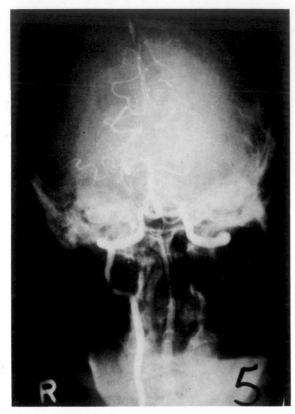

▶ **Figure 10–12**

An anteroposterior vertebral angiogram.

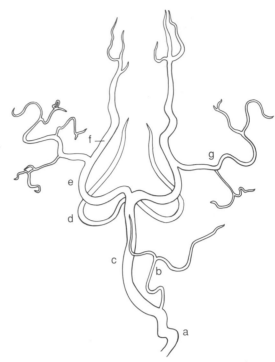

▶ **Figure 10–13**

Diagram of an anteroposterior vertebral angiogram half axial projection of the vertebrobasilar system. (a = vertebral artery; b = posterior inferior cerebellar artery; c = basilar artery; d = superior cerebral artery; e = posterior cerebral artery; f = occipital branch of posterior communicating artery; g = temporal branch of posterior communicating artery.) (Redrawn from an illustration by Martha J. Dane.)

occluded area in an attempt to revascularize. This important vascular phenomenon is called *collateralization* (Figs. 10–16 and 10–17).

Venous Circulation

Blood from the brain, superficial parts of the face, and the neck drain into the *jugular* vein. This vein commences in that part of the *transverse sinus* situated in the groove on the mastoid portion of the temporal bone. This groove is the *sigmoid sinus*.

The veins grouped together as those of the diploë, brain, and venous sinuses of the dura mater include veins from three subdivisions. The *diploic* veins in the channels of the diploic layer of the cranial bones communicate with the *meningeal* veins and with the *sinuses* of the dura mater.

The veins of the brain can be divided into two primary systems: the *cerebral* and *cerebellar* veins. The cerebral veins generally parallel the terminal portion of the arterial tree in the pial layer. They extend through the arachnoid membrane and meningeal layer of the dura mater to open into the cranial *venous sinuses*.

The *cerebral* veins can be divided into *external* (*superficial*) and *internal* (*deep*) groups, simply according to the surfaces that they drain. The external

cerebral veins are the *superior, inferior,* and *middle* cerebral veins.

The *cerebellar* veins are found on the surface of the cerebellum and consist of two sets, the *superior cerebellar* and *inferior cerebellar* veins. The superior cerebellar veins drain into the internal cerebral veins and terminate into the *transverse* and *petrosal sinuses*. The inferior cerebellar veins drain into the *transverse, superior petrosal,* and *occipital sinuses*.

The *venous sinuses* of the dura mater include the *superior sagittal, inferior sagittal, occipital, straight,* and two *transverse sinuses*.

The *superior* and *inferior sagittal* sinuses are associated directly with the falx cerebri (the fold of dura mater that dips down into the longitudinal fissure between the right and left cerebral hemispheres). The superior sagittal sinus is located under the sagittal suture of the skull and drains into a *transverse* sinus. The inferior sagittal sinus (located between the two cerebral hemispheres) becomes the *straight* sinus, which drains into the other (second) *transverse* sinus.

The *straight* sinus is an extension of the inferior sagittal sinus. The *right* and *left transverse* sinuses (which are continuations of the sagittal sinuses) course transversely across the inner surface of the occipital bone in grooves that are visible on any axial

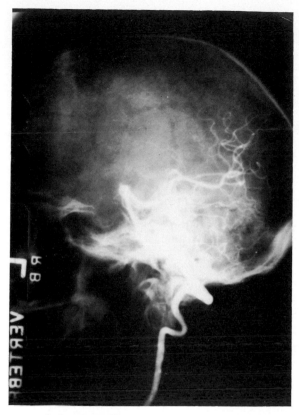

▶ Figure 10–14

Lateral view of the vertebrobasilar system.

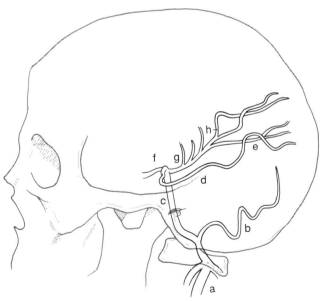

▶ Figure 10–15

Diagram of a lateral vertebral angiogram. (a = vertebral artery; b = posterior inferior cerebellar artery; c = basilar artery; d = superior cerebellar artery; e = temporal branch of posterior cerebellar artery; f = posterior part of circle of Willis; g = posterior cerebral artery; h = occipital branch of posterior cerebellar artery.) (Redrawn from an illustration by Martha J. Dane.)

projection of the skull. These sinuses turn downward toward the petrous portions of the temporal bone (pars petrosa) as the *sigmoid* sinuses.

The *right* and *left sigmoid* sinuses, as continuations of the transverse sinuses, pass down in the posterior cranial fossa bilaterally and leave the skull by way of the internal jugular foramina close to the foramen magnum as the *right* and *left internal jugular* veins.

The *internal jugular* veins are continuations of the sigmoid sinuses of the dura. Each jugular vein courses down the neck to join a *subclavian* vein and form the *brachiocephalic* (innominate) vein. The blood in the brachiocephalic vein then flows into the *superior vena cava* (Fig. 10–18). Table 10–5 lists the primary venous structures of the brain.

▶ PATIENT CARE PROCEDURES

Patient care management during cerebral angiography is the responsibility of the technical staff (technologists) or the radiologic nurse. The caregiver should be aware of the specific needs of the patients who are at a higher risk during an angiographic procedure. These include children and young females whose arteries tend to go into spasm and thus increase the incidence of thrombosis. Also, patients who are hypersensitive, who suffer from renal disease, and who are dehydrated are at increased risk. Geriatric patients suffering from the effects of "aging" are at increased risk owing to changes in their respiratory and cardiac status. Geriatric patients are subject to radical fluid shifts, and sodium and potassium levels are most often affected. The older patient is also at higher risk for acute renal failure (nephrotoxicity) when contrast agents are administered.

Nursing management is similar throughout all invasive procedures. It is best to attain a medical, physical, and emotional baseline on the patient before the procedure begins. This enables the caregiver to better assess the patient as the procedure progresses.

Overall, physical status, including any changes in vital signs, mental status, behavior, speech, and mood, should be observed and reported to the vascular surgeon, neuroradiologist, radiologist, or cardiologist. Nursing management requires maintenance of cardiovascular vital signs, adequate ventilation, fluid balance, and administration of medications as ordered by the appropriate medical specialist.

Restraints should be utilized only when needed. Most patients cooperate if the requirements in breathing and angiographic positioning are explained. If restraints are required, they should be applied with the patient's physical and emotional comfort and cooperation in mind. Explanations before, during, and after the procedure should be presented so that the patient knows what to expect before it happens. The patient should be allowed to be part of his or her

► Table 10–4
ARTERIES AND BRANCHES OF THE VERTEBROBASILAR SYSTEM

Right subclavian	**Left subclavian**
Right vertebral	**Left vertebral**
Anterior spinal	Anterior spinal
Right posterior inferior cerebellar	Left posterior inferior cerebellar
Right posterior spinal	Left posterior spinal
Right anterior-inferior cerebellar	Left anterior-inferior cerebellar
Basilar	
Right pontine branches	Left pontine branches
Right superior cerebellar	Left superior cerebellar
Right posterior cerebral	Left posterior cerebral
Right posterior communicating	Left posterior communicating

procedure and should be given verbal positive reinforcement following serial runs or injections (Fig. 10–19).

► EQUIPMENT

The angiographic equipment used in a given vascular suite should be tailored specifically to the types of procedures performed. For example, equipment needs in a dedicated cardioangiography suite vary considerably compared with the components utilized in a cerebral or peripheral-vascular suite. Cerebral angiography requires equipment that can allow for the rapid transit time of contrast media through the cerebrovascular network while imaging the arterial, capillary, and venous phases of cerebral circulation. Therefore, specialized high-capacity generators and x-ray tubes with fractional focal spots are necessary for neuroangiography.

Generators

The requirements for a neurovascular suite starts with the selection of a generator. The generator of choice would be a three-phase (12-pulse) unit with

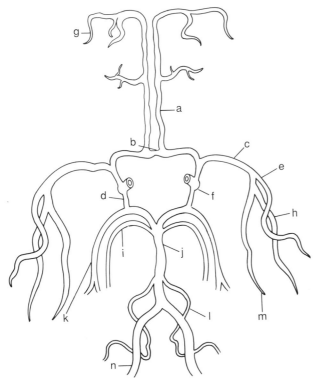

► **Figure 10–16**
Diagram of the circle of Willis. (a = anterior cerebral artery; b = anterior communicating artery; c = middle cerebral artery; d = posterior communicating artery; e = posterior parietal artery; f = internal carotid artery; g = frontopolar artery; h = angular artery; i = superior cerebellar artery; j = basilar artery; k = posterior cerebral artery; l = posterior inferior cerebellar artery; m = posterior temporal artery; n = vertebral artery.) (Redrawn from an illustration by Martha J. Dane.)

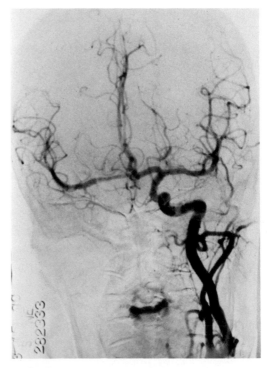

► **Figure 10–17**
An anteroposterior projection of a cerebral angiogram. The patient has a total occlusion of the right internal carotid artery with cross-filling by way of the anterior communicating artery.

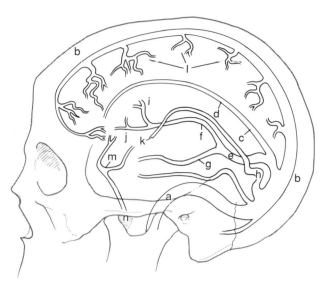

▶ **Figure 10–18**

Diagram of lateral cerebral venous return. (a = transverse sinus; b = superior sagittal sinus; c = straight sinus; d = inferior sagittal sinus; e = vein of Galen; f = internal cerebral vein; g = basal vein of cerebrum; h = inferior anastomotic vein of cerebrum; i = thalamostriate vein; j = septal vein; k = venous angle; l = superior cerebral veins; m = sphenoparietal sinus; n = cavernous sinus.) (Redrawn from an illustration by Martha J. Dane.)

1000- to 1500-mA (milliampere) capacity. The transition from single-phase to three-phase power during the last decade can be attributed to the demand in radiology for shorter exposure times. The constant potential capacity produces a more homogeneous x-ray beam, resulting in an image with less noise and minimal dose of radiation to the patient.

All types of angiography (including neuroangiography) require high mA, the shortest possible exposure factors available, and the lowest kilovolt (kV) setting

▶ **Table 10–5**

VENOUS CIRCULATION OF THE BRAIN

Cerebral veins
  Diploic
  Meningeal
    Superficial (external)
      Superior
      Inferior
      Middle
Cerebellar veins
  Deep (internal)
    Superior cerebellar
      Transverse sinus
      Petrosal sinus
    Inferior cerebellar
      Transverse sinus
      Superior petrosal sinus
      Occipital sinus
Dural (venous) sinuses
  Superior sagittal
  Inferior sagittal
  Occipital
  Straight
  Transverse (2)

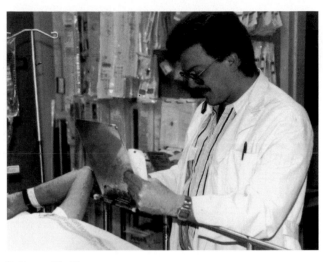

▶ **Figure 10–19**

The technologist is reviewing the patient's chart and is discussing the expectations for the examination with the patient.

in order to produce a radiograph with optimum contrast.

High mA maximizes the number of usable photons, thus decreasing the overall noise attributed to quantum mottle. Fast exposure times decrease subjective patient motion and minimize the loss of recorded detail that is commonly the result of vessel motion or spasm. Fast exposure times give the angiographic technologist a great deal of flexibility in establishing the programming sequence, which may include single or biplane filming. We prefer to utilize exposure factors in the range of 50 msec for cerebral angiography.

X-Ray Tubes

In most hospitals in which neuroangiography is performed, x-ray tube focal spots of between 0.6 and 1.2 mm are quite standard. In a dedicated cerebral angiography suite, recorded details of the vascular anatomy depend on the utilization of the smallest focal spot size. For nonmagnification cerebral angiography, a 0.6-mm focal spot is satisfactory. For the purposes of serial magnification, a focal spot of 0.3 mm is recommended. The 0.3-mm focal spot produces an image that quite easily can be enlarged to a ratio of $2:1$ or $2\frac{1}{2}:1$. Although focal spots are available in sizes smaller than 0.3 mm, their cost is appreciably higher. The combination of a high-capacity generator and an x-ray tube with a 0.3-mm focal spot yields high-quality neuroangiographic studies at a reasonable cost.

Rapid Serial Film Changer

Currently many types of serial film changers are marketed worldwide by several manufacturers. We have found that the cut-film changer is currently the changer of choice in many hospitals in Chicago and its surrounding community medical centers. Roll-film changers largely have been replaced by cut-film changers.

The advantage of cut-film is its ease in handling and processing following injection and exposure. This becomes important when the findings of the initial injection dictate the next angiographic step. The technologist can take the receiver to the darkroom and "count-down" in order to process the arterial, capillary, and venous films in proper order to determine if the study is complete or requires further intervention.

Biplane Serial Filming

In cerebral angiography, it is customary to use a method of serial filming that yields radiographs that are at right angles to each other (AP and lateral).

Rapid serial film changers are available for biplane use with two changers mounted on individual stands. The advantage of biplane filming is that the exposures can be made in each plane on a single injection without the procedural delay of setting the lateral changer and injecting a second time.

The disadvantage or objectionable aspect of biplane filming is scatter radiation that is produced during the x-ray exposure of the patient. The scatter radiation is the result of the exposure of the patient's head, which is in the AP position. The head is quite dense from front to back, and a significant amount of scatter radiation reaches the vertical film changer, causing fogging of the film. To offset this problem, a linear grid (usually an 8:1 ratio) is used in the horizontal film changer. The vertical changer employs a crossed, 8:1 grid. The grid in the vertical changer should absorb the radiation that is produced as a result of the biplane operation (Fig. 10–20).

An important consideration in selecting film changers is film capacity, or the number of usable films per magazine, and the maximum filming rate, or films exposed per second.

In cerebral angiography, the film rate should be set at a minimum of 2 films/sec during the arterial phase of injection for a period of 4 seconds followed by a rate of 1 film/sec for 4 seconds. This allows for 12 films to demonstrate the arterial-capillary-venous phases of circulation in both planes (Figs. 10–21, 10–22, and 10–23).

The goal of a grid is to provide adequate "cleanup" of secondary/scatter radiation while preventing artifactual grid lines from appearing on the finished radiograph. High-quality grids should be used in serial film changers for angiography, and especially when cerebral angiography is being performed. The grids used for cerebral angiography usually are 8:1 or 10:1, 100 line/inch grids with aluminum spacing.

Table 10–6 lists the standardized and optional features of a rapid serial film changer.

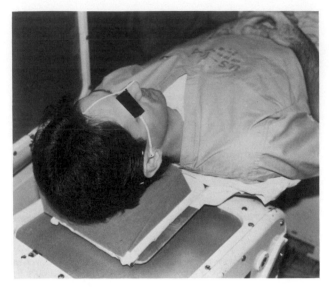

▶ Figure 10–20

Arrangement of serial changers for biplane filming.

Programming Device

The programming device allows the technologist to select the number of films desired per second (film rate) for a selected period of time. The faster the film rate, the shorter the exposure time. The manufacturers recommend a maximum exposure time for a given film rate. This refers to the requirement of high mA factors (high-capacity generators) in order to decrease exposure times for rapid serial changer use. Program selecting devices vary according to the manufacturer. Currently seen on the market are IBM punch cards, knob-selected programmers, and

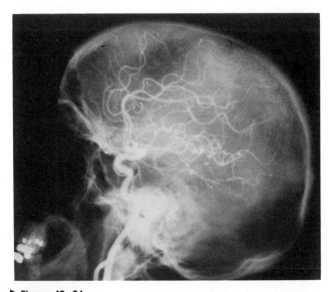

▶ Figure 10–21

Lateral view of the anterior cerebral circulation in the arterial phase.

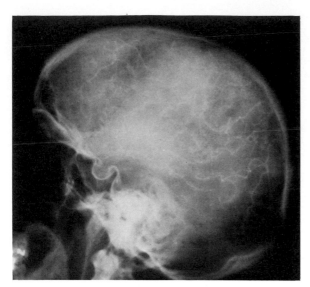

► **Figure 10–22**
Lateral view of the anterior cerebral circulation in the capillary phase.

► **Table 10–6**
RAPID SERIAL FILM CHANGER

Standard Features	Optional Features
Changer and mounting stand	Programmer
Supply magazine	Automatic shut-off
Receiving magazine	Crossed grids
Program selector	Microprocessor
Manual knife	Increased memory
Pressure plate	C-arm attachment
Intensifying screens	
Grid	

matic injectors are available for purchase. These injectors have many standard features as well as optional components. However, in most cases, both the serial changer and contrast medium injector are arranged to function synchronously with the programming device (Figs. 10–24 and 10–25). Table 10–7 lists the standard and optional features for an automatic contrast medium injector.

digital-selected, keyboard-operated program storage systems.

Automatic Contrast Medium Injector

The automatic injector is designed to deliver a predetermined quantity of contrast medium under pressure into the cerebral circulation. The amount of contrast medium delivered per unit of time is referred to as *flow rate* or *delivery rate*. As with serial changers, several types of electromechanical auto-

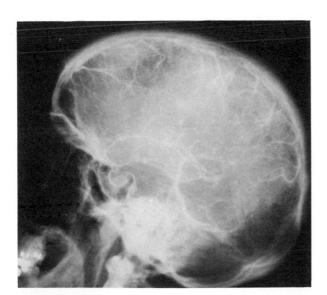

► **Figure 10–23**
Lateral view of the anterior cerebral circulation in the venous phase.

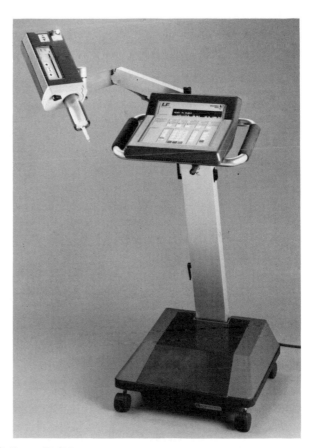

► **Figure 10–24**
An Angiomat 6000 contrast medium injector. (Courtesy of Liebel-Flarsheim Co., Cincinnati, OH.)

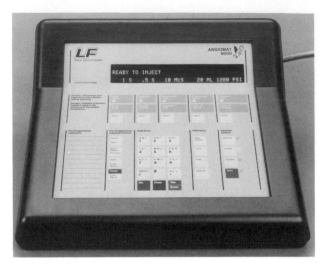

▶ **Figure 10–25**

An Angiomat 6000 contrast medium injector, programming console (Courtesy of Liebel-Flarsheim Co., Cincinnati, OH.)

Needles, Guidewires, and Catheters

Following selection of the arterial puncture site, the area is shaved and prepared, and a sterile barrier is set around the site. The technique generally used for selective cerebral angiography was described by Seldinger in 1953. Widely used today are the femoral, axillary, and brachial arteries and occasionally the direct-stick/puncture of carotid method (Fig. 10–26).

The choice of needle, guidewire, and catheter system usually depends on the individual neuroradiologist's experience and preference as well as on the condition of the patient's vascular system. The neuroradiologist's or radiologist's selection should be dictated by the system that produces a diagnostic angiogram while minimizing complications during the procedure.

The focus of catheterization techniques during the last 20 years is that "smaller is better." Whereas early angiographers used 15-gauge needles, 0.052″ guidewires and No. 8 French catheters, current philosophy dictates 18-gauge needles, 0.038″ guidewires, and catheters in the range from No. 4 to 7 French in outer diameter (Fig. 10–27).

The measurements used in catheterization equip-

▶ **Table 10–7**

FEATURES FOR AUTOMATIC CONTRAST MEDIUM INJECTOR

Standard Features	Optional Features
Control panel	Electrocardiogram triggering device
Syringe	Strip chart recorders
Heating device	Oscilloscope monitors
High-pressure mechanism	Detachable injector head
	Double-syringe assembly
	Safety devices

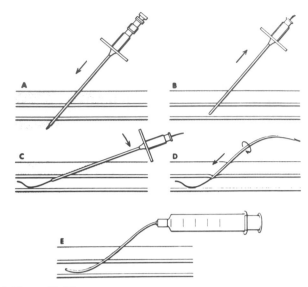

▶ **Figure 10–26**

Application of the Seldinger technique of arterial puncture. A, Puncture of both walls of the vessel. B, Retraction of the tip of the cannula into the arterial lumen after withdrawal of the needle insert. C, Passage of the guidewire through the cannula into the artery. D, Passage of the smoothly tapered catheter tip over the guidewire into the artery; gentle rotation of the catheter facilitates the entry. E, The catheter is in the lumen of the artery after the guidewire is withdrawn. (From Curry JL and Howland WJ: Arteriography. Philadelphia, WB Saunders, 1966.)

ment can be confusing to the apprentice angiographer or student technologist. Needle sizes are measured by *gauge,* guidewire sizes are indicated as a decimal in thousandths of an inch, and catheters are classified by the *French Catheter Scale* in their outer diameter. These individual systems must be compatible, result-

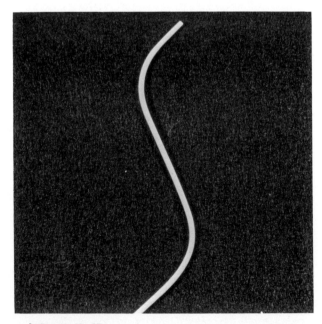

▶ **Figure 10–27**

A Simmons selective cerebral angiographic catheter.

ing in a smooth fit between the needle and the guidewire and between the guidewire and the catheters (Fig. 10–28).

Needles. There are several generally accepted needle systems used for the Seldinger technique. For children a thin-walled 19- or 21-gauge is utilized, and for adults a thin-walled 18-gauge needle is used. These thin-walled needles result in a smaller needle puncture and still allow the use of the same diameter of guidewire. Angiographic needles can vary and are generally classified as Amplatz, Potts-Cournand, Seldinger, and pediatric (Fig. 10–29). A 19-gauge butterfly needle will accept a 0.025″ guidewire.

Guidewires. The guidewire simply does what its name implies, it *guides* the catheter as the catheter traverses through the skin (tissue) at the injection site, through the arterial wall into the artery lumen. It also provides a guide or path to follow through often tortuous and plaque-laden arteries. Pediatric guidewires are often 125 cm in length, and adult guidewires are at least 145 cm in length.

Guidewires can be classified also according to the shape of the tip, from a straight end to those with a "J" configuration (Fig. 10–30). The J tip is measured by the radius of the tip and is in millimeters. Commonly used J tips are as follows: 1.5, 3.0, 7.5, and 15 mm. These guidewires are manufactured with a "fixed" or "movable" core. This design serves to increase the flexibility of the J tip. The selection or exchange of a guidewire is often dictated by its ease of passage through an artery. The angiographer closely observes the passage of the guidewire on the fluoroscopic television monitor. The J-shaped guidewire that encounters an atheromatous plaque on the intimal wall will gently bounce off the atheroma, and the physician can easily manipulate the wire so as to

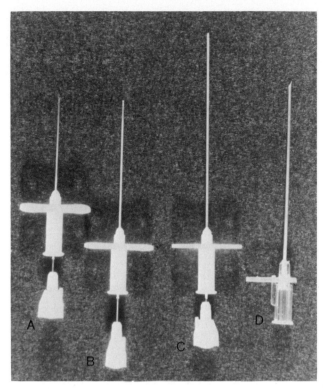

▶ **Figure 10–29**

Examples of common angiographic needles: *A,* pediatric; *B,* Potts-Cournand; *C,* Amplatz; *D,* Seldinger sidewall.

negotiate stenotic or tortuous vascular pathways. *Teflon-coated* wires are widely used in reducing both friction and the formation of an adhering thrombus.

Catheters. The catheters commonly used for selective cerebral arteriography are generally termed *multiple-curved* or *shaped catheters.* Catheter vendors often identify the specific type of curves such as

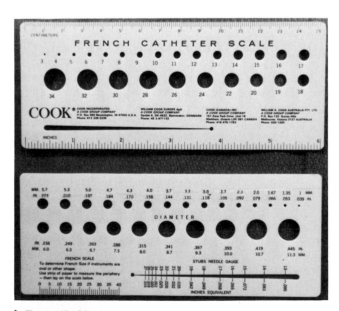

▶ **Figure 10–28**

A French Catheter Scale Card. (Courtesy of Cook Inc., Bloomington, IN.)

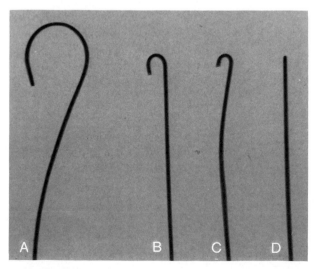

▶ **Figure 10–30**

Examples of angiographic guidewires. *A,* J curve with large radius. *B* and *C,* J curves with a tight radius. *D,* Straight guidewire.

cobra, headhunter, and sidewinder (Figs. 10–31 and 10–32).

An important factor in selective catheterization of the cerebral arteries is the outer diameter French size, compared with the inner diameter of the artery. The more a given catheter occludes a given artery, the higher is the probability of producing an intravascular thrombus.

Selective catheters have end holes only, with no side holes for better distribution and opacification of contrast material.

Angiographic technologists must always be aware of the potential hazards created by catheters, guide-wires, and needles due to their thrombogenicity. Although the creation of emboli is always a possibility, clot formation is most common with procedures that are lengthy. Procedures that extend for more than a 2-hour time period substantially increase the risk of clot production. The use of systemic heparinization to provide for the continuous flow of anticlotting agents in the vascular system throughout the procedure is recommended. An infusion pump–pressurized system of 1/2000 units of heparin to 500 ml of solution (5% dextrose and water or normal saline solution) works well. This method of systemic heparinization provides for a continuous flow of solution that will irrigate the vascular pathways and minimize the production of blood clots and potential emboli. Another method is intermittent heparinization. This method requires a hand injection every 2 minutes without interruption during the entire procedure.

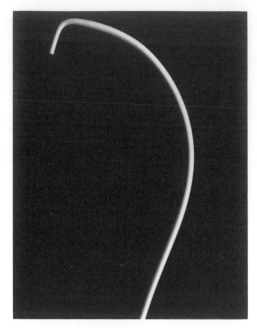

► Figure 10–32
A cobra III catheter.

Film-Screen Combinations

Film-screen combinations vary depending on the types of procedures dedicated to a given vascular laboratory. From my experience, it is possible to "marry" a film-screen system to provide the fine detail needed in cerebral angiography and also to provide the optimum subject contrast latitude and higher kilovolts peak (kVp) levels used in abdominal aortography. For cerebral angiography, a short-scale (high-contrast, high-mA, low-kVp) image is realized when a desirably fast film-screen combination is employed.

A slower-speed system of course results in better resolution, but it requires a higher kVp level, thus resulting in a longer scale of contrast (low-contrast, low-mA, high-kVp) image that is usually suboptimal. We recommend a relative film-screen combination of between 600 and 850 film-screen speed. The film-screen combination should provide the best possible diagnostic radiograph with the lowest possible radiation exposure to the patient.

► RADIOGRAPHIC TECHNIQUE

Kilovoltage determines the overall contrast on an image. The ideal range for cerebral angiography is 65 to 70 kVp. This provides adequate penetration for most projections and allows for a diagnostic scale of subject contrast and latitude within the K level of absorption for iodinated contrast.

Milliampere-seconds (mAs) determine the density of the image. Radiographic density is the overall "blackness" of a radiograph. Density is the amount

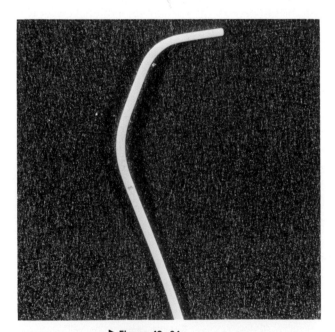

► Figure 10–31
A headhunter catheter.

of silver halide crystal that is exposed within the latent image and that is reduced (by development) to "black metallic silver." Density is also influenced by kilovoltage, because kilovoltage levels determine the amount of radiation that reaches the film. Scatter is fog. Scatter absorbed by the radiograph decreases the contrast and reduces film quality. As a general rule, the highest current (in mA) and shortest exposure time (in seconds) should be employed. The maximum exposure time should not be greater than 0.1 second (100 msec) in order to minimize patient and vessel motion artifacts.

► PROCEDURAL CONSIDERATIONS

Indications for Transcatheter Cerebral Angiography

1. Diagnosis of vascular occlusive disease (atherosclerosis), thrombosis, emboli, aneurysms, AVM, and fistulas
2. Diagnosis and localization of vascular tumors
3. Preoperative mapping of vascular anatomy (e.g., tumor resection and peripheral revascularization procedures)
4. Performance of vascular therapeutic interventional procedures (e.g., embolization, angioplasty, drug infusion)
5. Diagnosis and treatment of vascular complications of disease and surgery
6. Anatomic presentation of the arterial, capillary, and venous systems (vascular mapping)

Advantages of the Transcatheter Method

1. All brachiocephalic vessels including the arch can be examined via a single percutaneous catheter puncture.
2. The arterial puncture is at a site where local complications tend to be less urgent and more easily managed.

Direct Puncture Method

The direct puncture method has both advantages and disadvantages in comparison with the transcatheter method utilizing the Seldinger technique.

1. Bilateral examinations require puncture of both the right and left common carotid arteries.
2. Direct puncture of the common carotid and extension, pressure, and manipulation of the neck can produce often unpleasant and frightening experiences for the patient. General anesthesia, administered and monitored by an anesthesiologist, is often used with the direct puncture method.
3. The puncture is at a site where any local compli-

cations that may occur can become life threatening (e.g., spasm, intimal dissection/injection, hematoma, contrast medium extravasation, emboli, dislodgment of plaque, and puncture of the wrong vessel).
4. Selective injections are difficult.

► CONTRAST MEDIUM SELECTION

Evaluation of the patient's clinical history most often helps to determine the selection of a contrast agent for a cerebral angiogram. According to the current literature, the type of contrast medium for healthy patients should not necessarily be dependent on whether it is ionic or nonionic. This selection has very little influence on morbidity in a healthy patient. Low osmolar contrast agents do not eliminate adverse reactions, but they do cause less discomfort.

The ideal contrast material has the lowest iodine concentration yet provides adequate opacification on the radiograph and has the least osmolar load.

When selecting a contrast agent, radiologists often pay particular attention to two commonly used chemicals in the agent's cation contrast formulation: (1) *Citrates* can result in increased calcium binding and thus increase the risk of myocardial depression and increase chances of arrhythmias, and (2) *sodium salts* increase peripheral discomfort and are not well tolerated by the brain. The radiologist's selection is therefore dictated by viscosity, iodine content, and potential toxicity as well as by catheter length and diameter.

► SUBTRACTION TECHNIQUE

Subtraction is often used in cerebral angiography to better define and improve vessel visualization. This technique is especially helpful when areas of overlying dense bony structures obscure fine vascular detail. It is also readily used in pathologic findings of vascular tumors and intracerebral hemorrhage.

The critical requirement in subtraction technique is that there is absolutely no patient motion. Patient motion can result in the creation of artifactual lesions and the loss and blurring of important pathology.

Subtraction parameters would include the fastest possible exposure factors, optimal well-penetrated radiographic technique, and patient head restraints when needed. Film technique should provide for a scout or base film at the beginning of the serial run. This can be attained by delaying the injection via the injector itself or by allowing for a delay on the film programmer (Figs. 10–33 and 10–34).

► POSITIONING AND FILMING PROTOCOL

The first step in cerebral angiography is to take a preliminary or scout film in both projections (AP and

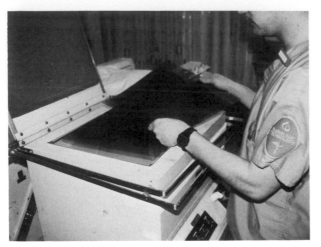

▶ **Figure 10–33**

The technologist is utilizing a Dupont subtraction unit. He is preparing to superimpose the scout film and the mask film.

Anteroposterior (Semiaxial) Projection

The AP projection provides an image in which the roofs of the orbits (supraorbital ridges) are superimposed over the roofs of the petrous pyramids (pars petrosa). From the scout film, positioning can be adjusted in one of two ways. The x-ray tube in its caudal angulation can be increased or decreased. The tube angle is usually determined by the patient's body habitus. Patients who are lying in the supine position and who are of the sthenic, hyposthenic, or asthenic habitai can comfortably be adjusted so that the orbitomeatal line (OML) of the skull is perpendicular to the horizontal plane of the film changer. Patients who are hypersthenic have less mobility of the head and neck; thus, the infraorbital meatal line (IOML) is the positioning base line of choice. If a technologist desires to build up the head (with an angled sponge) to line up a particular positioning baseline, he or she must be aware that he or she is creating an increase in the object-image-receptor distance (OIRD) and a subsequent increase in part magnification and a loss of the recorded detail. Another consideration is patient comfort. If the patient is not comfortable and secure, there is likely to be movement and subsequent motion on the finished radiograph. The angled sponges can provide a reasonable OIRD while providing patient comfort. In addition, the use of sponges provides elevation of the head for the lateral projection. Generally, these types of decisions are made on a patient-by-patient basis (Fig. 10–35).

A caudal tube angulation of 15 to 20 degrees is used to visualize the carotids during a cerebral arteriogram. The central ray enters the skull just superior to the glabella. The head should be symmetric in its position with the median sagittal plane, parallel to the changer grid and the tube centering light. If keyhole collimation is being utilized (Figs. 10–36 and 10–37),

lateral). This serves several purposes and always results in a better angiographic study and often reduces the need for repeat exposure and injection caused by technical errors.

The scout film allows the technologist and radiologist to establish proper radiographic positioning and also to define optimal film and subject contrast. The body habitus varies from one patient to another and influences positioning and imaging procedures. The proper subject contrast must be produced for each patient, regardless of differing anatomic characteristics.

The two standard projections utilized in cerebral angiography or carotid arteriography are the AP (semiaxial) and lateral projections.

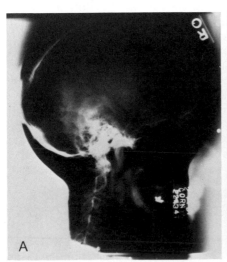

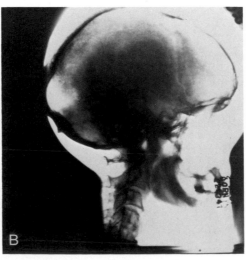

▶ **Figure 10–34**

Examples of an angio film (A) and a final subtraction print (B). Notice the result of the leaded keyhole collimation devices.

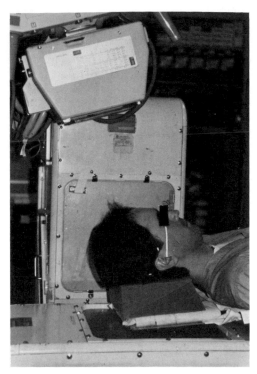

▶ **Figure 10–35**
Routine anteroposterior axial projection cerebral angiogram.

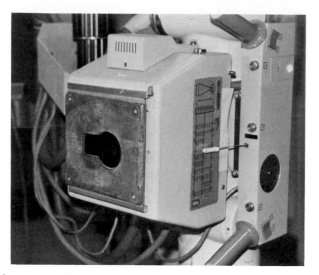

▶ **Figure 10–37**
A leaded keyhole collimation device fits into the provided slot on the lower end of the collimator.

Lateral View

For the lateral view, in a carotid arteriogram the median sagittal plane is parallel to the lateral changer. The central ray passes horizontally through the head to a point just superior and anterior to the external auditory meatus for cerebral arteriography. For vertebral arteriography, the central ray is directed to a point 3 cm posterior of the external auditory meatus. It should be noted that the radiographic technique (exposure) may have to be increased in order to better portray the vertebrobasilar system through the thick petrous and mastoid areas of the skull (Fig. 10–38).

We routinely increase the lateral source-image distance (SID) to 50″ to provide for a better projection of the cerebral and carotid arteries on the lateral image.

the head will simply need to be positioned in the light field projected on the changer field surfaces. I cannot emphasize enough the use of proper coning during cerebral angiography to reduce scatter and to improve angiographic technique.

If the vertebrobasilar circulation is of interest, the caudal tube angulation is increased from 25 to 30 degrees. The head and the chin can also be tucked in, in order to throw the posterior vasculature above the foramen magnum. The vertebral projection often requires additional radiographic exposure because the position is different from the routine 15-degree scout view. The central ray enters at the bregma (where the frontal bone meets both parietal bones).

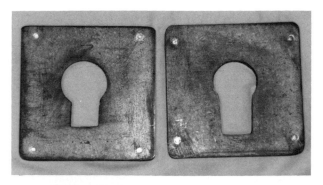

▶ **Figure 10–36**
Two configurations of keyhole collimation.

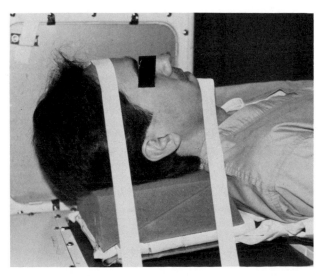

▶ **Figure 10–38**
A routine lateral projection cerebral angiogram.

This is especially helpful in patients of hypersthenic habitus. The increase of 10″ in SID does not affect radiographic technique in a substantial manner but does visualize more vasculature, including the carotid bifurcation on the angiogram (if the shoulders are depressed).

Special Positions and Projections

In some cases, it may be necessary to use alternative positioning to demonstrate specific areas and pathology of interest. This may often apply to vessels that appear tortuous or superimposed in the AP (semiaxial) position.

Oblique Supraorbital Position

The oblique supraorbital position is used for demonstrating pathology involving the anterior communicating artery, especially aneurysms. In this position, the patient's head is rotated 30 degrees *away* from the side being injected. The central ray is directed 15 to 20 degrees caudal and enters just superior to the supraorbital margin (Fig. 10–39).

Straight and Oblique Intraorbital Positions

In these positions the middle cerebral artery and its branches are projected into the center of the bony orbit. In the straight intraorbital position, the head is straight in a true AP position or can be rotated slightly (5 to 10 degrees) toward the injected side. The central ray is directed through the middle of the orbit.

The oblique intraorbital position shows both the anterior communicating artery and the middle cerebral artery. The head is rotated 30 degrees away from

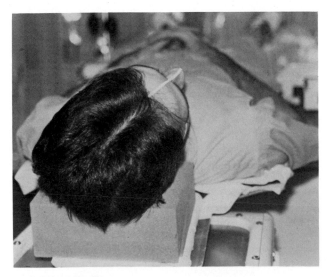

▶ **Figure 10–39**

An oblique supraorbital position of the patient's head.

the side being injected. The central ray is directed perpendicular through the middle of the orbit or is angled 5 degrees cephalad.

If imaging the neck or cervical portion of the carotid artery is desired, additional positioning requirements may be needed. In AP and lateral projections, the central ray should be directed to the bifurcation area, C3 to C5. The skull can be rotated 15 to 20 degrees away from the injected side. This rotation reduces the chance of superimposition of the mandible over the common carotid artery and bifurcation.

▶ PATHOLOGY

There are several diseases and conditions involving the cerebrovascular system that are imaged and diagnosed via carotid arteriography, cerebral angiography, and vertebral angiography.

Atherosclerosis is probably the leading illness that results in symptomatic disease. As the disease progresses, the lumen of the carotid artery becomes narrow, thus resulting in diminished blood flow to the brain. The carotid bifurcation is the location where the intima is most likely to be narrowed. This disease, affecting mostly persons older than 50 years of age, could be asymptomatic or could result in a CVA or stroke. Affected individuals experience "little strokes" or *transient ischemic attacks* (TIAs). Most TIAs produce sensory neurologic symptoms that last for only a few minutes, and the effects are completely resolved within 24 hours.

A *reversible ischemic neurologic deficit* (RIND) usually affects the patient for 24 to 48 hours before it resolves. The patient may also experience an event in which a "curtain" or "shade" seems to cover one or both eyes for a few moments. This is called *amaurosis fugax*. However, other incidents may also occur. Autopsies conducted on persons succumbing to a fatal stroke have revealed the presence of multiple infarcts of the brain, indicating that most persons have had numerous "little strokes" over a period of years. A high percentage of persons with this history will suffer a fatal CVA. Persons who are symptomatic are often examined by the duplex scanning technique or Doppler method prior to angiography. Sounds created by stenotic blood vessels and the turbulent blood flow in them are thus made audible. Turbulent blood flow can also be detected when a stethoscope is placed at or near the carotid bifurcation. These audible sounds are called *bruits*. Atherosclerotic disease is often bilateral, and many forms of treatment are available. Endarterectomy is a procedure that essentially scrapes out plaque from the carotid system, thus permitting the resumption of reasonable blood flow. Figures 10–40 and 10–41 demonstrate a man with bilateral carotid atherosclerotic disease. This examination utilized digital subtraction angiography and revealed total occlusion of the right internal carotid artery (RICA) and a 95% stenosis of the left internal carotid artery (LICA).

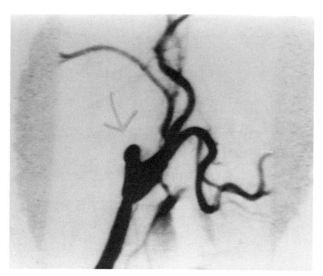

▶ Figure 10–40

Total occlusion of the right internal carotid artery.

An *aneurysm* is described as a sac formed by the localized dilatation of the wall of an artery, vein, or heart. Although aneurysms are most commonly found in the distal aorta, they are frequently found as individual or multiple lesions within the brain. Arteries have three distinct layers or coverings. If a person is born with a congenital weakness of a wall of an artery, an aneurysm may develop. However, some cerebral hemorrhages occur simply by vessel rupture where there is a defect or weakness in the vessel wall. This can occur with normal blood flow. With a congenital aneurysm, the aneurysm involves all layers of the vessel wall. All aneurysms occurring with other etiologies are considered to be false or pseudoaneurysms. Conditions such as hypertension, infection, dissection, and AVM are examples of aneurysms that are

considered to be false. When a false aneurysm occurs, only two walls of the vessel are involved. Regardless of the cause, most cerebral aneurysms can prove fatal. Figures 10–42 and 10–43 demonstrate a cerebral angiogram of a 58-year-old woman who came to the hospital emergency room with a severe headache. AP and lateral projections revealed the presence of a large aneurysm of the right middle cerebral artery.

Figures 10–44 and 10–45 demonstrate a cerebral angiogram of a 62-year-old man with a long history of hypertension and diabetes. The angiogram revealed a giant "leaking" aneurysm of the anterior cerebral artery. The patient suffered convulsions shortly after the angiogram was completed. The patient lapsed into a coma and died only a few moments later.

Figures 10–46, 10–47, 10–48, 10–49, and 10–50 depict a cerebral angiogram of a 57-year-old man who had a long history of exacerbating headaches. Standard lateral views of the anterior cerebral circulation are shown, and the presence of a huge aneurysm is revealed at the origin of the midcerebral artery.

Figures 10–51 and 10–52 represent a very unusual patient history and pathologic finding. A 47-year-old stable worker was kicked in the neck by a horse 6 years previously. The patient discovered a swelling in the right side of his neck, with the progressive enlargement of what was thought to be a carotid pseudoaneurysm. Selective catheterization of the carotid artery was performed. The final diagnosis was a pseudoaneurysm of the internal jugular vein.

A 27-year-old man was involved in an automobile accident in which he sustained a depressed fracture of

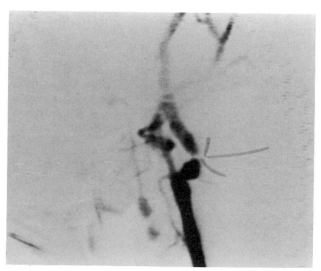

▶ Figure 10–41

Stenosis of 95% of the left internal carotid artery of the same patient as in Figure 10–40.

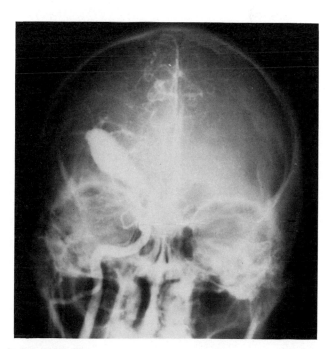

▶ Figure 10–42

Anteroposterior axial projection revealing a giant aneurysm of the right middle cerebral artery in a 58-year-old woman.

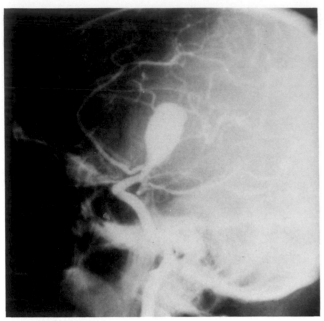

▶ **Figure 10–43**
Lateral view of a giant aneurysm of the right middle cerebral artery in the same patient as in Figure 10–42.

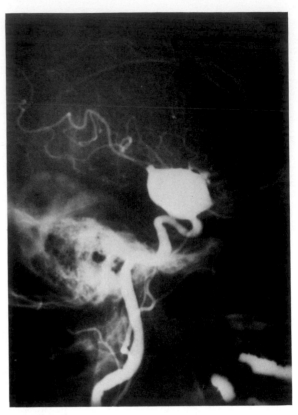

▶ **Figure 10–45**
Lateral view of a huge aneurysm of the left middle cerebral artery in the same patient as in Figure 10–44.

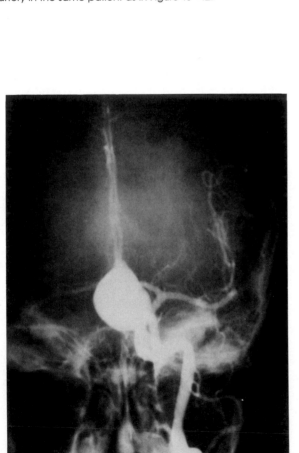

▶ **Figure 10–44**
Anteroposterior axial projection revealing a huge aneurysm of the left middle cerebral artery in a 62-year-old man.

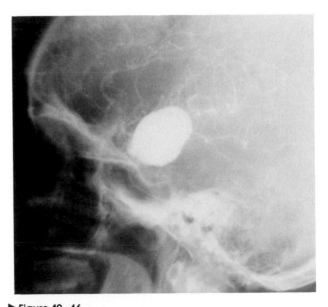

▶ **Figure 10–46**
Right lateral view of a large leaking aneurysm at the origin of the right middle cerebral artery in a 57-year-old man.

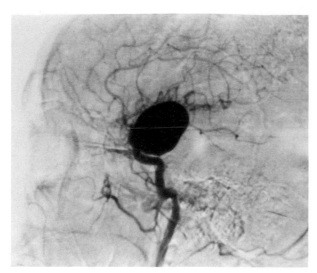

▶ **Figure 10–47**
Right lateral subtraction image of the same patient as in
Figure 10–46.

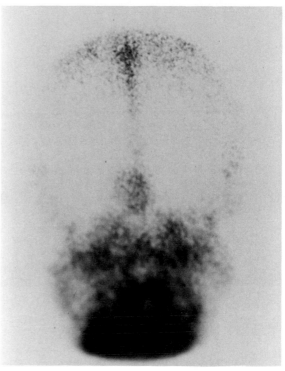

▶ **Figure 10–49**
A radioisotope scan of the brain of the same patient as in
Figure 10–46.

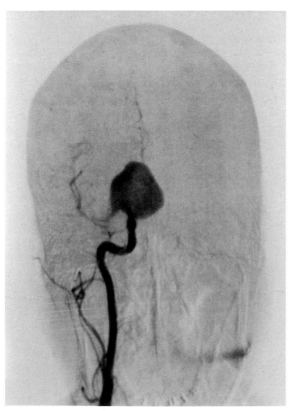

▶ **Figure 10–48**
Anteroposterior subtraction image of the same patient as in
Figure 10–46.

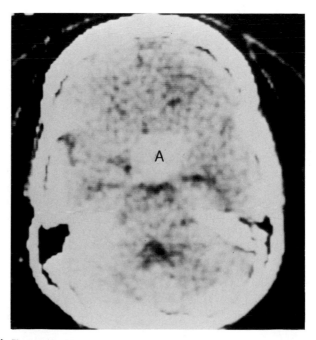

▶ **Figure 10–50**
Computed tomography scan of the brain of the same patient
as in Figure 10–46.

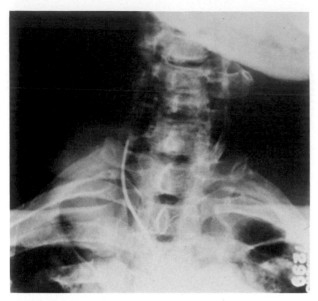

▶ **Figure 10–51**

A man who was kicked in the right side of the neck by a horse 6 years before. A soft tissue mass was visualized.

the occipital bone. After 48 hours of hospitalized observation, the patient was released without any further incident. Two weeks later, the patient was examined at the emergency room because of constant, worsening headaches. Bilateral cerebral angiography was performed. The subtraction mask film is shown in Figure 10–53. This film clearly delineates the depressed fracture fragment in the occipital region. Figure 10–54 is a lateral view in venous circulation that reveals occlusion of blood flow due to compression of

the fracture fragment upon the superior sagittal sinus. The situation was corrected surgically by reducing the fracture and by relieving the pressure on the sagittal sinus.

Subdural hematoma occurs beneath the dura mater, between the tough casing and the more delicate arachnoid membrane. This injury occurs when the skull bluntly strikes an immovable object, such as occurs in automobile accidents. Fractures of the skull are most often absent in the presence of a subdural hematoma. The hematoma accumulates after a bridging vein is torn at the point where the vessel leaves the subdural space to enter the dura. The leaking of blood can be acute as well as chronic. Most are found in the temporoparietal region and can occur bilaterally. Subdural hematomas are associated with a shift of midline brain structures, which can be identified on CT scans as well as with angiography. Figures 10–55 and 10–56 demonstrate a left temporoparietal subdural hematoma and midline shift on AP cerebral angiogram and subtraction films. Figure 10–57 is an unenhanced CT head scan demonstrating a midline shift and displacement of lateral ventricles.

AVMs are usually *congenital dysplasias*. When present at birth, they are difficult lesions to correct. These malformations develop early in embryonic development, perhaps as early as between the fifth and 16th day of gestation. The malformation usually involves one or more parts of a vessel, usually an artery. In many cases, the blood flow is from the artery directly to the vein and bypasses capillary circulation. However, the tangled webb of vessels that represent the lesion can involve the artery, capillary, or vein. Figures 10–58, 10–59, and 10–60 demonstrate an arteriovenous fistula or AVM in a 2-week-old male infant who presented signs of neurologic dysfunction at birth. This infant has a lesion that was being fed by the MCA. An arteriovenous fistula is frequently pro-

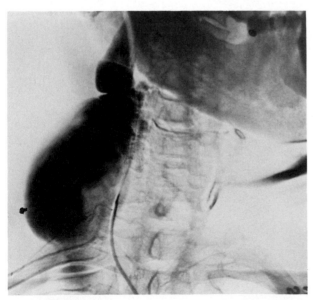

▶ **Figure 10–52**

Anteroposterior projection—subtracted image of an aneurysm of the internal jugular vein in the same patient as in Figure 10–51.

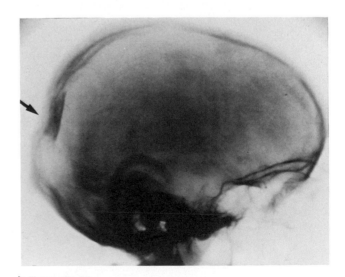

▶ **Figure 10–53**

A left lateral subtraction mask film of a man who sustained a depressed skull fracture (*arrow*) in an automobile accident.

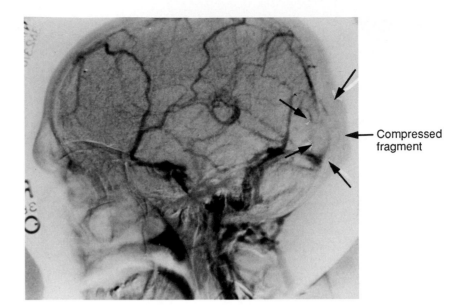

Compressed
fragment

► **Figure 10–54**

A right lateral subtracted venous phase
cerebral arteriogram revealing an
occlusion of the superior sagittal sinus
by a compressed fractured fragment
found in the same patient as in Figure
10–53.

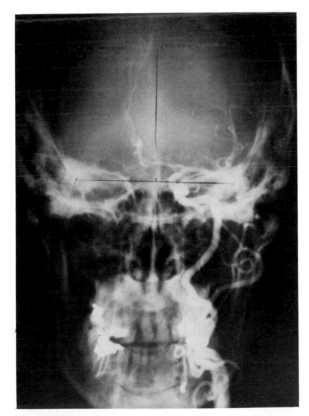

► **Figure 10–55**

This man sustained a head injury in an automobile accident.
An anteroposterior axial projection reveals a subdural
hematoma in the left parietal region with a midline shift of
the anterior cerebral artery to the right.

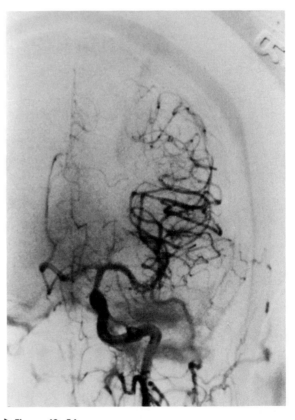

► **Figure 10–56**

Subtracted image of the same patient as in Figure 10–55.

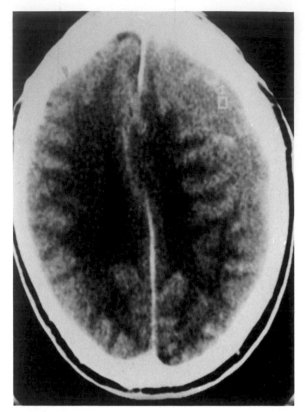

▶ **Figure 10–57**

This computed tomography scan reveals a midline shift and ventricular compression. This is the same patient as in Figure 10–55.

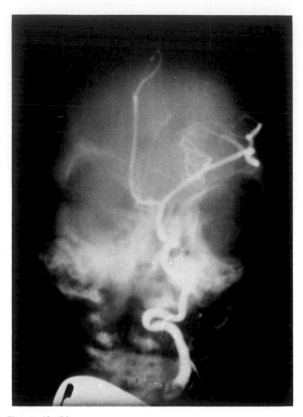

▶ **Figure 10–58**

An anteroposterior projection of a 2-week-old male infant who was born with an arteriovenous malformation involving the left middle cerebral artery. This is the early arterial phase.

duced as a secondary complication to a head injury, especially when there is a direct blow to the frontal region of the skull. This fistula is the result of a disruption of the internal carotid artery where it passes through the lamina of the cavernous sinuses. Once the arteriovenous fistula has been formed, the veins in this area become engorged with arterial blood. Figures 10–61 and 10–62 are AP and right lateral projections of an arteriovenous fistula involving the MCA that was produced when this adult male was involved in an automobile accident and struck the frontal region of his skull on the steering wheel. This fistula was produced as a secondary result of the primary trauma.

A CVA or stroke is the third leading cause of death, exceeded only by heart disease and cancer. *Thrombosis, embolism,* and *hemorrhage* are the three leading causes of a stroke. The cerebral embolism is a moving clot and is the second leading cause of stroke. Figure 10–63 is a lateral view of a cerebral angiogram. A filling defect is noted in the internal carotid artery (ICA) just below the birfurcation and subsequent reduction in blood flow to the MCA. The MCA is a direct continuation of the ICA; thus, lesions present just proximal to the bifurcation usually affect the flow into the MCA.

Cerebral angiography is useful in determining the location and relationship of the vascular blood supply to any lesion, especially a tumor. Most brain tumors

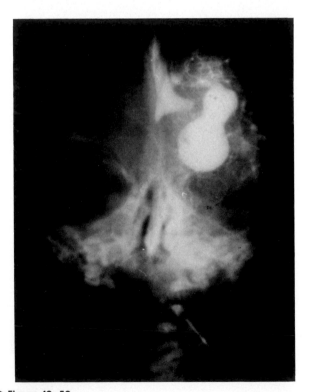

▶ **Figure 10–59**

An anteroposterior projection of the same patient as in Figure 10–58. This later arterial phase reveals advanced filling of the arteriovenous malformation.

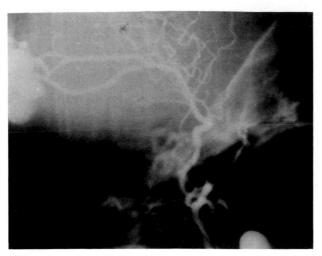

▶ **Figure 10–60**

A left lateral view of the same patient as in Figure 10–58. This reveals an excellent demonstration of the left middle cerebral artery feeding malformation.

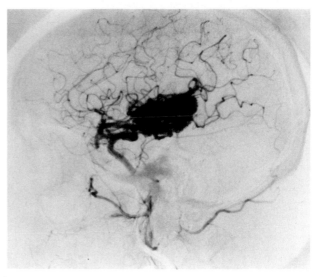

▶ **Figure 10–62**

A right lateral view of a fistulous formation involving the middle cerebral artery. The same patient is shown as in Figure 10–61.

have the same density as normal brain tissue (exceptions include some *craniopharyngiomas* found in the suprasellar region and most *meningiomas*, which are usually calcified) and as a result are not visible on plain skull radiographs or angiograms. Angiography

is useful in determining vessel displacement and whether the tumor contains any vascular components or is being fed by an anomalous vessel. Figure 10–64 demonstrates an AP cerebral angiogram with a large, dense, calcified tumor appearing over the left orbit. In most patients, meningiomas are found on the surface of the dura mater. Thus, they are very superficial in addition to being benign. Figure 10–65 demonstrates a lateral view, revealing a large calcified meningioma over the left parieto-occipital region. Figure 10–66 shows a very dense tumor that is described as a calcified meningioma. Meningiomas can also be of vascular origin. The subtraction technique has proved to discriminate these lesions better than routine contrast-enhanced angiography. With the subtraction

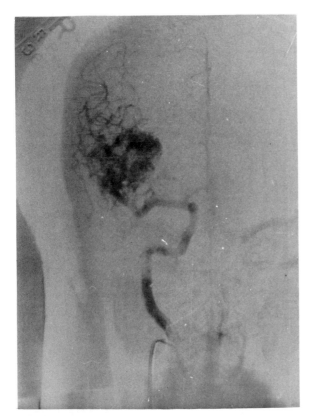

▶ **Figure 10–61**

An anteroposterior axial projection of a cerebral angiogram, reveals an arteriovenous fistula of the middle cerebral artery. The patient was injured in an automobile accident. A tangle of vessels is seen in the right temporoparietal region.

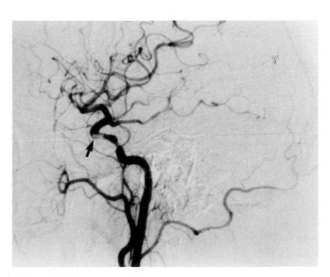

▶ **Figure 10–63**

A cerebral embolism of the right internal carotid artery (*arrow*).

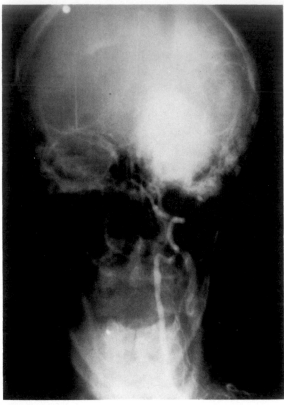

▸ **Figure 10–64**

Anteroposterior axial projection of a cerebral angiogram. A large calcified meningioma is seen over the left orbitofrontal region in this projection.

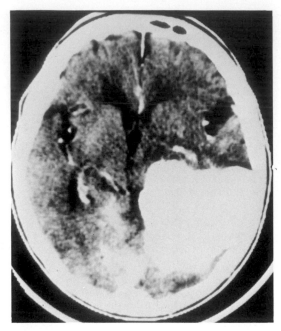

▸ **Figure 10–66**

This computed tomography scan verifies the presence of a calcified meningioma. The same patient is shown in Figures 10–64 and 10–65.

technique, a meningioma may be described as a "tumor blush" or dark-appearing lesion, as seen on the following angiogram.

Figure 10–67 shows a subtracted AP projection demonstrating a tumor blush in the right parietal re-

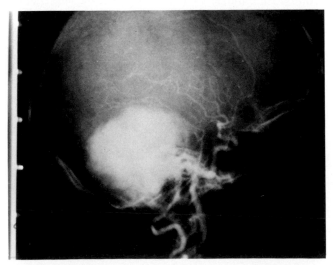

▸ **Figure 10–65**

This lateral projection identifies a calcified meningioma in the left temporo-occipital region. The same patient is shown in Figure 10–64.

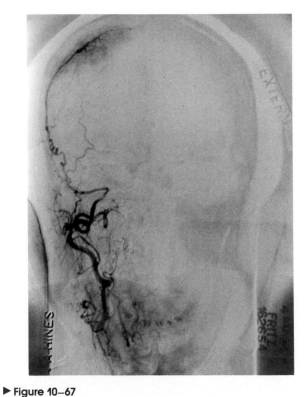

▸ **Figure 10–67**

Anteroposterior axial subtraction cerebral angiogram of a 64-year-old man. A tumor blush is observed with anomalous communication of the middle cerebral artery to the vascular meningioma.

gion. This vascular meningioma appears to be fed by an anomalous vessel arising off the MCA. Figure 10–68 presents a right lateral view of the meningioma with an excellent demonstration of the primary vessel feeding the tumor. Figure 10–69 presents a coned-down, magnified view of the meningioma and its vascular components. Figure 10–70 gives a different demonstration of the lesion as seen on lateral view (angiogram), venous phase. The meningioma and its vascular remnants appear to be located superficially, on the outside of the brain rather than within the brain itself.

Cavernous hemangiomas are benign congenital tumors that consist of a network of newly formed blood vessels on or near the surface of the skin. The term *cavernous* pertains to hollow spaces. These tumors should be treated as soon as possible. The lesions have a tendency to grow, and there is the possibility of severe hemorrhage if the lesion is injured and starts to bleed. Treatment is by irradiation, injection of a sclerosing agent, or surgery. Figure 10–71 is an AP coned-down, soft tissue projection of the occipital region of the skull. Figure 10–72 is a plain right lateral view of the skull revealing a posteroinferior occipital scalp swelling (*straight arrow*) and an adjacent cavernous hemangioma (*curved arrow*).

Figure 10–73 is an angiographic lateral view revealing the network of twisting anomalous vessels. Note that primary anomalous filling is within the scalp. The expanded hemangioma is located somewhat superiorly in the occipital region.

One may occasionally see an uncommon tumor. A *chemodectoma* is any tumor of the chemoreceptor system. The *carotid body tumor* is a prime example. The chemoreceptor system involves cells or organs that are adapted for stimulation by chemical substances and that are located outside the central nervous system. Chemoreceptors in the large arteries of

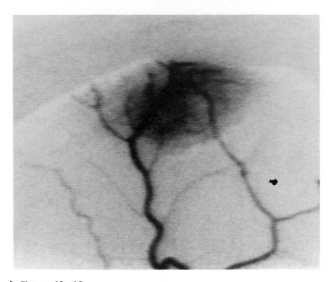

▶ **Figure 10–69**

A coned-down, magnified subtraction image of a vascular meningioma. The same patient is shown in Figure 10–67.

the thorax and neck are called carotid and aortic bodies. These receptors respond to changes in the oxygen, carbon dioxide, and hydrogen ion concentration in the blood. When the oxygen concentration falls below normal in the arterial blood, the chemoreceptors send impulses to stimulate the respiratory center (in the medulla oblongata) so that there will be an increase in alveolar ventilation and consequently an increase in the intake of oxygen by the lungs. Figure 10–74 is an AP axial (projection) carotid arteriogram of a male patient taken in response to the evidence of a visible mass on the right side of the neck. With the patient in the supine position, the head is turned to the left away from the affected side. A small area of in-

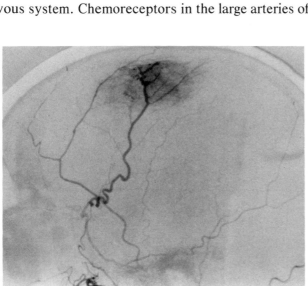

▶ **Figure 10–68**

A right lateral view more accurately describes an anomalous feeding of this vascular meningioma. The same patient is shown in Figure 10–67.

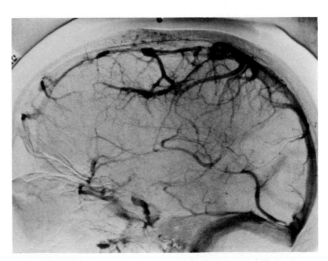

▶ **Figure 10–70**

Subtraction image of the venous phase, demonstrating the superficial nature of a meningioma with visibility of its vascular components. The same patient is shown in Figure 10–67.

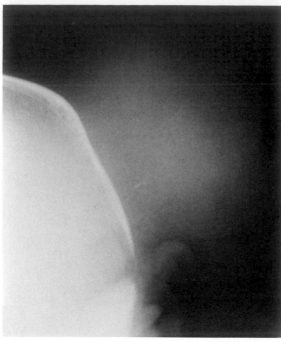

▶ **Figure 10–71**

An anteroposterior plain film of the skull with a tangential projection. A large soft tissue swelling is shown adjacent to the calvarium. This is a 6-day-old male infant with a congenital cavernous hemangioma.

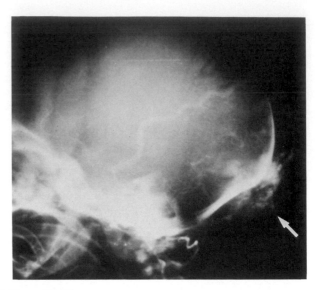

▶ **Figure 10–73**

This angiographic view reveals a network of twisting vessels in the soft tissues adjacent to the skull. The same patient is shown in Figure 10–71.

creased density is noted just above the carotid bifurcation on this subtraction print. The mass is extravascular. Figure 10–75 shows the patient in the same position as in Figure 10–74, but the dense mass appears much larger. In Figure 10–76, the mass is demonstrated in a right lateral perspective. Minimal opacification of the carotid system but increased density of the mass is still apparent on this subtracted image. The final image of this carotid body series presents the encircled lesion on a CT scan (Fig. 10–77).

Cerebral angiography, in addition to demonstrating abnormal vascularity, can illustrate variations of normal anatomy. These different or atypical anatomic variants must be distinguished from abnormal vasculature and physiology. The following study not only illustrates one type of normal variant but also demonstrates the advantages of subtraction imaging. Figure 10–78 shows a four-vessel arch study, presented with conventional contrast-enhanced angiography. Figure 10–79 shows a subtraction study and identifies the

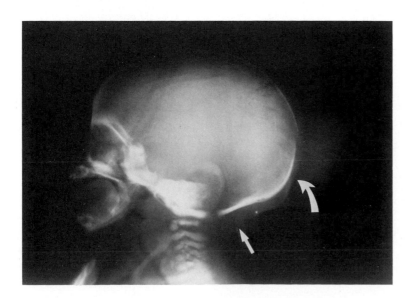

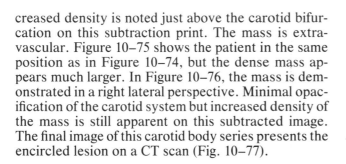

▶ **Figure 10–72**

This right lateral plain skull film shows a swelling of the soft tissues on the undersurface of the occipital bone (*straight arrow*) that is just inferior to the hemangioma (*curved arrow*). Some cortical destruction of the outer table of the occipital bone is also noted. The same patient is shown in Figure 10–71.

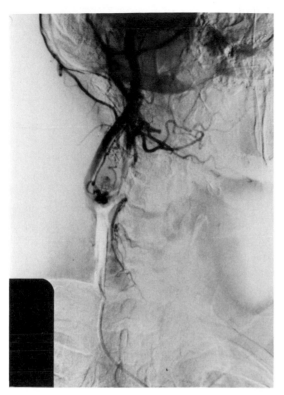

▶ **Figure 10–74**

An anteroposterior axial projection (subtraction) with the patient's head turned away from the side of the injection. A selective injection of the common carotid artery reveals an early image of an extravascular carotid body tumor containing vascular components.

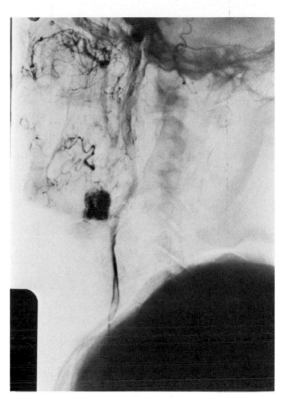

▶ **Figure 10–76**

A subtracted right lateral image with a carotid body tumor that is well visualized. The same patient is shown in Figure 10–74.

innominate or brachiocephalic artery arising off the left side of the aortic arch instead of its usual origin on the right side. The right subclavian artery arises independently off the right side of the arch. The most graphic aspect of this variant is the emergence of both

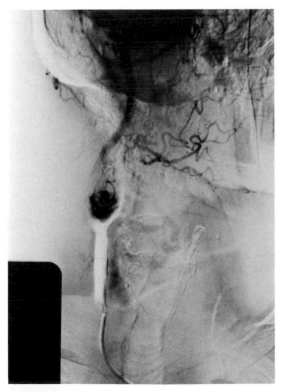

▶ **Figure 10–75**

Later vascular filling of a carotid body tumor is shown. The same patient is shown in Figure 10–74.

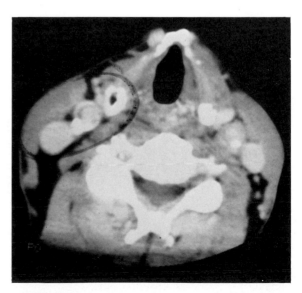

▶ **Figure 10–77**

A computed tomography scan showing the involved area of carotid body tumor, which is encircled. The same patient is shown in Figure 10–74.

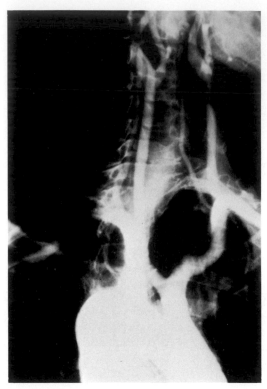

▶ **Figure 10–78**

An anteroposterior arch arteriogram reveals several vascular normal variants. The right subclavian artery originates directly off the right side of the aortic arch; the innominate artery originates off the left side of the arch; two common carotid arteries form a bifurcation off the innominate origin.

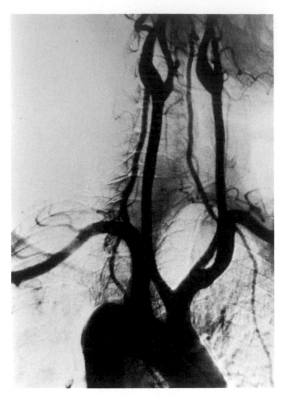

▶ **Figure 10–79**

Anatomic variants are greatly enhanced by the subtraction technique. The same patient is shown in Figure 10–78.

common carotids, arising as a bifurcation off the innominate artery. The subtraction print more clearly demonstrates this remarkable variation of normal carotid vasculature at both proximal and distal sites. It is not known whether this normal variant was of significance to the patient's clinical history and subsequent diagnosis.

▶ BIBLIOGRAPHY

Abrams HL: Angiography, 3rd ed. Boston, Little, Brown, 1983.

Curry TS, Dowdey JE, and Murray RC: Christensen's Introduction to the Physics of Diagnostic Radiology. Philadelphia, Lea & Febiger, 1984.

Johnsonrude IS, Jackson DS, and Dunnick NR: A Practical Approach to Angiography, 2nd ed. Boston, Little, Brown, 1989.

Kadir S: Diagnostic Angiography. Philadelphia, WB Saunders, 1986.

Kandarpa K: Handbook of Cardiovascular and Interventional Radiographic Procedures. Boston, Little, Brown, 1987.

Laudicina P: Applied Pathology for Radiographers. Philadelphia, WB Saunders, 1989.

Meschan I: Radiographic Positioning and Related Anatomy. Philadelphia, WB Saunders, 1978.

Newton TH and Potts DG: Radiology of the Skull and Brain, Vol 1, Books 1 and 2. St Louis, CV Mosby, 1971.

Thompson T: A Practical Approach to Modern X-Ray Equipment. Boston, Little, Brown, 1978.

Williams P and Warwick R: Gray's Anatomy. London, Churchill/Livingstone, 1980.

▶ SELF-ASSESSMENT QUIZ

1. Who first performed carotid arteriography?
   a. Moniz
   b. Seldinger
   c. Forsmann
   d. Sones

2. The aortic arch contains _____ primary branch(es).
   a. one
   b. two
   c. three
   d. four

3. The brachycephalic/innominate branch originates at what aspect of the aortic arch?
   a. right
   b. middle
   c. left

4. The internal carotid arteries supply oxygenated blood to the
   a. face only
   b. frontal, parietal, and temporal lobes of the brain
   c. neck, face, and mouth

5. The ophthalmic artery is a primary branch of the _____ artery.
   a. external carotid

b. anterior cerebral
c. internal carotid
d. vertebral

6. The two primary terminal branches of the internal carotid arteries are the
   a. anterior and posterior communicating
   b. vertebral and basilar arteries
   c. anterior and middle cerebral
   d. anterior choroidal and posterior communicating

7. The sylvian triangle
   a. describes a rare vascular disease
   b. is an important anatomical landmark
   c. is the terminal portion of the carotid bifurcation
   d. is the dividing point of the anterior and middle cerebral artery

8. The vertebrobasilar system supplies oxygenated blood to which aspect of the brain?
   a. anterior only
   b. anterior and midbrain
   c. posterior and inferior
   d. inferior only

9. Both vertebral arteries originate from the _____ arteries.
   a. carotid
   b. innominate
   c. basilar
   d. subclavian

10. The basilar artery is formed by the union of the
    a. anterior and middle cerebral arteries
    b. anterior cerebral and anterior communicating arteries
    c. vertebral arteries
    d. carotid arteries

11. An indirect communication between one cerebral hemisphere and another is by way of the
    a. venous system
    b. anterior and posterior cerebral arteries
    c. sylvian triangle
    d. circle of Willis

12. The vein of Galen drains into the
    a. superior sagittal sinus
    b. cavernous sinus
    c. cerebral and cerebellar veins
    d. straight sinus

13. The superior vena cava receives venous blood from the
    a. internal jugular veins
    b. collateral vessels
    c. superior cerebellar veins
    d. petrosal sinuses

14. Which of the patients are considered "high risk"?
    1. those who are allergic to iodine
    2. those with severe, advanced arteriosclerosis
    3. those of advanced age
    4. those with renal dysfunction
    a. 1 only
    b. 1 and 2
    c. 1, 2, and 3
    d. 1, 2, 3, and 4

15. What type of equipment is preferred in neuroangiography?
    a. single-phase 6-pulse
    b. single-phase 12-pulse
    c. three-phase 6-pulse
    d. three-phase 12-pulse

16. What technique combination(s) is or are preferred in neuroangiography?
    1. the lowest possible kVp setting
    2. high mA and short exposure time
    3. the highest possible kVp setting
    4. low mA and long exposure time
    a. 1 only
    b. 1 and 2
    c. 1, 2, and 3
    d. 1, 2, 3, and 4

17. For purposes of serial magnification a _____ focal spot is required.
    a. 0.3-mm
    b. 0.3-cm
    c. 0.6-mm
    d. 1.2-cm

18. Most hospitals prefer the _____ changer as the changer of choice for neuroangiography.
    a. roll-film
    b. cut-film
    c. cassette

19. In biplane angiography, the goal(s) of the grid is to
    1. provide adequate clean-up of scatter radiation
    2. eliminate grid line artifacts
    3. speed up the exposure time
    4. increase the number of films taken per second
    a. 1 only
    b. 1 and 2
    c. 1, 2, and 3
    d. 1, 2, 3, and 4

20. The most common type of automatic contrast medium pressure injector is
    a. one that is driven with gas cartridges
    b. one that is operated with compressed gas
    c. one that is electromechanical
    d. one that is atomic powered and suspended from the ceiling

21. Seldinger described his percutaneous needle puncture technique in
    a. 1910
    b. 1927
    c. 1953
    d. 1965

22. Which arteries are most frequently employed for neuroangiography?
    1. brachial
    2. common femoral
    3. axillary
    4. common carotid
    a. 1 only
    b. 1 and 2
    c. 1, 2, and 3
    d. 1, 2, 3, and 4

23. The focus of catheterization techniques during the last 20 years is that
    a. shorter is better
    b. smaller is better
    c. longer is better
    d. bigger is better

24. The names Potts-Cournand and Amplatz are associated with

a. types of Teflon catheters
b. techniques of injection
c. types of angiographic needles
d. techniques of subtraction

25. What shape is the typical guidewire tip?
a. J
b. Y
c. L
d. O

26. The ideal kVp range for cerebral angiography is
a. 50 to 60 kVp
b. 65 to 70 kVp
c. 75 to 80 kVp
d. 85 to 90 kVp

27. For cerebral angiography, the exposure time should not exceed
a. 100 msec
b. 150 msec
c. 200 msec
d. 300 msec

28. Which technique is used to better define and improve vessel resolution?
a. magnification
b. stereo
c. subtraction
d. breathing

29. What is the enemy of subtraction?
a. fog
b. secondary radiation
c. too high of contrast
d. motion

30. Which base line would be best for a cerebral angiogram when the patient is hypersthenic?
a. IOML
b. AML
c. OML
d. GAL

31. For a lateral projection to demonstrate posterior cerebral circulation, the central ray would enter
a. anterior of the EAM
b. anterior and superior of the EAM
c. directly to the EAM
d. behind the EAM at the mastoid process

32. Which position best demonstrates pathology of the anterior communicating artery?
a. AP
b. lateral
c. axial
d. oblique supraorbital

33. The leading disease that results in symptomatic disease is
a. aneurysm
b. atherosclerosis
c. AVM
d. hypertension

34. What percentage of stenosis of the carotid artery is considered hemodynamically significant and requires surgery?
a. 10%
b. 25%
c. 50%
d. 75%

35. A localized dilatation or saccular enlargement of an artery describes a (an)
a. stenosis
b. occlusion
c. plaque
d. aneurysm

36. A venous leaking of blood that takes place between the dura and arachnoid membrane is referred to as _____ hematoma.
a. subdural
b. epidural
c. intracerebral
d. subarachnoid

37. Which is the correct sequence of cerebral circulation?
a. arterial, venous, capillary
b. venous, arterial, capillary
c. arterial, capillary, venous
d. capillary, arterial, venous

38. The term "tumor blush" usually refers to what type of tumor?
a. calcified meningioma
b. craniopharyngioma
c. sellar adenoma
d. vascular meningioma

39. _____ are benign congenital tumors consisting of a network of newly formed blood vessels on or near the surface of the skin.
a. medulloblastomas
b. meningiomas
c. cavernous hemangiomas
d. carotid body tumors

40. When we discuss a "four-vessel" study, what four vessels are being focused on?
a. carotids and subclavians
b. subclavians and vertebrals
c. carotids and vertebrals
d. brachiocephalic, both carotids, and left vertebral

▶ **STUDY QUESTIONS**

1. List the radiologic procedures that are performed in neuroangiography.

2. List the indications for carotid arteriography, cerebral angiography, and vertebral angiography.

3. List the contraindications for carotid arteriography, cerebral angiography, and vertebral angiography.

4. List the major arteries that supply the brain.

5. List the major venous structures that drain the brain.

6. List and describe the types of equipment that are necessary to perform neuroangiography.

7. Describe three ways that subject contrast can be improved when performing neuroangiography.

8. Describe the applications of magnification radiography and subtraction technique to neuroangiography.

9. Describe the advantages and disadvantages of biplane filming as it applies to neuroangiography.

10. List and describe three special patient positions that are used in neuroangiography.

11. Describe five lesions that are demonstrated in neuroangiography.

12. Describe the duties of the radiographer with regard to patient care procedures in the neuroangiographic suite.

13. What types of catheters and guidewires are used in neuroangiography?

14. Describe the primary components of a rapid-film serial changer.

15. Describe three optional components that could be found in an automatic contrast medium injector.

► SECTION FOUR

► **INTERVENTIONAL PROCEDURES**

► CHAPTER ELEVEN

► VASCULAR INTERVENTIONAL PROCEDURES

► CHAPTER OUTLINE

► CHAPTER OBJECTIVES

Upon completion of Chapter 11 the technologist will be able to:

1. Describe three ways of reducing arterial hemorrhage
2. List and describe five materials used to accomplish percutaneous vascular embolization
3. Distinguish between temporary and permanent embolic media
4. Explain the action of vasoconstrictors
5. Describe seven methods of treatment that increase blood flow
6. List the diseases and conditions that may alter blood flow

In the early to mid-1970s, computed tomography (CT) and ultrasound were finding wider application in special procedures. The number of angiographic procedures began to diminish. This new trend caused many people to express some doubt with regard to the future of angiography. During that era, "special procedures," as we used to call it, involved a wide range of vascular as well as nonvascular procedures. Practically all of these procedures were performed for diagnosis.

It was during the early 1970s that great strides were being made in a type of angiography that became known as *vascular interventional procedures,* a radiologic specialty that interfaced diagnostic radiology with therapeutic radiology. Instead of joining the proponents of CT, many physicians explored the realm of therapeutic angiography.

Many important events took place in the formative era of therapeutic angiography and culminated in the development of the *balloon dilatation* catheter in 1974.

The first of many milestones in therapeutic angiography was achieved in 1959 by Rastelli and associates, who were the first to demonstrate gastrointestinal (GI) bleeding in the experimental animal.

In 1960, two significant events took place. Lussenhop and Spence performed an artificial embolization of a cerebral arteriovenous malformation (AVM), and Margulis and associates demonstrated intraoperative mesenteric angiography showing cecal AVM.

In 1963, one of the greatest milestones was achieved when Nusbaum and Baum demonstrated a method of localizing a GI bleeding site via percutaneous angiography. This was followed in 1964 by a technique referred to as *transluminal arterial recanalization,* which was first performed by Dotter and Judkins and was designed to recanalize stenotic femoral arteries; it later became known by its current name, *percutaneous transluminal angioplasty* (PTA).

Although Dotter and Judkins' accomplishments were the talk of diagnostic radiology, this procedure was not without complications. The coaxial system was used to open up stenoses and occlusions. Regrettably, the resultant arteriotomy matched the diameter of the vessel lumen produced. These large catheters induced damage to the vascular endothelium, leading to significant rates of early thrombosis, restenosis, and poor long-term performance.

In 1967, Nusbaum and associates were the first to administer vasopressin into the vascular system for variceal bleeding. This was followed in 1969 by *intraarterial vasopressin* for arterial GI hemorrhage.

In 1972, two important events took place: Rosch and associates utilized *transcatheter embolization* in GI bleeding, and Margolies and associates demonstrated the application of transcatheter embolization in trauma.

In 1974, Gruntzig and Hopff took the work of Dotter and Judkins to the next step when they developed the balloon dilatation catheter. This catheter had a double-lumen balloon sheath that was designed to improve the recanalization procedure while reducing procedural complications. This was accomplished by inflating the balloon to a predetermined size and by not continuing to inflate beyond that point.

Gruntzig's success allowed for PTA to be utilized at other arterial sites, including the coronary arteries. As a result of Gruntzig's work, PTA is now widely used as an adjunct to surgery or even as an alternative to bypass surgery. Table 11–1 lists some milestones in therapeutic angiography.

► PERCUTANEOUS TREATMENT OF ARTERIAL HEMORRHAGE

Transcatheter Embolization

Percutaneous catheter embolization describes a mechanical method of stopping abnormal blood flow in arteries. The percutaneous catheter approach, via the *Seldinger technique,* makes possible the identification of the actual site of the bleed and, with this information, helps us to decide which method of embolization is best.

Indications

Uncontrolled bleeding occurs in situations in which medical therapy is unsuccessful or in situations in which vasoconstrictors have not arrested the hemorrhage. Embolic material can be injected through a

---

► **Table 11–1**
MILESTONES IN THERAPEUTIC ANGIOGRAPHY

1959	Rastelli et al	Radiographic demonstration of GI bleeding in the experimental animal
1960	Lussenhop and Spence	Artificial embolization of cerebral arteriovenous malformation
1960	Margulis et al	Intraoperative mesenteric angiography shows cecal arteriovenous malformation
1963	Nusbaum and Baum	Percutaneous angiography localizes GI bleeding sites
1964	Dotter and Judkins	Transluminal arterial recanalization
1967	Nusbaum et al	Intra-arterial vasopressin for variceal hemorrhage
1969	Nusbaum et al	Intra-arterial vasopressin for arterial GI hemorrhage
1972	Rosch et al	Transcatheter embolization in GI hemorrhage
1972	Margolies et al	Transcatheter embolization in trauma
1974	Gruntzig and Hopff	Balloon dilatation catheter

GI = gastrointestinal.

catheter selectively into the bleeding artery. The emboli are carried peripherally by the blood flow and occlude the branches of the artery being embolized, including the bleeding branch.

There are situations in which a vascular tumor is present and the surgeon desires to decrease blood flow to the affected organ. When performed preoperatively, embolization causes tumor vessels to collapse, resulting in a decrease in operating time and blood loss. In patients with inoperable tumors, it is undertaken to relieve symptoms and to reduce tumor size. In many situations, the patient's age and clinical history dictate the actions of the surgeon. If the patient's condition contraindicates surgery, embolization can be performed on a temporary basis until the patient is better stabilized. However, in some situations in which the patient's status puts him or her at risk, the surgeon may choose to do surgery and permanently embolize, occlude, or *kill* the organ. Two examples of tumor ablation include renal cell carcinoma or primary and metastatic carcinoma (Figs. 11–1 and 11–2). In tumor palliation, the objective is to decrease pain, reduce ectopic hormones, or control the effects of the tumor.

Transcatheter embolization is one of the more successful methods of dealing with AVMs. Embolization of AVMs can help control or reduce vascularity, control arteriovenous shunting, and in some cases effec-

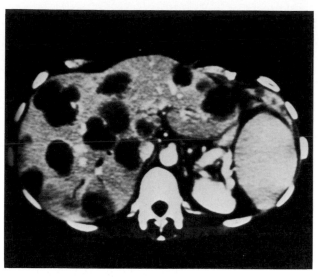

► Figure 11–2

Metastatic liver carcinoma.

tively control the size of certain AVMs present in the soft tissues of an extremity or bone or in a solid organ.

Miscellaneous functions of transcatheter embolization include control of hypertension, combination embolic and chemotherapy, or radioactive particle therapy for malignancy. Table 11–2 lists the primary indications for percutaneous catheter embolization.

Contraindications

Nontarget embolization can cause infarction elsewhere in the body. The embolic material can be erroneously delivered into systemic circulation. Spinal cord infarction during bronchial artery embolization and hepatic infarction have been reported, with paraplegia, hemorrhagic shock, and death as the tragic results. Other potential sites of nontarget embolization include the gallbladder, stomach, small bowel, and bladder.

In addition to nontarget embolization, a complication of transcatheter embolization is the *postembolization* syndrome, which is characterized by fever, leukocytosis, and discomfort. Close observation of the patient is necessary to ensure that no infection is present. Because it is difficult to clinically differentiate the postembolization syndrome from infection in the embolized area, it is advised that patients receive

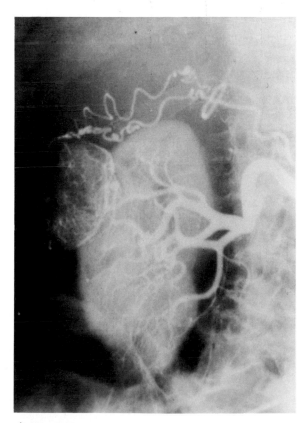

► Figure 11–1

Renal cell carcinoma of the right kidney, upper pole.

► Table 11–2

PRIMARY INDICATIONS FOR PERCUTANEOUS
CATHETER EMBOLIZATION

1. Uncontrolled bleeding
2. Tumor ablation
3. Tumor palliation
4. Arteriovenous malformations
5. Miscellaneous

prophylactic antibiotic therapy before the procedure is done. Blood cultures should be obtained if the patient exhibits signs and symptoms of infection. Table 11–3 lists the primary contraindications for percutaneous catheter embolization.

Embolic Media Classification

A wide variety of embolic agents are available for clinical application. These materials can be classified according to their chemical and physical properties. *Particulate* and *liquid* materials and *absorbable* and *nonabsorbable* materials are included in this grouping. Embolic media can also be classed according to the term of occlusion—*temporary, intermediate,* or *permanent.* For example, GI bleeding and tumors that are embolized preoperatively require only short-term occlusion, whereas AVMs require permanent occlusion. Materials may be also be selected based on the site or level of occlusion—proximal or peripheral.

Embolic Media Criteria

Transcatheter embolization is an invasive procedure that can be accomplished utilizing a wide variety of embolic agents. Radiologists and cardiologists, while having a wide selection, must make that choice according to valid criteria. The embolizing agent must be nontoxic, easy to deliver, safe to inject, and radiopaque for easy localization. The agent must be utilized in both primary and collateral vessels, produce no adverse reaction, have a low failure and recurrence rate, produce no pain for the patient, be convenient to obtain from the manufacturer, and be inexpensive.

Toxicity of the embolic material is an important consideration. Certain tissue adhesives are designed to rapidly and permanently occlude vessels. When injected forcefully, these adhesives may penetrate deeply into the microcirculation, induce a perivascular response, and cause subsequent tissue infarction.

Of concern is the pathologic nature of the circulation being embolized, its collateral supply, and the effects of acute occlusion of tissues beyond the site of embolization. Total occlusion of the vascular bed of a tumor requires microparticles or a liquid polymer. A focal occlusion of a single vessel or an arteriovenous fistula (AVF) may require a detachable balloon or metallic coil.

The patient's ability to form a clot varies. A deficiency of clotting factors requires an exogenous embolic agent.

▶ **Table 11–3**
CONTRAINDICATIONS FOR
TRANSCATHETER EMBOLIZATION

Absolute:	Unacceptably high risk of nontarget organ embolization for the expected potential benefit
Relative:	Lesions of the small bowel and colon

Delivery System

The delivery system must be able to accommodate the various sizes and consistencies of embolic material required for a given vascular bed. The catheter must be long enough to allow the embolic material to pass with ease, and the catheter's shape should allow its tip to stabilize within the orifice of the target vessel.

Embolic Materials

The use of therapeutic embolic media was first noted in 1930 when Brooks utilized muscle tissue in the treatment of a carotid cavernous fistula. Autologous materials were used exclusively until 1966, when Luessenhof utilized silicone spheres to embolize a cerebral AVM. Numerous embolic agents are currently in use. Table 11–4 lists the materials used for embolization.

Particulate Materials

In the late 1970s and early 1980s, autologous materials were introduced through standard angiographic catheters. Autologous and particulate materials tend to

▶ **Table 11–4**
MATERIALS USED FOR EMBOLIZATION

Particulate Materials
Autologous Materials
  Clot
    Native
    Modified
  Tissue
    Muscle
    Fat
    Dura
    Fascia lata

Absorbable Materials
  Surgical gelatin sponge (Gelfoam)
  Oxycel cellulose (Oxycel)
  Microfibrillar collagen (Avitene)
  Collagen flocculi (Tachotop)
  Occlusion gel (Ethibloc)

Nonabsorbable Materials
  Polyvinyl alcohol (Ivalon)
  Silicone spheres
  Plastic and metallic pellets and spheres

Liquid Materials
  Bucrylate:isobutyl-2-cyanoacrylate (IBCA)
  Silicone
  Absolute ethanol
  Sclerosing agents
  Hot contrast medium
  Hypertonic glucose solution
  Barium sulfate

Mechanical Devices
  Stainles-steel coils

Balloon Catheter Systems
  Nondetachable balloon catheters
  Detachable balloon catheter systems

Chemoembolization Agents

Electrocoagulation (Electrothrombosis)

occlude a catheter. For this reason, vascular sheaths are commonly used in transcatheter embolization.

Catheters (No. 5 to 7 French) used with these procedures usually contain only an open end. The presence of side holes only creates additional hazards during injection because of the potential lodging of the material within the side hole. The type of embolic material determines whether the catheter has a tapered preformed tip or is untapered.

Detachable (occlusive) balloon catheters also can be employed to prevent reflux, to reduce flow during polymer introduction, and to temporarily occlude major vessels.

The *coaxial* catheter system is a popular method of delivering embolic materials. However, the mode of delivery is predicated on the nature of the lesion being treated, its location, and the arterial anatomy that is involved.

The term *autologous* is defined as "belonging to the same organism." *Native* clot is whole blood (20 to 50 ml) that is withdrawn from the patient (at the time of embolization) and is allowed to stand in a glass tube until the cellular proteins aggregate and a solid clot is formed. In 1972, Rosch and associates were the first to utilize clotted whole blood as an embolic material into the vascular system. Native clots usually provide moderately long-term occlusion of a vessel, usually from 6 to 12 hours. In 1974, Bookstein and associates and Reuter and Chuang attempted to prolong the clot by mixing it with epsilon-aminocaproic acid. When the clot is altered to increase its effectiveness, it is referred to as *modified*. A commercially prepared product called *Amicar* (epsilon-aminocaproic acid) is an amino acid that is a potent inhibitor of plasminogen and plasmin and indirectly of fibrinolysis. This amino acid is used as a hemostatic agent. The Amicar-enhanced clot is firmer, and serum can be expressed from it. The compressed clot can then be cut into workable bits or pieces and injected with a tuberculin syringe. Despite the improvement of the clot with Amicar, it has a short half-life; thus, autologous clots are not employed as often as are other materials that have a longer life. Amicar increases the longevity of the clot from 12 to 24 hours. One milliliter (250 mg) of Amicar may be added to 10 ml of the patient's blood.

Dura mater, fascia lata, fat, and *muscle* provide a longer lasting occlusion and are relatively easy to handle. However, these tissues have a distinct disadvantage in that they must be harvested from other body sites. Because of the availability of other types of embolic materials and the difficult task of harvesting body tissues, radiologists usually select other embolic agents for transcatheter embolization.

Absorbable Materials

Surgical Gelatin Sponge or Gelfoam. Surgical *gelatin sponge* is the most commonly used intermediate embolic material. *Gelfoam* is very accessible and is inexpensive. Gelfoam is available in a powder, in a block-sponge form, and in small sheets. It is nonir-

ritating and nonantigenic and occludes vessels by forming a matrix for developing a clot. The substance is biodegradable, and occlusions usually last from 7 to 21 days. Partial recanalization occurs between 21 and 23 days, and complete recanalization occurs after 30 to 35 days. Gelfoam has been found to be nontoxic.

Powdered Gelfoam produces peripheral occlusions and should not be used for GI hemorrhage because of its propensity to cause *ischemia* or *infarction*. Gelfoam powder can be mixed with water-soluble contrast media. Skin necrosis, neural injury, and gallbladder infarction have been reported with the use of Gelfoam powder.

Gelfoam in particulate form is easily used. Once the site of hemorrhage has been identified, the Gelfoam is cut into small *cubes* about 2 to 3 mm on a side or *strips* of about 8 to 10 mm in length and 2 to 3 mm across (*torpedos*). The strips are used when bleeding is not controlled with the small cubes. The cubes or strips are soaked in a nonheparinized saline or iodinated contrast agent. They then become very pliable. The Gelfoam is then drawn into a tuberculin syringe and injected along with saline through the catheter to the site of hemorrhage. An additional option with particulate Gelfoam is to combine it with a sclerosing agent (e.g., sodium tetradecyl) that enhances clot formation.

Extreme care must be taken when injecting particulate Gelfoam to prevent inadvertent embolization. Care must be exercised to avoid forceful flushing or injection of contrast media. During *diastole*, emboli move in a retrograde direction, particularly when enough emboli have been injected to slow the blood flow in the vessel being occluded. These *refluxing* emboli may occlude other arterial branches. When a piece of Gelfoam occludes the catheter, it can be gently advanced with a guidewire (Figs. 11–3 and 11–4).

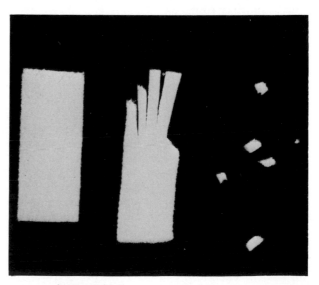

► **Figure 11–3**
Gelfoam is being made ready for use.

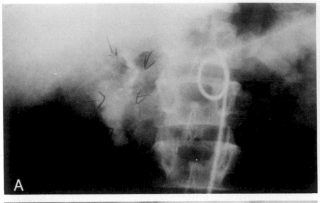
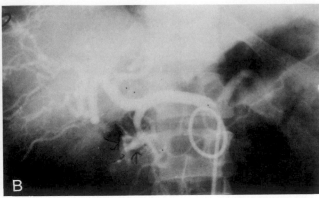
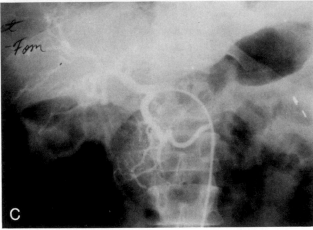

▶ **Figure 11–4**

A, Gastric artery bleed. B, Introduction of Gelfoam.
C, Postembolization.

Oxycel. Other absorbable particulate materials are available, such as oxidized cellulose (*Oxycel*). Oxycel is a hemostatic agent. Clotting takes place via platelet aggregation, producing a material-like matrix similar to Gelfoam. Oxycel can be combined with the patient's whole blood. This produces a solid clot that can be cut into small pieces. Oxycel produces an occlusion of intermediate duration (days).

Microfibrillar Collagen. *Avitene* is a *microfibrillar bovine collagen* and is utilized to achieve peripheral embolization. Avitene is usually mixed with a water-soluble contrast agent, forming a low-viscosity suspension that is easily injected through a lumen as small as a No. 3 French selective catheter. Avitene can also be utilized as an adjunct to a proximal embolization with steel coils, in the renal vasculature in the presence of hypervascular tumors, and in vascular tumors of the head and neck. The occlusion produced by Avitene lasts from days to weeks.

Collagen Flocculi. *Tachotop flocculi* are prepared from *equine collagen*. This foam-like material is transformed into clusters of many sizes, ranging from 1.8 to 4 mm and from 3 to 7 mm. Tachotop can be suspended in contrast media or normal saline and can be easily injected through standard balloon catheters. This injection is enhanced by Tachotop's lubricating properties. Tachotop is utilized for preoperative and palliative embolization of malignant renal tumors, for malignancies of the urinary bladder, and for patients with *malignant hypertension* (300+ systole and 120+ diastole).

Occlusion Gel. *Ethibloc* is a viscous (emulsion) version of zein, sodium amidotrizoate tetrahydrate, oleum papaveris, and propylene glycol and is available in a ready-to-inject syringe.[1] A water-soluble medium is added to ensure opacification. For best results, this emulsion is injected through a balloon catheter. Ethibloc functions like bucrylate (Crazy Glue) and precipitates (after 5 minutes) when coming in contact with ionic substances. Ethibloc solidifies in 5 minutes. This is an advantage, because it allows a greater time for placing the material and for removing the catheter tip. Ethibloc is indicated for preoperative embolization of hypervascular renal tumors.

Nonabsorbable Particulate Materials

Polyvinyl Alcohol (PVA)—Ivalon. Ivalon is a particulate nonabsorbable material (inert plastic foam) that provides permanent embolization and is available in sheets or as small particles. PVA is also available in radiopaque form, with the addition of 60% barium sulfate or tantalum powder.[1] Ivalon expands when exposed to blood or other fluids. Ivalon is frequently affixed to the end of a guidewire in a dry form (after being soaked in saline solution) and compressed (in a vice, and allowed to dry) and can be transported to the desired location. In this form, Ivalon is reduced 15 times in size; it returns to its original size in 3 minutes when replaced in a solution. Because of this characteristic, smaller Ivalon *pellets* may pass through standard diameter catheters to produce vascular occlusion when they make contact with blood. The particles are available in many sizes, from 0.25 to 1 mm in diameter. The PVA is first injected into the catheter and is then propelled into the artery using a second saline-filled tuberculin syringe. Ivalon, like Gelfoam, is radiolucent, so it is necessary to mix it with a positive contrast agent. Ivalon is especially effective when used to occlude varices during a transhepatic portal venous study. Ivalon has the disadvantage of being difficult to inject, because it traps air and the particles have a high surface tension. The flow of particles to the lesion are monitored fluoroscopically, while the system is flushed with controlled injections of 30% contrast medium (Figs. 11–5 and 11–6).

Silicone Spheres. Silicone spheres are nonresorbable embolic agents that are available in several sizes and are impregnated with barium sulfate. The spheres are an excellent means of embolizing AVMs, carotid cavernous sinus fistulas, and juvenile angiofibromas.

Plastic and Metallic Pellets and Spheres. These embolic agents are used to occlude many lesions, including meningiomas, dural AVMs, renal tumors, bone metastases, lesions of multiple myeloma, and peripheral angiomas.

The spheres are manufactured into many different types of material, including *acrylic* spheres, *methylmethacrylate* spheres, *Sephadex* particles, and *polystyrene* microspheres.

Liquid Materials

Isobutyl-2-cyanoacrylate (Bucrylate). This liquid-embolizing agent is a polymer or tissue adhesive that

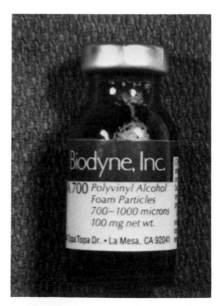

► **Figure 11–5**
A vial of polyvinyl foam particles.

is sometimes referred to as *Crazy Glue*. It has not yet been released for unrestricted clinical usage (controlled substance). *Bucrylate* has been classified as a "suspect" carcinogen and is currently used only in life-saving situations. In clinical trials, this polymer is introduced as a liquid through a small catheter or open-ended guidewire and solidifies almost immediately upon coming to rest at the target site. The rate of solidification is proportionate to the amount of contrast medium that is added to the material. Bucrylate is otherwise a radioparent material. In controlled clinical trials, bucrylate has been used to embolize renal tumors, cerebral AVMs, splenic lesions, and other selective vascular abnormalities. Bucrylate is usually introduced by way of a coaxial catheter system. Complications include infarction of tissue with necrosis or abscess formation; embolization of nontarget areas; and adhesion of the catheter within the vessel wall.

Other polymers that are nonadhesive are available. *Silicone rubber* and *polyurethane* are examples of nonadhesive polymers. These nonadhesive polymers are less reactionary with tissues compared with bucrylate; however, their nonadhesive tendency increases the potential for nontarget embolization.

Silicone. Silicone rubber mixture consists of a medical-grade preparation of the dimethylpolysiloxane (Silastic elastomer 382) and silicone fluid 360.[1] Silicone is a medium that is used to embolize capillary beds and has the advantage of being an inert substance that has no antigenic or carcinogenic properties and is basically nontoxic. The primary disadvantages of silicone include its highly viscous properties and the fact that total occlusion of small vessels may result in organ infarction.

Silicone has been utilized to ensure organ ablation, embolotherapy of extracranial vascular tumors, and dural malformations. Low-viscosity mixtures have been used for embolization of spinal cord malformations and neoplasms of the spine.

Absolute Ethanol. Ethanol produces direct tissue necrosis and permanent vascular occlusion via an induced infarct. The vessel is essentially "killed." During this process, arterial spasms are produced as the blood flow to the vessel is slowed. Reflux may be produced at this point if further amounts of ethanol are injected. Thus, balloon occlusion catheters can be used to prevent reflux.

Ethanol has been most successful in the treatment of AVMs and hypervascular renal tumors. Ethanol has the advantage of being relatively inexpensive and easily available. It is also nonviscous and, therefore, is easily delivered.

Sclerosing Agents. Some of the sclerosing agents currently in use include sodium tetradecyl sulfate (Sotradecol), sodium morrhuate (Varicocid), and aethoxysklersol (Polidocanol). These agents have been utilized in sclerotherapy of the spermatic veins.

Hot Contrast Media. Contrast agents may be heated to boiling and injected directly into the venous system. This induces intimal damage and an inflammatory response with subsequent thrombotic occlu-

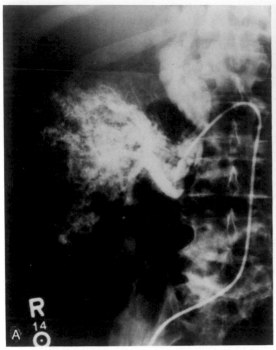
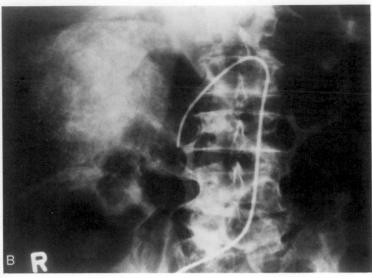

▶ **Figure 11–6**
A, Pre-embolization: renal cell carcinoma of the right kidney.
B, Postembolization with polyvinyl alcohol.

sion. Hot contrast media as a venous occlusion substance were first used experimentally in superficial veins and in spermatic veins and have also been utilized for renal ablation.[1] Hot contrast media used for *thermal sclerotherapy* of spermatic veins effectively occlude the primary vein and collaterals. The primary fault with the injection of hot contrast media is the extreme pain felt by the patient.

Hypertonic Glucose Solution. Hypertonic glucose solution has been used almost exclusively in the treatment of esophageal varices. Complete obliteration of the varices is the goal of this solution.

Barium Sulfate. Barium sulfate is used to make silicone spheres radiopaque.[1] It is also used as an intra-arterial embolic agent for the treatment (occlusion) of tumor vessels.

Mechanical Devices

Metallic Coils. Stainless-steel coils or occluding spring emboli, which were first introduced by Gianturco, Anderson, and Wallace in the mid-1970s, were designed initially to embolize large vessels. Today, coils are the most inexpensive permanent embolic medium and are utilized in numerous sites.

Coils are available in helix diameters of 3, 5, 8, 12, and 15 mm and can be introduced through most No. 5 to 6 French tapered catheters using a standard 0.038″ guidewire (Fig. 11–7). The coil size should be equal or slightly smaller than the diameter of the artery being embolized. The radiologist must pay close attention to the manufacturer's specifications and instructions for embolization. Complications could arise with improper-sized coils. A coil that is too small will fail to embolize properly, and one that is too large

could inadvertently project into a feeder artery. AVFs may require large coils. To enhance the occlusive effectiveness of a coil in a large fistula, a metallic *spider* coil may be employed. Spider coils are available in 10- and 15-mm diameters and contain "barbed" feet that affix the coil to the vessel wall. A special threaded guidewire is available to permit precise positioning before releasing the spider coil.

During the manufacturing process, the coils are housed in an *introduction sheath,* which is placed in the hub end of a catheter, and the coil is slid into the catheter with the aid of a guidewire. The coil is advanced to a point at which the catheter begins to curve and is pushed carefully out of the sheath by the guidewire. The coil then reassumes its original shape at the desired location.

At first, the metallic coils had *wool fibers* attached to the coil tip to facilitate thrombosis. Wool was found to promote granulomatous formation. *Dacron* was selected as the alternative material and is currently the fabric of choice.

Stainless-steel coils are widely used in treating *GI hemorrhage.* The coils are especially effective when bleeding originates from a major visceral artery. Coils are also widely used in the embolization of malignant vascular tumors of the kidneys.

The use of coils is not without complication. Coils may become wedged in the catheter. The strands of fabric material may become impacted and stick in the tip of the catheter. A coil may become unraveled, jammed, and difficult to displace from the catheter larger than the recommended diameter (thin-walled No. 5 or standard wall No. 6.5 French). If the coil is caught in the catheter tip and is only partially ejected, it may be dislodged into the target artery by injecting

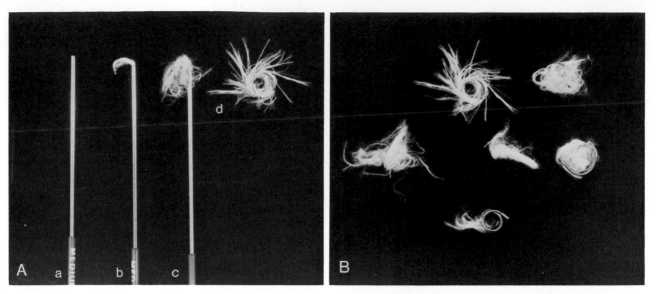

▶ **Figure 11–7**

A, Gianturco coils. (a = introducer; b = coil partially exposed; c = fully exposed with Dacron threads; d = fully detached from the introducer.) *B,* Assorted sizes of Gianturco coils.

normal saline at high pressures. Bunching of the Dacron threads at the catheter tip may cause withdrawal of the coil from its intended position when the catheter is removed. The coil must then be retrieved.

Despite the potential difficulties, complications are rare, and coils are an excellent way to permanently embolize vessels in a very precise focal area.

Figure 11–8 shows a 62-year-old man diagnosed with a malignant vascular tumor of the left kidney. Because the patient was not a good surgical candidate, an attempt was made to permanently occlude the vessel feeding the tumor.

Figure 11–9 depicts a patient with bilateral renal disease and evidence of marked hematuria. Both kidneys are nonfunctioning. Because this 57-year-old man was a poor surgical risk, both kidneys were permanently embolized.

Balloon Catheter Systems

Nondetachable Balloon Catheters. Nondetachable balloon catheters are utilized for occlusion arteriography and phlebography. Injection of particulate and liquid embolic agents can take place with these catheters. Nondetachable balloon catheters can also be used for treating inoperable aneurysms of the carotid artery.

Detachable Balloon Catheters. The detachable balloon is often used as an alternative to metallic coils and is most often utilized in the control of AVFs that are complications of traumatic incidents. One distinct advantage of this detachable balloon is that the radiologist can determine the position and competency of the occlusion before the balloon is detached. Many balloon systems are available, and all must be utilized

properly to ensure proper embolization and safety. The balloon must be delivered safely into the peripheral circulation and positioned accurately before being detached. Certain precautions have to be taken when using detachable balloons. The correct concentration of contrast medium must be used. When inadequately visualized, the balloon can be detached prematurely. If improperly placed, the balloon should be deflated completely before it is withdrawn and repositioned.

Chemoembolization Agents

Chemoembolization agents utilize the combination of intra-arterial infusion of a chemotherapeutic agent with intra-arterial embolization.[1] The purpose of this combination is to provide a prolonged drug release while decreasing the systemic toxicity of chemotherapy.

Electrocoagulation

Transcatheter electrocoagulation or electrothrombosis is the process of producing blood clots at a targeted intravascular site. Transcatheter electrocoagulation has been used successfully to occlude vessels clinically. A guidewire is extended through a selectively placed catheter at the target site, and a constant current is applied with a neutral electrode attached to the body. Direct current is safer than alternating current, because alternating current acutely disrupts the vessel's wall. Low amperage (<50 mA) is required to produce the clot safely. This method is advantageous, because the site of occlusion can be accurately determined and there is little risk of reflux or nontarget embolization. The primary disadvantage is that the

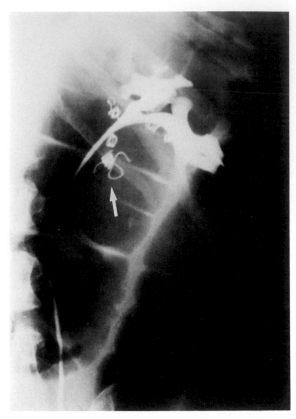

▶ **Figure 11–8**

A 62-year-old male patient with hypernephroma of the left kidney. Note the "spider" occluding coil (*arrow*).

procedure is very time consuming (up to 20 to 30 minutes in vessels with a 4- to 5-mm diameter). Typically, the procedure may take up to 1 hour to achieve adequate occlusion.

Transcatheter electrocoagulation is employed to treat AVMs, to control hemorrhage, and to embolize vascular tumors.

Complications of Embolization.

There are complications that are specific to each method of embolization. The most serious complication is reflux of emboli with occlusion of a nontarget vessel. Reflux is the result of the rate of flow of the circulation as well as the rate of injection. Emboli enter freely at the onset of injection, but as resistance in the vascular bed increases, the speed and quantity of injection must be decreased. Reflux occurs from *overinjecting* and from not terminating the embolization procedure sufficiently early. This complication can be prevented by (1) careful monitoring with fluoroscopic guidance; (2) using a small syringe, thus allowing a more controlled injection; (3) actually seeing the emboli by mixing them with dilute contrast medium or tantalum; and (4) both preceding and flushing the emboli with dilute contrast medium.

Infusion of Vasoconstrictors

Arterial infusion of vasopressin has been used in the treatment of GI hemorrhage and esophageal varices. Vasopressin is an aqueous solution of the pressor component of the posterior pituitary gland and is presently the vasoconstrictor agent of choice. It causes contraction of smooth muscle of the GI tract and acts on the capillaries, small arterioles, and venules. Vasopressin produces a significant and sustained reduction in visceral blood flow that is particularly intense in areas where it is selectively infused. Prolonged vasoconstriction results in a stable clot formation in the area of bleeding.

Vasopressin has been most effective in controlling bleeding of gastric and mesenteric origin. Vasopressin is highly successful in lower GI bleeding in the elderly. Reported success rates of intravascular embolization with vasopressin have exceeded 82%. Emergency colonic surgery is enhanced by the ability of vasopressin to control hemorrhage. Vasopressin is contraindicated in patients with ischemic heart disease, recent myocardial infarction, advanced peripheral and cerebral vascular disease, congestive heart failure, and renal failure with fluid retention.

In terms of preparation, vasopressin is diluted in normal saline or 5% dextrose into a 0.2 μg/ml concentration and is delivered with an arterial infusion pump. The dose is determined by the size of the selected artery.

Figure 11–10 describes a patient with a hemorrhage of the midcolic artery following surgical resection. Figure 11–10*A* reveals gross colonic hemorrhage. Figure 11–10*B* shows the reduction in bleeding following infusion of vasopressin. Figure 11–10*C*, taken following the administration of vasopressin, shows a complete cessation of colonic hemorrhage.

▶ PERCUTANEOUS TREATMENT OF ALTERED BLOOD FLOW

Twenty-seven years have passed since peripheral angioplasty was first described. At that time, it was not possible to recanalize small vessels below the level of the popliteal arteries. Catheter and guidewire science did not permit exploration into the smaller vessels without high risk for intimal damage. In 1964, Dotter and Judkins successfully recanalized atherosclerotic arteries that were significantly stenosed. Other improvements in this technique followed during the next 10 years. It was not until 1974 that Gruntzig and Hopff provided new excitement with the development of the *double-lumen balloon sheath catheter*. Investigators began to realize that atherosclerotic plaques of the intima were not as malleable as was once thought; these dry lesions were actually hard. Thus, improvements in guidewire and catheter science led to the development of the balloon catheter and to the application of *balloon angioplasty*, thera-

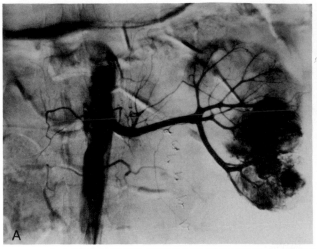
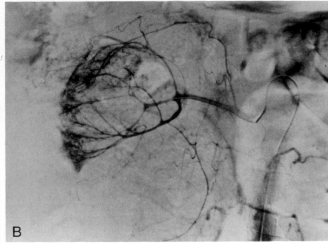
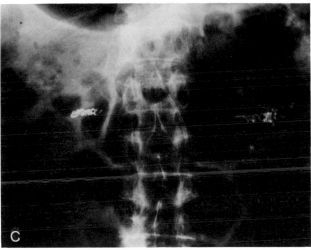

► **Figure 11–9**

A and *B*, A 57-year-old man with bilateral renal disease. *C*, Bilateral renal embolization.

peutic angiography, and the birth of interventional procedures in 1976.

In current interventional radiology, procedures such as intravascular thrombolysis are now used with balloon angioplasty. Stents, which were once limited to nonvascular sites, are now being utilized in the vascular system.

It is now possible to retrieve vascular foreign bodies and extract emboli from the pulmonary vascular system.

Advancements in mechanical design have made possible atherectomy devices that are much improved over the previous designs of the early to middle 1980s.

Lasers are being refined for vascular use, and only time will determine their future applications.

Percutaneous Transluminal Angioplasty

Indications

The primary indication for PTA is *atherosclerosis*. Angioplasty can be applied to almost any location within the vascular system. The application of coronary angioplasty was discussed in Chapter 7. Narrowing of the vessels of the pelvis and lower limbs often produces symptoms referred to as *intermittent claudication*. Intermittent claudication can be described as a complex of symptoms characterized by an absence of pain or discomfort in a limb when the patient is at rest, followed by the commencement of pain, tension, and weakness upon resumption of exercise (walking). These symptoms intensify until the patient can no longer walk. Once the person is at rest, the pain subsides. These symptoms are indicative of occlusive arterial disease of the limbs (usually lower) (Fig. 11–11). Table 11–5 lists the primary indications for PTA.

Angioplasty is also indicated when a patient suffers pain while at rest, or when there are worsening vascular changes such as is seen with nonhealing ulcers or lesions with gangrenous potential (Fig. 11–12).

Renal artery angioplasty has the ability to control or resolve renovascular hypertension and thus avoid the complications associated with surgical revascularization or nephrectomy.

Angioplasty is also employed preoperatively when

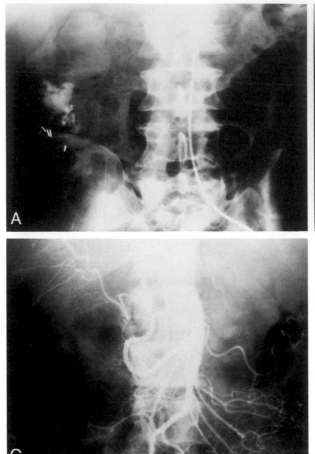

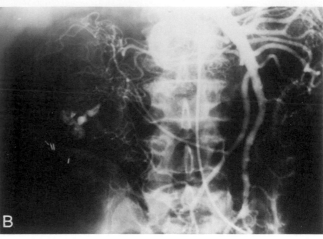

► **Figure 11–10**

A, An active hemorrhage of the midcolic artery. *B,* A reduced hemorrhage after the administration of vasopressin.
C, Complete cessation of a colonic hemorrhage after the administration of vasopressin.

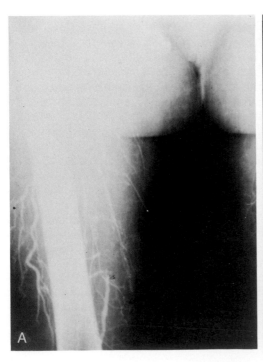

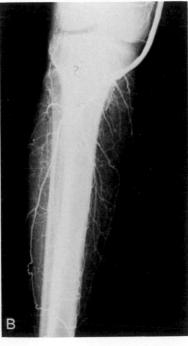

► **Figure 11–11**

A, This 66-year-old male patient revealed a complete occlusion of the right superficial femoral artery. *B,* Distal runoff showing collateral circulation of the right lower leg in the same patient.

► **Table 11–5**
INDICATIONS FOR PERCUTANEOUS
TRANSLUMINAL ANGIOPLASTY

Extremity
Intermittent claudication
Rest pain in extremity
Nonhealing ulcer or gangrene
Need to improve inflow prior to distal surgical bypass
Graft anastomotic stenoses

Renal
Renovascular hypertension
Renal insufficiency
Renal transplant arterial stenosis
Renal artery saphenous vein bypass graft stenosis

► **Table 11–6**
CONTRAINDICATIONS FOR PERCUTANEOUS
TRANSLUMINAL ANGIOPLASTY

Extremity
Medically unstable patient
Stenosis that is not hemodynamically significant
Long-segment arterial occlusion
Long-segment iliac (>4 cm) or superficial femoral (>10 cm)
    stenoses
Lesions in essential collateral vessels
Contrast medium hypersensitivity

Renal
Medically unstable patient
Stenosis that is not hemodynamically significant
Long-segment total occlusion
Ostial renal artery lesion
Contrast medium hypersensitivity

there is a need to improve inflow prior to distal bypass and when there is occlusive disease at or within a graft anastomotic site. Angioplasty is also indicated for hemodynamically significant stenoses (75% or greater), if a 15-mm Hg pressure gradient exists across the stenosis at rest, or if a 20 mm Hg gradient exists across it after peripheral vasodilatation.

PTA is a relatively safe procedure with an extremely low morbidity rate and usually produces favorable long-term results. In comparison with alternative surgical procedures, the term of hospitalization is much less with angioplasty.

Contraindications

The hazards for PTA are basically the same as for angiography and include sensitivity to the contrast agent, nephrotoxicity, and vascular injury related to catheterization and infection (Table 11–6).

Complications

Overall, the incidence of complications for extremity angioplasty is between 7 and 12%. The rate of renal artery restenosis within 1 year is 27 to 33%. Table 11–7 lists the primary complications associated with extremity and renal angioplasty.

Vascular Sheaths

Vascular sheaths are valuable because they limit the amount of puncture site trauma from manipulation and permit the reinsertion of a smaller angiographic catheter after balloon removal for postangioplasty arteriography.[2]

► **Table 11–7**
COMPLICATIONS OF PERCUTANEOUS
TRANSLUMINAL ANGIOPLASTY

Extremity
Death
Continued response to contrast medium reaction
Restenosis
Acute thrombus occluding arterial lumen
Puncture site hematoma
Nontarget embolization
Intimal damage by a guidewire
Vessel perforation
Vasospasm
Pseudoaneurysm

Renal
Death
Continued response to contrast medium reaction
Localized thrombus formation
Nonocclusive dissection
Arterial rupture
Peripheral renal embolus
Guidewire-related dissection
Renal failure
Segmental renal infarction
Emboli to extremities
Puncture-site trauma

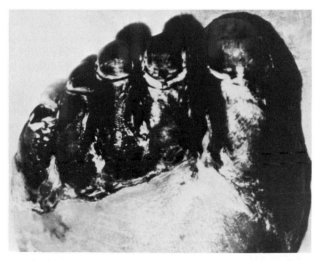

► **Figure 11–12**
Gangrene of the distal foot including the toes in this 55-year-old diabetic patient who has advanced peripheral vascular disease.

Digital Subtraction Imaging

Digital *roadmapping* is helpful in guiding remanipulation of the guidewire or catheter and allows for contrast injections that reveal catheter placement. These images can be stored for later fluoroscopic manipulation.

Guidewires

Many guidewires are available today. One of the newer instruments is the torquable guidewire, which comes with a stiff shaft and a soft, safer (less traumatic) tip design that is indicated exclusively for vascular use (see Fig. 5–46).

The advantage of the soft tip is that the wire can safely negotiate the most stenosed pathway without injury to the vessel. Torquable wires can move in narrow areas and also have enough stiffness for a balloon to be advanced through the lesion without buckling. Thus, we now have a wire that will significantly increase the success rate of the examination. A negative aspect of the soft-tipped wire, however, is the cost. Soft-tipped wires are three to four times more expensive than wires with a standard tip (degree of stiffness). Of course, like standard wires, the torquable wires are heparinized and coated in Teflon. Some radiologists utilize these expensive wires only in high-risk cases.

Catheters

As discussed in Chapter 9, it is not unusual for patients to have occlusive disease in many areas from the distal aorta, to the iliac vessels, to superficial femoral and popliteal arteries, and so forth. Radiologists are frequently faced with tortuous pathways in addition to the occlusions. One can perform the procedures from different sites with a retrograde femoral, translumbar, or axillary artery approach. Thus, with all these variables in mind, one should have several different types of balloon catheters available. Some catheter types are polyvinyl chloride, standard polyethylene, high-pressure, and low-profile. Specific information regarding each type of catheter is beyond the scope of this text. Many types of balloon catheters are available to the radiologist; however, although many radiologists seem to prefer an all-purpose balloon catheter, the type made of polyethylene seems to be the overwhelming favorite. On the other hand, the low-profile balloon catheter represents the latest in technologic advancements in balloon catheter design. This type is very flexible and easy to manipulate in some of the smallest distal vessels beyond the tibial vessels. As expected, the low-profile balloon catheters are at least twice as expensive as the standard balloon catheters (Fig. 11–13).

Balloon Inflator and Pressure Gauge

It is not absolutely necessary that the radiologist should utilize a specialized balloon inflator and pres-

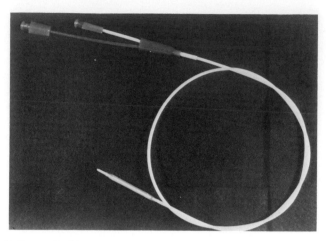

▶ **Figure 11–13**

Blu-Max 7 French No. 5 balloon catheter. (Courtesy of Meditech/Boston Scientific Corporation, Watertown, MA.)

sure gauge. Any standard 10-ml syringe will suffice; however, unless the radiologist is an extremely experienced angiographer, the chance of inadvertent bursting of the balloon is greatly increased.

When any balloon is used near its pressure limit, a pressure gauge enables maximum dilatation pressure just below the bursting pressure of the balloon catheter to be achieved.[3]

When it is necessary to provide precise, incremental pressure increases, the balloon inflation device provides the most exact screw advancement of the syringe piston and can increase the margin of safety, particularly if combined with an inflation pressure that measures the gauge (Fig. 11–14).[4]

Intravascular Thrombolysis/Fibrinolysis

Spontaneous thrombolysis of blood was first described by Hunter in his *Treatise on the Blood* in 1794. Tillet and Garner discovered the exogenous thrombolytic activity of a streptococcal extract.[5] Additional investigation resulted in the isolation of streptokinase from β-hemolytic streptococci. Urokinase was isolated from human urine and was tested for thrombolytic activity. The first clinical application of streptokinase was reported in 1955,[6] followed by clinical trials using urokinase a short time thereafter.

The use of thrombolytic agents for local vascular infusion date back to the early 1960s. Dotter and associates formalized the angiographic application of thrombolytic infusion in 1974.

The human body has the natural ability to preserve vascular integrity and patency. This unique system can be activated by *endogenous* factors within the vascular system. Activation occurs by conversion of the inactive *plasminogen,* present in circulating blood, or bound to *fibrin* in clot, to the active proteolytic enzyme plasmin, which hydrolyzes a solid clot into peptide fragments called fibrin degradation prod-

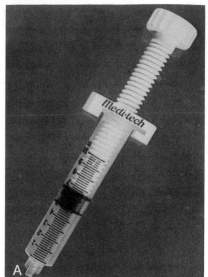

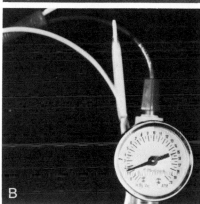

▶ **Figure 11–14**

A, Leveen inflator. *B,* A Leveen pressure gauge and a Blu-Max 7 French balloon catheter. (*A* and *B,* Courtesy of Medi-tech/ Boston Scientific Corporation, Watertown, MA.)

ucts. Plasminogen is synthesized rapidly and, if depleted during thrombolytic activity, returns to normal within 24 hours of cessation of therapy. *Plasmin* has a very short half-life due to its nearly immediate inactivation in the blood by *antiplasmin,* which is a specific inhibitor. In a *thrombus,* the presence of fibrin prevents plasmin inactivation, allowing plasmin acidity and fibrin breakdown. Activation of the fibrinolytic mechanism is normally controlled by specific inhibitors at various steps to maintain hemostasis and prevent fibrinolysis, except in areas of high fibrin concentration (e.g., a thrombus).[3]

Indications

Current projections indicate that 5% of men older than 50 years of age develop intermittent claudication. In 1 to 5% of patients with claudication, limb amputation will eventually be necessary. Patients with atherosclerotic disease present in the coronary and cerebral vascular systems suffer an accelerated mortality rate of 30% at 5 years and 50% at 10 years after presentation. Patients who are diabetic and who smoke have a much worse prognosis. *Thrombolysis* is used in the presence of native artery or bypass graft occlusions and frequently in patients with clot formation in the renal artery. Thrombolysis for bypass occlusion, when utilized in combination with balloon angioplasty, facilitates the rate of graft salvage.

Most long occlusions are caused by one or two critical lesions (thromboses) with *antegrade* and *retrograde* thrombosis to the nearest patent collateral vessels. Table 11–8 lists the indications and contraindications for thrombolysis.

Contraindications

The most significant situations in which thrombolysis is avoided include *active internal bleeding,* signs of irreversible *limb ischemia, recent stroke, intracranial neoplasm,* or recent *craniotomy.* Other contraindications include recent major surgery (10 days), history of GI hemorrhage, recent trauma, coagulopathy, advanced cerebrovascular disease, and diabetic hemorrhagic retinopathy.

Streptokinase and Urokinase

Currently, the choice of thrombolytic agent depends on the preference of the radiologist and cardiologist; many cardiologists seem to prefer *streptokinase* when the patient presents symptoms of pulmonary embolism and coronary artery thrombosis. The benefits of streptokinase therapy that are seen soon after acute myocardial infarction are maintained for at least 3 years,[7] according to a study from Germany that was published in 1991. Improvements in left ventricular function (both global and regional) are still apparent 3

▶ **Table 11–8**

INDICATIONS AND CONTRAINDICATIONS FOR THROMBOLYSIS

Indications	Contraindications
Coronary artery thrombosis	Active internal bleeding
Cerebral artery atherosclerosis	Recent (2 months) cerebrovascular accident
Atheromatous arterial plaque of the upper and lower limbs	Recent (2 months) intracranial or intraspinal surgery
Venous thrombosis	Intracranial neoplasm
Pulmonary embolism	Irreversible limb ischemia
Occlusion of bypass grafts	Recent trauma
	Coagulopathy
	Diabetic hemorrhagic retinopathy

years later in patients who receive streptokinase within 6 hours of the onset of an anterior myocardial infarction. For patients whose myocardial infarctions are inferior, however, streptokinase therapy gives only minor, insignificant benefits over short and long periods.[7]

Streptokinase is an antigenic protein of β-hemolytic streptococci and is associated with a wide range of antibodies. Almost all patients have some antibodies to streptococci, and much of the irregular dose response to systemic streptokinase therapy can be traced to neutralizing antibodies.

When combined with human plasminogen, streptokinase acts to form plasmin, which dissolves fibrin in the reparative framework and prevents the infection from being walled off.

Urokinase is more reliable than streptokinase, results in faster recanalization, and presents fewer complications. These factors outweigh the cost of urokinase, which is about six times greater than that of streptokinase. Unlike streptokinase, urokinase is a *nonantigenic*, proteolytic enzyme obtained from the kidneys of human embryos. It has a plasma half-life of 16 minutes, and because it is an *endogenous human protein*, it elicits no immune (allergic) response. It acts by converting *plasminogen* into *plasmin*, which breaks down *fibrin*, *fibrinogen*, and other plasma proteins in the clot.

When an infusion of urokinase is considered, the femoral puncture takes place on the unaffected side.

Leakage of blood at the catheter site can produce a large hematoma, which can compress the artery and further compromise blood flow.

To prepare 500,000 units of urokinase in 250 ml of 0.9% NaCl, the two vials of urokinase powder are mixed in 10 ml of sterile water, with 5 ml in each vial. Sterile water that has no preservatives is used to prevent microfilaments from forming in solution. The stream is directed against the inner walls of the vial in order to avoid foaming of the solution.

Before the reconstituted urokinase is added to the saline bottle, 10 ml of saline is withdrawn to ensure that it contains exactly 2000 units/ml.

In 1985, McNamara and Fischer described a method of urokinase infusion that has gained widespread popularity in the United States.[2] The infusion catheter is placed near the obstructing clot, and a straight guidewire is passed as far as possible into the thrombus. Urokinase (500,000 units in 200 ml of saline) is infused directly into proximal clot at a rate of 4000 units/min. The treatment response is checked every 2 hours via arteriography. Once there is restoration of retrograde flow, infusion is slowed to a rate of 1000 units/min. Infusion is stopped when the clot lyses, and the catheter is removed 1 hour after therapy with heparin and urokinase is discontinued (Fig. 11–15).

Table 11–9 lists some comparisons between streptokinase and urokinase.

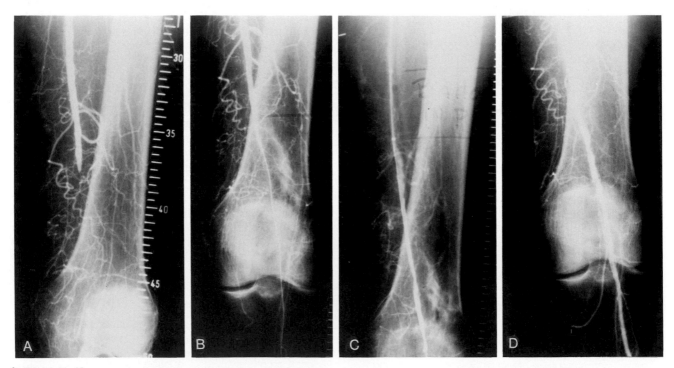

▶ **Figure 11–15**

A, Complete occlusion of the right superficial femoral artery in a 54-year-old man as demonstrated on a distal runoff. Note the corkscrew collateral vessels. *B,* The same patient after balloon angioplasty. *C,* The same patient 15 minutes after the infusion of urokinase (Abbokinase). *D,* The same patient 60 minutes after the infusion. Note the recanalization of the previously occluded area of the superficial femoral artery.

▶ **Table 11-9**

STREPTOKINASE VERSUS UROKINASE

Streptokinase	Urokinase
Foreign and antigenic protein	Human derived
Produces ill effects	No ill effects
Slightly pyrogenic	Nonpyrogenic
10- to 12-Minute half-life	11- to 16-Minute half-life
Higher fibrinolytic ratio	Lower fibrinolytic ratio
More hemorrhagic complications	Less hemorrhagic complications
Stable at room temperature	Must be stored at 4° C until use
Less expensive per unit	More expensive per unit (6 times)
Requires less quantity for low-dose local regimens	Requires 4 times more quantity for low-dose local regimens
Requires less quantity for systemic or IV regimens	Requires 3 to 4 times more quantity for systemic or IV regimens

IV = Intravenous.

Tissue Plasminogen Activator

One of the newer agents currently under study is tissue plasminogen activator (tPA). This material is an endogenous activator of plasminogen that was first prepared from human uterine tissue and is now being manufactured by biogenetic engineering techniques. Tissue plasminogen activator can be found in many tissues and activates plasminogen only in the presence of fibrin.

Although the use of tissue plasminogen is in its formative period, it has been suggested that it may be administered intra-arterially at the rate of 0.05 mg/kg/hr.

Infusion of Vasodilators

Patients with nonocclusive (stenotic) disease should be treated with intra-arterial infusion of vasodilatory drugs. The conditions that warrant treatment with vasodilators include vascular spasm and acute nonocclusive mesenteric ischemia. Many patients with ischemia also present with vasospasms. The infusion therapy opens up collateral pathways.

Several vasodilators are currently available for intra-arterial infusion, including phenoxybenzamine, tolazoline, diltiazem, prostaglandin E, Laevadosin (a mixture of adenosine diphosphate and triphosphate), and papaverine.

Embolectomy

Indications

Embolectomy is indicated when a massive pulmonary embolism is apparent. Catheter embolectomy is currently the preferred procedure when the patient's life is at stake. Catheter embolectomy (utilizing a special suction device) can be performed when the patient is in shock or in cardiopulmonary distress (Fig. 11-16).

Removal of Intravascular Foreign Bodies

Indications

Percutaneous intravascular intervention takes place when foreign bodies are present within the vascular system. A nonsurgical technique for the removal of intravascular foreign bodies was first introduced by Thomas in 1964. This technique described the removal of foreign bodies such as catheter and guidewire fragments, intravenous polyethylene catheters for central venous pressure measurements, and cardiac pacemaker wires. Intravenous polyethylene catheters introduced for parenteral feeding or central venous pressure monitoring account for the majority of intravascular foreign bodies (79.4%).[8] Foreign bodies frequently lodge in the right side of the heart or in major pulmonary branches. Patient mortality is extremely high in the absence of retrieval of the foreign body. Many types of catheters are utilized to extract the foreign body. Regardless of which catheter type is selected, great care must be taken to avoid further damage to the vascular walls (Fig. 11-17).

Forceful maneuvers during selective catheterization and faulty materials may produce fragmentation and detachment of the distal ends of guidewires. Repeated sterilization with ionizing radiation and chemical sterilization can cause structural changes in catheters and guidewires.

Dislodgment of Gianturco coils can occur during percutaneous embolotherapy.

Complications

The helical loop basket and guidewire snare usually do not present serious complications when used appropriately under fluoroscopic guidance. The multipurpose forceps, which is a three-pronged snare, is typically utilized for nonvascular interventional procedures and can present a significant risk when employed within the vascular system (Fig. 11-18).

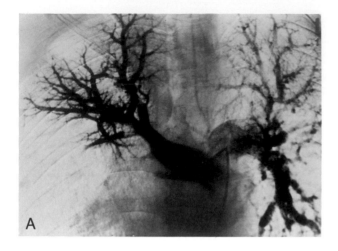

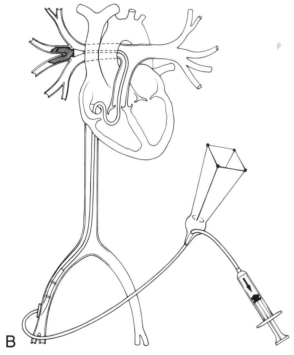

▶ **Figure 11–16**

A, Massive pulmonary embolism of the primary branch of the pulmonary artery supplying the right lower lung lobe in a 44-year-old man. This is an example of the type of embolism that might be treated by an embolectomy. *B,* This illustration describes a Greenfield suction cup and catheter that have been inserted by way of a surgical cut-down. Suction is usually applied with a 50-ml syringe in order to retrieve the thrombi.

Intraluminal Vascular Stents

In 1969, 5 years after he introduced transluminal angioplasty, Dotter described the application of coiled springs as *endovascular stents.* Although his theories produced some interest, little progress was made due to the emergence of transluminal angioplasty. It was not until 1982 that Maass expanded on Dotter's original idea and began to develop various materials that led to the development of a rough version of an *expandable* stent in 1985.

Even today, although in use, the vascular stent has a lot of room for refinement. Since Dotter's first use of a coil in 1963, vascular stents of different materials and unique shapes continue to evolve. Stents are employed following balloon angioplasty for the purpose of preventing restenosis. An adjunct to the vascular stent is the vascular graft, which is useful in older patients who have atherosclerotic aortic aneurysms and who are poor surgical candidates. Stents for nonvascular application continue to develop and are being quickly refined.

Indications

Vascular stents are designed to hold open stenotic blood vessels following unsuccessful angioplasty. Acute vessel restenosis can occur during or immediately after angioplasty. These abrupt arterial restenoses or reclosures may be the result of extensive dissection, which is frequently associated with spasm or thrombosis and elastic recoil. Abrupt restenosis occurs in 1 to 2% of peripheral angioplasties, and less extensive dissections occur at a rate of 4 to 5% during iliac angioplasty. Overall, restenosis occurs on an average of 25 to 75%, depending on the vessel being treated.

Stent technology will soon be undergoing Food and Drug Administration (FDA) clinical trials and is not approved for routine application. Most research that has been completed involves lesions of the iliac arteries. Other vessels under current study include the renal, coronary, and femoral arteries; the venae cavae; the portal veins; and other systemic veins.

Conditions such as the vena cava syndrome involve venous congestion, resulting in increased pressure to the venous system. Treatment of vena caval occlusion is often resistant to dilatation; thus, the stent appears to present a reasonable alternative, but much more investigation needs to be completed before conclusions can be drawn.

Research studies have produced favorable results on treatment of iliac lesions; however, as of this writing, adequate long-term results are not yet available. It is predicted that intravascular stenting will have application for patients with complex peripheral, coronary, and even vertebrobasilar and carotid occlusive disease.

Four types of vascular stent have dominated clinical trials: the Palmaz, Strecker, and Gianturco stents and the Schneider or Wallstent stent. The Palmaz and Strecker stents are balloon-expandable, whereas the Gianturco and Schneider stents are self-expanding. Further, the Palmaz and Gianturco stents are relatively rigid compared with the Strecker and Schneider stents, which retain some longitudinal flexibility.

Early results of iliac lesions utilizing the Palmaz stent revealed that 89% improved clinically initially. Improvement was maintained in 93% at 1 year and 86% at 2 years after installation. The Palmaz balloon-expandable intraluminal stent is the first permanent implant approved by the FDA (Fig. 11–19).

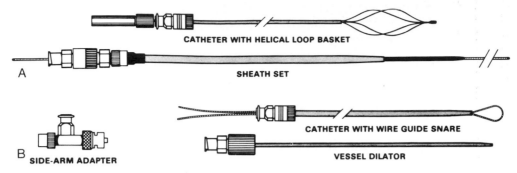

▶ **Figure 11–17**

A, The Dotter Intravascular Retriever Set. B, The Curry Intravascular Retriever Set. (A and B, Courtesy of Cook, Inc., Bloomington, IN.)

The Palmaz vascular stent is made of a single piece of·stainless-steel tubing with staggered rows of rectangular slots etched into the stent wall. The stent is mounted and crimped into an angioplasty balloon and is deployed at the desired site through a protective sheath that (following appropriate positioning) is withdrawn to expose the stent. The stent is 3 cm in length but shortens to 2 cm when fully expanded.[9] The Palmaz stent is deployed by inflation of the balloon, and the balloon is removed after deflation. Once expanded, the initial rectangular slots form diamond-shaped slots that are easily seen with fluoroscopy. The balloon may be inflated from 8 to 12 mm (Fig. 11–20).[10]

Complications

The complications associated with vascular stenting are associated with the delivery of the stent. Complications include hematoma, thromboembolytic episodes, extravasation, and puncture site pseudoaneurysms. The complication rate is expected to diminish with additional procedural experience of the radiologist combined with improvements in the technology of the delivery device.

Percutaneous Atherectomy

Transluminal devices have been developed for the purpose of disrupting or removing atheromatous plaque.

Simpson and Kensey are names given to two of several types of rotational atherectomy devices. The majority of these devices have been approved for atherectomy, but we consider these to be recanalization devices, because they generally do not function as stand-alone instruments for treatment of atheromatous disease.

Both the Simpson and Kensey atherectomy devices have received FDA approval, but the Simpson device has been used more frequently in clinical trials. Which device is better remains to be seen. Both have advantages and disadvantages that go beyond the scope of this text. The atherectomy devices are performed in conjunction with balloon angioplasty, which is performed following atherectomy.

Indications

The purpose of atherectomy is to debulk or remove as much atheromatous material as possible. Atherectomy usually precedes PTA.

Complications

In general, percutaneous mechanical atherectomy is a time-consuming, expensive procedure that has the potential risks of distal embolization and intimal perforation (Fig. 11–21).

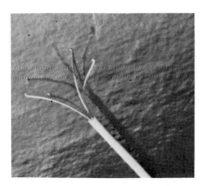

▶ **Figure 11–18**

MPF 20/55 multipurpose forceps. (From Snopek AM: Fundamentals of Radiographic Special Procedures, 3rd ed. Philadelphia, WB Saunders, 1992, p 348.)

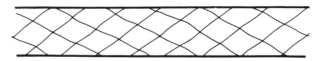

▶ **Figure 11–19**

An example of a vascular stent.

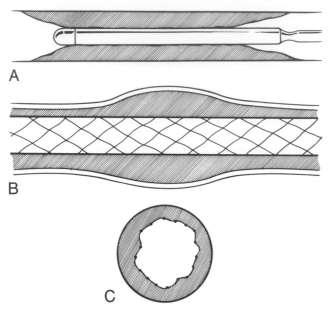

► **Figure 11–20**

A, The unexpanded stent is placed in a stenotic artery. *B,* The stent is mounted on an angioplasty catheter and expanded by inflation of the balloon. *C,* Once expanded, the catheter is withdrawn and the expanded stent remains in place, improving the cross-sectional diameter of the lumen.

Percutaneous Laser-Assisted Angioplasty

Atherosclerotic cardiovascular disease is the leading cause of death today in the United States and accounts for four of every 10 deaths. Treatment with pharmacologic agents has not been effective or permanent. Surgical intervention via an endarterectomy or vascular bypass has been the mainstay of therapy.

There are many types of laser systems designed for therapeutic application. Laser systems differ in wavelength and energy levels; whether they are pulsed or continuous; and in the amount of tissue penetration and interaction that they produce.[11]

Most recently, laser-assisted angioplasty, utilizing laser technology combined with optical fibers, has been integrated with percutaneous transluminal balloon angioplasty for the treatment of vascular atherosclerosis.

A laser can be described as a device that converts electromagnetic radiation (light) of varying frequencies into one or more separate frequencies of highly amplified and coherent radiation. The high-intensity, nearly monochromatic light output is essential for the laser's application to intravascular treatment of atherosclerosis. Optical fibers, combined with the laser

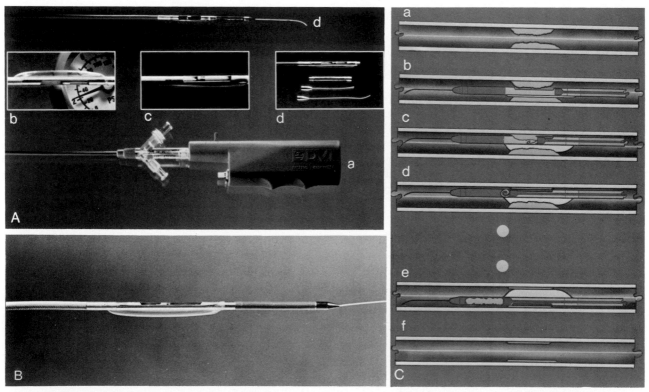

► **Figure 11–21**

A, The Simpson Peripheral AtheroCath. (a = motor drive unit, flush port and shaft; b = balloon, window, and pressure gauge; c = window, cutter, and balloon; d = flexible collection chamber and guidewire.) *B,* Close-up of a Simpson atherectomy catheter window, cutter, balloon, collection chamber, and guidewire. *C,* The Simpson atherectomy catheter technique. (a = stenotic blood vessel; b = the AtheroCath is near the lesion; the housing is positioned so that the atheromatous material protrudes toward the window of the housing; the balloon is inflated to 10 to 40 psi; c = the cutter is advanced; d = atheromas are excised; e = excised atheromas are captured inside the distal housing; f = recanalization of the blood vessel.) (*A, B,* and *C,* Courtesy of DVI, Inc., Redwood City, CA.)

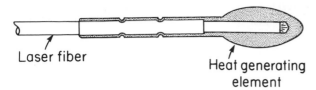

► Figure 11–22

The basic laser probe design. (From Topol E: Textbook of Interventional Cardiology. Philadelphia, WB Saunders, 1990.)

system and balloon angioplasty, have added a new dimension to the treatment of the atherosclerotic lesion. However, no laser system has been documented to have better initial or long-term patency rates than does balloon angioplasty alone.

Indications

Laser-assisted angioplasty is designed to treat atherosclerotic peripherovascular lesions and cardiovascular disease not successfully treated with conventional treatment methods. Specifically, laser-assisted angioplasty is used to treat areas of concentric and eccentric stenosis and occlusion that compromise or prevent blood flow to the body tissues (Fig. 11–22).

The laser is designed to *vaporize* plaque, improve initial patency rates, and reduce restenosis by debulking the lesion.

Complications

The complications of laser-assisted angioplasty are very similar to those of balloon angioplasty. With laser angioplasty, the patient may experience pain in the treatment area. Acute thrombosis and vascular spasm are possible. The most severe complication is vascular perforation, which is usually related to technical or human factors. Distal embolization is a potential risk for any form of laser application. Currently, the long-term effects of laser therapy are unknown.

► REFERENCES

1. Dondelinger RF, Rossi P, et al (eds): Interventional Radiology. New York, Thieme Medical Publishers, 1992.
2. Kadir S: Diagnostic Angiography. Philadelphia, WB Saunders, 1986.
3. Cassarella W: Percutaneous transluminal angioplasty below the knee: New techniques, excellent results. Radiology 169:271, 1988.
4. Collen D: On the regulation and control of fibrinolysis. Haemostasis 43:77, 1980.
5. McNamara TO and Fischer JR: Thrombolysis of peripheral arterial and graft occlusions: Improved results using high-dose urokinase. Am J Radiol 144:769, 1985.
6. Schwarten DE and Cutcliff W: Arterial occlusive disease below the knee with percutaneous transluminal angioplasty performed with low-profile catheters and steerable guide wires. Diagn Imaging 68:63, 1991.
7. Tillet WS, Johnson AJ, and McCarthy WF: The intravenous infusion of the streptococcal fibrinolytic principle (streptokinase) into patients. J Clin Invest 34:169, 1955.
8. Bloomfield DA: The nonsurgical retrieval of intracardiac foreign bodies: An international survey. Cathet Cardiovasc Diag 4:1, 1978.
9. Cope C, Burke D, and Meranze S: Interventional Radiology: Percutaneous Balloon Angioplasty. New York, Gower Medical Publishing, 1989.
10. Katzen BT: Refinements widen utility of interventional devices. Diagn Imaging 68:13, 1991.
11. Snopek AM: Fundamentals of Special Radiographic Procedures, 3rd ed. Philadelphia, WB Saunders, 1992.

► BIBLIOGRAPHY

Kandarpa K: Handbook of Cardiovascular and Interventional Radiologic Procedures. Boston, Little, Brown, 1989.
Tillet WS and Garner RL: The fibrinolytic activity of hemolytic streptococci. J Exp Med 58:485, 1933.
Vitello-Cecclu L: Thrombolytic therapy. J Cardiovascular Nurs 2:59, 1987.
Voth E, Tebbe U, Schicha H, et al: Intravenous streptokinase in acute myocardial infarction (I.S.A.M.) trial: Serial evaluation of left ventricular function up to 3 years after infarction estimated by radionuclide ventriculography. J Am Coll Cardiol 18:1610, 1991.
Wojotowycz M: Interventional Radiology and Angiography. Chicago, Year Book Medical Publishers, 1990.

► SELF-ASSESSMENT QUIZ

1. Nusbaum and Baum are noted for what achievement in interventional procedures?
   a. first to demonstrate GI bleeding in animals
   b. developed the coaxial catheter
   c. first to demonstrate a method of localizing a GI bleeding site via percutaneous angiography
   d. utilized transcatheter embolization in the treatment of GI bleeding

2. Who was responsible for the development of the double-sheath balloon dilatation catheter?
   a. Gruntzig and Hopff
   b. Dotter and Judkins
   c. Rastelli and Seldinger
   d. Nusbaum and Baum

3. The terms "native" and "modified" refer to
   a. liquid embolic media
   b. autologous embolic materials
   c. polymers
   d. silicone spheres

4. Polyvinyl alcohol (Ivalon) is what classification of embolic material?
   a. autologous
   b. absorbable
   c. nonabsorbable
   d. liquid

5. Which of the following are examples of liquid embolic media?

1. bucrylate
2. silicone
3. absolute ethanol
4. barium sulfate
   a. 1 only
   b. 1 and 2
   c. 1, 2, and 3
   d. 1, 2, 3, and 4

6. Which of the following is an example of a "permanent" embolic medium?
   a. fascia lata
   b. Avitene
   c. Oxycel
   d. coils

7. Surgical gelatin sponge is otherwise known as
   a. aminocaproic acid (Amicar)
   b. Oxycel
   c. Avitene
   d. Gelfoam

8. Avitene is most related to which term(s) below?
   a. Oxycel
   b. aminocaproic acid (Amicar)
   c. microfibrillar collagen
   d. Gelfoam

9. Tachotop is a nonabsorbable particulate material?
   a. true
   b. false

10. What is the major disadvantage of a hot contrast medium when used as an embolic agent?
   a. very expensive
   b. very painful for the patient
   c. opacifies poorly
   d. short-lasting

11. What is meant by intermittent claudication?
   a. the length of time that it takes to embolize a blood vessel
   b. aneurysmal dilatation of a blood vessel
   c. lower limb pain during exercise and pain relief during rest
   d. the flushing of a catheter with a heparinized solution

12. Percutaneous transluminal angioplasty
   a. has a low complication rate
   b. has a moderate complication rate
   c. has a high complication rate
   d. is comparable in cost to surgery

13. Streptokinase and urokinase are pharmacologic agents used with what interventional procedure?
   a. electrocoagulation
   b. laser angioplasty
   c. foreign body extraction
   d. intravascular thrombolysis

14. Which thrombolytic agent is prepared from human uterine tissue?
   a. streptokinase
   b. urokinase
   c. tissue plasminogen activator
   d. fascia lata

15. Simpson and Kensey are names given to two of the most commonly utilized _____ devices.
   a. thrombolytic
   b. laser-assisted angioplasty
   c. atherectomy
   d. embolectomy

16. What is the name of the procedure that is described as a mechanical method of stopping abnormal blood flow in arteries?
   a. atherectomy
   b. percutaneous angioplasty
   c. intravascular thrombolysis
   d. transcatheter embolization

17. Which of the following complications are part of the postembolization syndrome?
1. fever
2. leukocytosis
3. discomfort
   a. 1 only
   b. 1 and 2 only
   c. 3 only
   d. 1, 2, and 3

18. Avitine is
   a. microfibrillar bovine collagen
   b. a product of fetal uterine tissue
   c. prepared from equine collagen
   d. a product of human urine

19. Arterial infusion of vasopressin has been used in the treatment of
   a. carotid artery stenosis
   b. renal hyperplasia
   c. GI hemorrhage
   d. iliac stenosis

20. The terms high pressure and low profile pertain to
   a. types of embolic media
   b. balloon catheters
   c. thrombolytic agents
   d. laser angioplasty

▶ STUDY QUESTIONS

1. What are the implications of "nontarget" embolization?

2. List at least four factors that are important when selecting an embolizing agent or material.

3. Select 10 embolic materials from the list in Table 11–3, and list one advantage and disadvantage for each.

4. Explain how stainless-steel coils (occluding spring emboli) are introduced into the intravascular target site.

5. What is the purpose of chemoembolization agents?

6. What is the primary advantage of electrocoagulation when used with transcatheter embolization?

7. What is vasopressin, and what is its action on the vascular system? For what pathologic conditions are vasopressin indicated?

8. Describe some of the advantages and disadvantages of PTA.

9. Compare streptokinase and urokinase. What are the indications and contraindications of each agent?

10. Describe two types of foreign bodies that may result from a vascular interventional procedure.

► CHAPTER TWELVE

► NONVASCULAR INTERVENTIONAL PROCEDURES

► CHAPTER OBJECTIVES

Upon completion of Chapter 12 the technologist will be able to:

1. List and describe the indications for percutaneous needle biopsy
2. Describe the indications for percutaneous abscess drainage
3. List those diseases and conditions of the hepatobiliary system that are examined via endoscopy
4. List and describe the indications for percutaneous nephrostomy
5. Describe patient preparation protocol for nonvascular interventional procedures
6. List the primary contraindications for percutaneous needle biopsy, endoscopic biliary procedures, and percutaneous nephrostomy

▶ PERCUTANEOUS NEEDLE BIOPSY

Percutaneous needle biopsy provides the shortest, simplest, and least invasive approach to a cytologic or histologic diagnosis.

Guidance by fluoroscopy, ultrasound, or computed tomography (CT) defines the most accessible route and verifies the position of the needle tip within the lesion. The use of magnetic resonance imaging (MRI) in percutaneous biopsy must still be determined.

Percutaneous needle biopsy has been performed for many years utilizing fluoroscopy. Angiography has the disadvantage of not being able to exactly locate and describe the extent of a tumor. It was not until the invention of CT and ultrasound that it was possible to produce cross-sectional images of pathologic processes that allowed the physician to safely locate and take a biopsy of many types of lesions.

Fluoroscopy is an inexpensive and quick method of localization for chest and bone biopsies. The only real risk is exposure to radiation.

Real-time ultrasound is currently the preferred method of localization, because it does not present any radiation hazards and is the most cost-effective means of needle-to-lesion guidance. Most abdominal lesions can be visualized well enough with ultrasound to allow precise needle placement.

CT must first be used to scan the area of interest and locate the lesion. Usually four or five images are taken during this procedure, which takes longer to complete than does ultrasound. This may be a disadvantage in the case of a patient who is ill.

MRI technology continues to increase its applications. From the beginning, MRI was able to image brain pathology better than any other modality; thus, methods have been developed in which MRI stereotaxic systems are employed. The development of nonferromagnetic needles made it possible to perform needle biopsies under MRI control. At approximately the year 2000, MRI is expected to surpass computed tomography for needle biopsy of brain lesions.

Indications

Percutaneous needle biopsy is used to confirm the presence and extent of a lesion or disease process that cannot be diagnosed by other noninvasive methods. These disease processes can be neoplastic or inflammatory, or they can represent infections. Differentiation of benign and malignant lesions by way of a biopsy can clearly identify the treatment plan of choice. Decisions regarding surgery, radiation therapy, and chemotherapy can be made using the information provided by needle biopsy.

With several imaging choices for needle localization, a biopsy can be taken at almost any site in the body. Lesions found in the chest, abdomen (organs), or brain can be investigated without surgical intervention. Percutaneous needle biopsy has an extremely high success rate in the diagnosis of abdominal epithelial lesions. Table 12–1 lists the indications, contraindications, and complications of percutaneous needle biopsy.

Contraindications

There are several contraindications of the needle biopsy procedure. One contraindication is when a vascular lesion, such as a hemangioma, is present. Any vascular lesion presents the potential of hemorrhage. This does not mean that needle biopsies of vascular lesions are not done, but that diagnosis of this particular lesion can be made solely with MRI, CT, and sonographic imaging, thus reducing the risks usually encountered with needle biopsy. A vascular lesion can also be confirmed with a technetium red blood cell (RBC) study (nuclear medicine) in which the hemangioma shows slow uptake but prolonged radionuclide accumulation.

Patients with severe pulmonary hypertension have an increased risk of bleeding. Patients with abnormal coagulopathy should not be considered for needle biopsy—for example, in the case of a patient with a

▶ Table 12–1

INDICATIONS AND CONTRAINDICATIONS FOR AND COMPLICATIONS OF PERCUTANEOUS NEEDLE BIOPSY

Indications	Contraindications	Complications
Neoplastic lesions	Vascular lesions	Hemorrhage
Abdomen	Pulmonary hypertension	Infection
Lymph nodes	Coagulopathy	Bile leakage
Chest	Cystic lesions with malignant potential	Pneumothorax
Pelvis	Pneumothorax	Hemoptysis (lung biopsy)
Brain	Bone tumors	Air embolism
Inflammation		Tumor seeding
Infection		

prothrombin time (PT) that is prolonged by 3 seconds or more or in whom the platelet count is less than 100,000/mm^3.

A biopsy should not be taken of a cystic lesion with a potential for malignancy because of tumor seeding into adjacent tissues.

Pneumothorax is a complication of chest biopsies and of liver biopsies that are near the dome of the diaphragm.

Percutaneous bone biopsy is usually contraindicated when primary bone tumors of the extremities are suspected. Tumor seeding is the greatest concern, especially in the presence of a primary malignant bone disease (see Table 12–1).

Biopsy Needle Selection

To date, more than 40 biopsy needles are available for percutaneous biopsy. Despite the types available, the final choice lies with the radiologist.

Biopsy needles have undergone significant improvement during the last 10 years. Until recently, the needles were quite large, and needles with a 14- to 18-gauge were not uncommon. Currently, 20- to 22-gauge needles are being utilized for biopsy as well as for fluid aspiration.

As with many types of equipment, both advantages and disadvantages exist. The larger the needle, the larger the specimen obtained, and the greater the potential for increased trauma and complication. The tips may be beveled, pencil- or diamond-shaped, blunt, hooked, spiraled, notched, or trephined (Fig. 12–1).

The needle that is chosen will depend somewhat on the method of placement and on the recovery of a specimen. Many variables are involved, and small samples are obtained. Multiple samples are usually necessary to obtain an accurate diagnosis. The choice of needle may be determined by the type and location of the lesion.

Complications

With the progress of biopsy needle science, morbidity is very low, mainly because of the decrease in the cross-sectional diameter, the sharp tip, and the disposability factor (one-time use). A disposable needle has the sharpest end possible and almost eliminates cross-contamination.

The latest current published mortality rate for percutaneous biopsy is 0.008%. The usual cause of death is a hemorrhage.

Whenever an invasive procedure is performed, there is always a chance of infection. A percutaneous needle biopsy is no exception. Although infection is a rare occurrence, it is recommended that, whenever possible, the path of the biopsy should not traverse the colon.

Bile leakage is a risk whenever a liver biopsy is performed. When this does occur, the patient presents with symptoms of peritonitis that have to be corrected with biliary decompression.

Pneumothorax is a potential complication whenever a biopsy crosses the pleural space, especially in lesions near the dome of the liver.

Hemoptysis is a primary complication of lung biopsy. The location of the biopsy is highly influential in the development of hemoptysis. This finding is more common when the lesion is more central than periph-

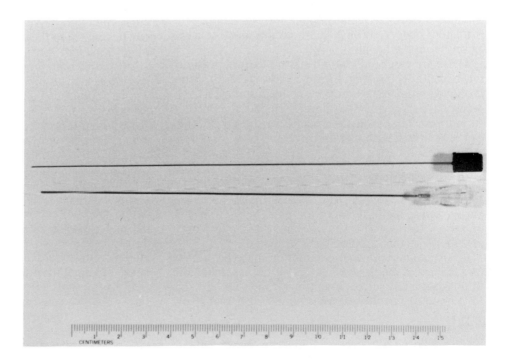

▶ **Figure 12–1**

Small-gauge biopsy needles.

eral, such as with lesions of the mediastinum. Incidence is rare.

Air embolism is a rare complication that can occur when needle placement is in a major central vessel. This is the reason why the needle hub should always be occluded if the central stylet has been removed from the needle.

Tumor seeding is most common in bone biopsy and is not usually a factor in a biopsy of the chest or abdomen (see Table 12–1).

Procedures

Lung Biopsy

Percutaneous transthoracic needle biopsy is a safe and conclusive method for the diagnosis and management of pulmonary nodules and masses.

Fine-needle biopsy of lung lesions can be accomplished with fluoroscopy, ultrasound, or CT guidance. Before the procedure is begun, the exact location of the lesion should be identified on chest x-ray films, tomograms, or CT scans. The patient rarely requires premedication.

The specific techniques of percutaneous lung biopsy have been described by many individuals during the last several years. However, these methods are selected according to the physician's preference and are beyond the scope of this text. An example of a technique of lung biopsy is shown in Figure 12–2 *A* through *F*. An example of percutaneous needle biopsy of a lung lesion utilizing CT guidance is described in Figure 12–3*A* and *B*.

Hemorrhage and pneumothorax are the most common complications that occur, and severe life-threatening situations are rare. Most complications are managed quite successfully. If the needle biopsy is being performed on an outpatient basis, the patient is usually observed for 2 to 3 hours before being released from the hospital.

There are essentially no absolute contraindications for percutaneous lung biopsy. Patients with compromised pulmonary function, coagulation disorders, pulmonary hypertension, and advanced age present an increased risk, but the benefits of the procedures usually outweigh the risks.

Mediastinal Biopsy

Many diseases involve the mediastinum, both primarily and secondarily. As with lung biopsy, a review of x-rays (especially the overpenetrated chest film) and scans by the radiologists is essential.

CT is capable of producing better anatomic details and images of mediastinal and hilar masses than plain film radiography and conventional tomography. This technique of needle biopsy is similar to that of lung biopsy.

The complications encountered in mediastinal biopsy are similar to those found in lung biopsy— namely, pneumothorax and hemorrhage. These findings can be confirmed following withdrawal of the biopsy needle and a repeat CT scan.

Bone Biopsy

Percutaneous bone biopsy was first utilized in the 1930s in the aspiration of bone marrow. The applications of bone biopsy have been expanded to include investigation of patients with osteomyelitis and metabolic bone disorders. Most recently, bone biopsy has included the harvesting of suspected metastatic lesions, especially lytic lesions that are present in the pelvic region. Conventional radiography is utilized for location and for the approach route of the needle. CT is useful when the lesion cannot be identified using conventional radiography.

There are no absolute contraindications for percutaneous bone biopsy. Pain is the most common and important complication. Tumor seeding is not a typical complication with this procedure.

Biopsy of Abdominal Viscera

Percutaneous needle biopsy of the abdominal viscera most frequently involves the pancreas and the liver. Many guidance methods are possible, including fluoroscopy, ultrasound, combined fluoroscopy and ultrasound, CT, and, most recently, MRI. Percutaneous sampling of solid tumors is the primary indication for needle biopsy. Figure 12–4 shows a 66-year-old male patient with a biopsy needle placed percutaneously into the tail of the pancreas under CT guidance.

▶ PERCUTANEOUS ABSCESS DRAINAGE

Advances in diagnostic and interventional cardiovascular radiology have made possible procedures that can be applied to the management of diseases in many other organs of the body.

Untreated abdominal abscesses may have a mortality rate as high as 80% when left untreated, despite the use of antibiotics. Traditional surgical treatment has an associated mortality rate of between 20 and 43%.

Although CT and ultrasound are utilized with the evaluation, diagnosis, and treatment of most abdominal lesions, conventional radiography (with or without contrast media) remains a method of preliminary investigation. Procedures such as an upper gastrointestinal series and intravenous urography are used to detect fluid collections in the abdomen. The KUB or flat plate, upright, and decubitus positions of the abdomen often reveal a soft tissue mass or possibly an air-fluid interface that can have an impact on the position of adjacent organs and structures.

Conventional radiography, however, has its limitations. It is not sensitive enough to detect subtle signs of abscesses because of its limitations in differentiating soft tissue densities. In addition, specific changes taking place in the postoperative patient will

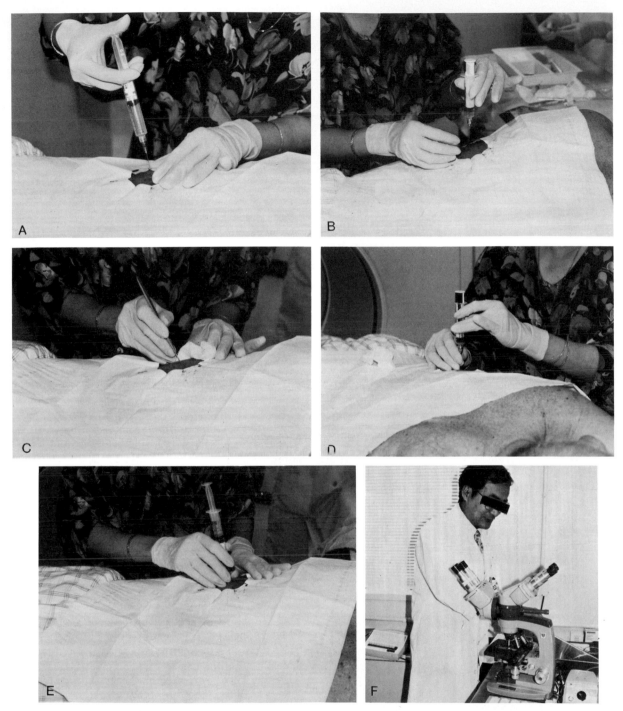

► **Figure 12-2**

An example of a percutaneous biopsy technique. *A,* Following a computed tomography scan and localization, the biopsy area is marked, prepared, and anesthetized. *B,* Deep infiltration of a localizing anesthetic agent. *C,* With a scalpel, a small area is exposed to facilitate needle puncture and passage. *D,* With the patient in a prone position, a biopsy needle and syringe are passed percutaneously into the suspected lesions. *E,* The specimen is aspirated. *F,* A pathology specimen is examined immediately by the pathologist to determine the quality of the specimen.

often obscure the presence of abdominal abscesses. Thus, conventional radiography is used as an adjunct to CT and ultrasound, but the latter methods are the most informative and accurate for an evaluation of abscess cavities.

The use of cross-sectional imaging procedures al-
lows for the accurate detection of abscess formations as well as for the drainage of these fluid-filled lesions. CT scanning and ultrasound provide accurate guidance of the needle or catheter into the abscess cavity and are associated with a success rate of between 80 and 85%. In addition to CT and ultrasound, radionu-

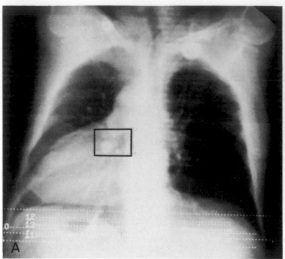
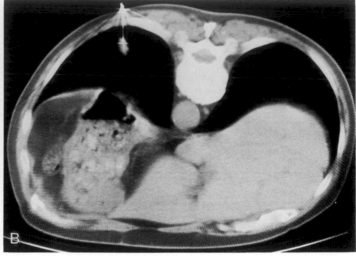

► **Figure 12–3**

A, A scout computed tomography (CT) image of a solid lung tumor. *B,* Using CT guidance, a biopsy needle is passed percutaneously through the lung and into the lesion.

clide scanning utilizing ^{67}Ga and ^{111}In-labeled leuko-cytes is frequently used for localization of abscess cavities.

Indications

Any abscess located in the abdomen or pelvis that cannot be approached by simple incision and drainage may be approached by the use of catheters. Table 12–2 lists the indications, contraindications, and complications of percutaneous abscess drainage.

Contraindications

The radiologist must avoid traumatizing vascular structures when manipulating aspiration instruments. Severe coagulopathy is a relative contraindication to catheter placement (see Table 12–2).

Complications

Infection, peritoneal spillage, and shock are possible complications (see Table 12–2).

Procedures

The Menghini aspiration biopsy set and the Sachs-Elecath one-step fluid drainage kit are two examples of the type of equipment used for percutaneous drainage of fluid collections (Figs. 12–5 and 12–6).

Figure 12–7 shows an ultrasound examination of a 19-year-old female patient who presented with pain in the lower anterior abdomen. Longitudinal and transverse images revealed a 9-cm mass (abscess) in the pelvis superior to the urinary bladder. Several hundred milliliters of pus were aspirated.

Figure 12–8*A* is a CT scout image of the abdomen of a 48-year-old man who presented with abdominal pain and a low-grade fever. This image reveals positive contrast material in the colon and urinary system. The left lower ureter appears to be displaced by a space-occupying lesion that was determined to be a flank abscess. Figure 12–8*B* shows the presence of a 10.3-French pigtail catheter positioned within the abscess cavity and attached to suction. Figure 12–8*C* reveals a CT image following suction and drainage of

► **Figure 12–4**

Percutaneous needle puncture of the tail of the pancreas utilizing guidance with computed tomography scanning.

▶ Table 12–2

INDICATIONS, CONTRAINDICATIONS, AND COMPLICATIONS OF PERCUTANEOUS ABSCESS DRAINAGE

Indications	Contraindications	Complications
Intraperitoneal and intrathoracic fluid collections	Noncooperative patient Coagulopathy Infected tumors and hematomas	Infection Peritoneal spillage Shock

the abscess. The size of the abscess is considerably reduced.

Figure 12–9A and B represents a study of a 58-year-old woman who had pain in her right leg and back and who also was constipated. Drainage of a retroperitoneal abscess was required. After percutaneous puncture, the puncture site was progressively dilated with a series of dilating catheters so that a No. 14 French catheter could be introduced. A sump catheter was introduced into the abscess, and 750 ml of purulent brownish material was aspirated. Some diluted positive contrast was irrigated into the abscess and revealed an abscess cavity that extended down into the iliopsoas region and up to the posterior perinephric region. The catheter was fixed to the skin using an ostomy disk and tape and was attached to a bulb syringe for drainage.

Figure 12–10A and B shows a CT scan and upper gastrointestinal series of a man with an acute pancreatic abscess that was causing stenosis of the duodenum and the abdominal wall.

Figure 12–11A through D represents four images of a localized collection of air under the right hemidiaphragm, with air-fluid levels representing a loculated subdiaphragmatic abscess.

▶ ENDOSCOPIC AND PERCUTANEOUS MANAGEMENT OF BILIARY DISEASE

Endoscopic procedures have emerged during the last 20 years in the diagnosis and treatment of biliary and pancreatic disease. For many years, percutaneous transhepatic cholangiography (PTHC) was the mainstay for biliary procedures. A combination of endoscopic retrograde cholangiopancreatography (ERCP) and cross-sectional imaging (using CT) has created a better method of biliary intervention. Fine-needle PTHC has been applied in patients with obstructive jaundice and to determine the resectability of neoplasms.

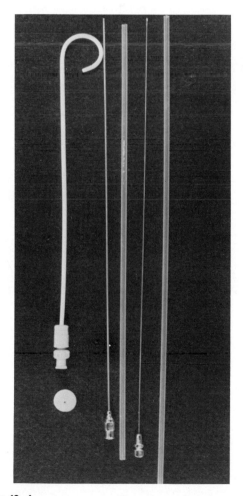

▶ Figure 12–6

An Elecath One-Step Fluid Drainage kit. (Courtesy of Electro-Catheter Corp., Rahway, NJ.)

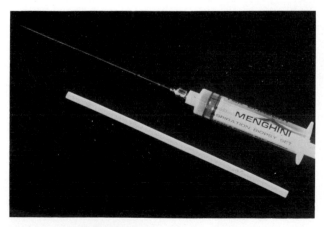

▶ Figure 12–5

A Menghini aspiration biopsy set.

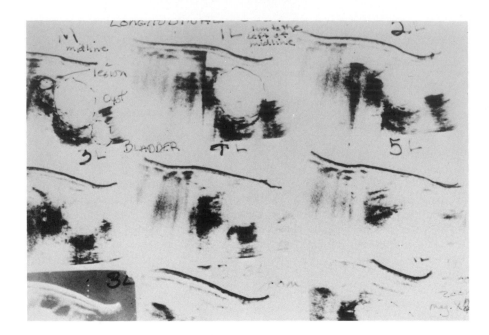

▸ **Figure 12–7**
An ultrasound examination of the abdomen demonstrating a 9-cm pelvic mass (abscess) that is located superior to the urinary bladder.

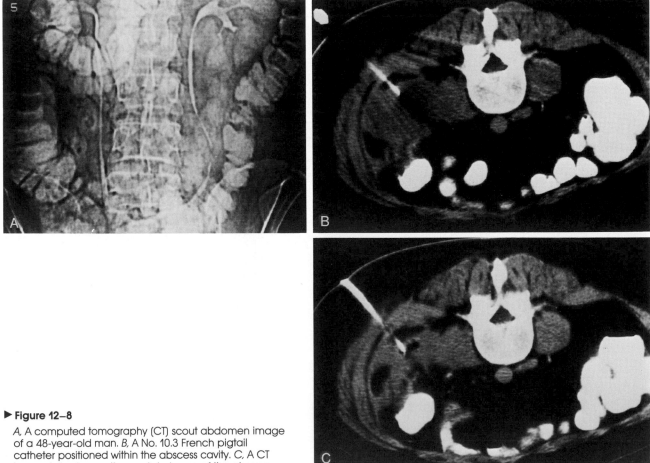

▸ **Figure 12–8**
A, A computed tomography (CT) scout abdomen image of a 48-year-old man. B, A No. 10.3 French pigtail catheter positioned within the abscess cavity. C, A CT image following suction and drainage of the abscess.

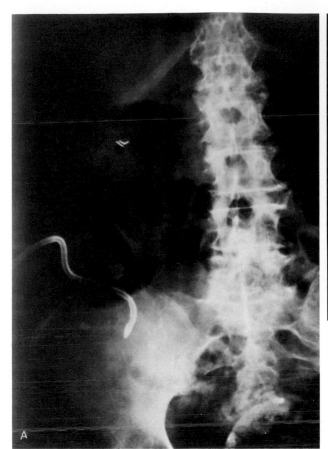

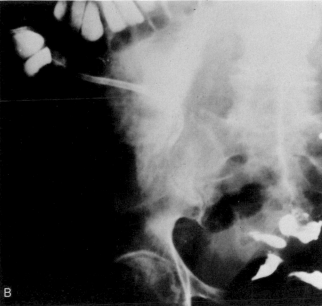

► **Figure 12–9**
A and *B,* Before and after drainage of a retroperitoneal abscess.

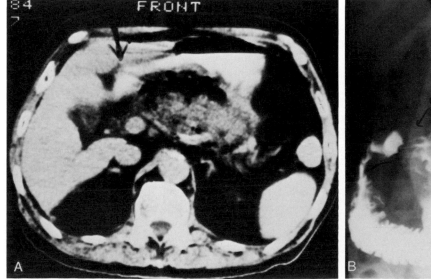

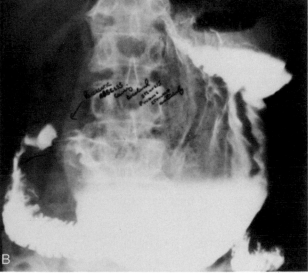

► **Figure 12–10**
A and *B,* A computed tomography scan and an upper gastrointestinal series of a man with an acute pancreatic abscess.

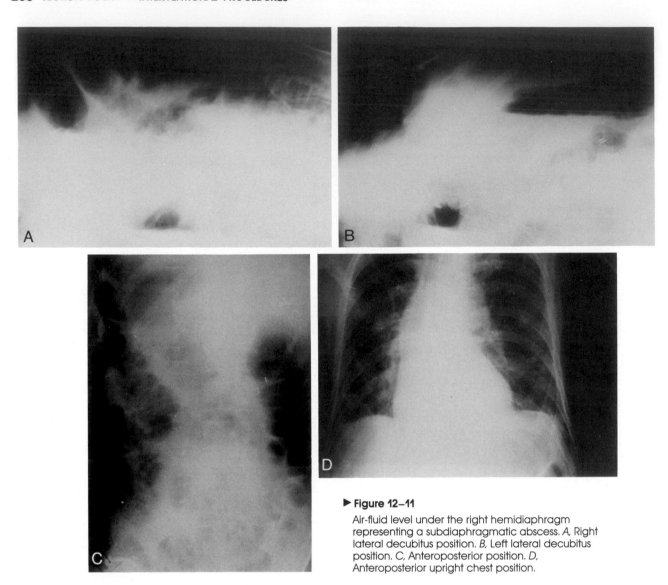

▶ **Figure 12–11**

Air-fluid level under the right hemidiaphragm representing a subdiaphragmatic abscess. *A,* Right lateral decubitus position. *B,* Left lateral decubitus position. *C,* Anteroposterior position. *D,* Anteroposterior upright chest position.

Indications and Contraindications

Table 12–3 lists the indications, contraindications, and complications for endoscopic and percutaneous management of biliary disease.

Although the specific techniques of PTHC and ERCP are beyond the scope of this text, the patient is usually in the supine position. Guidance in most cases is provided by fluoroscopy. The actual site of needle puncture depends on individual factors, such as obstructive lung disease and the size of the liver. Periodic injections of an iodinated contrast medium are done to determine flow patterns.

Complications

Complications of endoscopic and percutaneous management of biliary disease include infection, cholangitis, biliary peritonitis, and hemorrhage (see Table

12–3). Figure 12–12 shows the normal anatomy of the bile and pancreatic ducts by way of ERCP.

Figure 12–13 is a PTHC of a 65-year-old man with multifocal hepatobiliary pancreatic disease. The common bile duct is obstructed and dilated. The hepatic structures are dilated and irregular, suggesting fibrosis. There is an irregularly noted pancreatic duct (*arrow*).

Figure 12–14 shows a 56-year-old woman with severe abdominal pain and abnormal serum amylase. An ERCP revealed a markedly irregular pancreatic duct. She was diagnosed with acute pancreatitis.

Figure 12–15*A* and *B* shows a 66-year-old man with a common bile duct obstruction. Figure 12–15*A* demonstrates early filling of the biliary tree by way of PTHC. Figure 12–15*B* demonstrates the obstruction in a later filling image.

Palliative drainage for malignancy can be accomplished by way of a percutaneous transhepatic puncture and by the addition of a permanent stent

► Table 12–3

INDICATIONS, CONTRAINDICATIONS, AND COMPLICATIONS OF ENDOSCOPIC AND PERCUTANEOUS
MANAGEMENT OF BILIARY DISEASE

Indications	Contraindications	Complications
Obstructive jaundice	Bleeding disorders	Infection
Choledocholithiasis	Contrast media sensitivity	Cholangitis
Malignant strictures	Known hepatic vascular tumors or malformations	Biliary peritonitis
Tumor biopsy		Hemorrhage
Biliary drainage		
Stone extraction		
Stent placement		
Detection of congenital malformations		

placed into the bile duct. Figure 12–16 shows a patient
with a bile duct malignancy. Note the presence of a
stent tube.

Figure 12–17A and B shows a 73-year-old man with
an occlusion of the common bile duct in two areas. A
PTHC was performed with a double catheter placement draining two separate areas of the biliary system. Figure 12–17A shows the position of the catheter drainage system in the mid-axillary region.
Figure 12–17B shows the position of the second catheter.

Most tumors that are found within the biliary tree
produce an obstruction by ductal compression. Short,
irregular biliary strictures are seen on most bile duct
and pancreatic carcinomas.

Figure 12–18 shows a 69-year-old man who has a
complete occlusion of the common bile duct with
dilatation of the biliary system. He presented with a
history of squamous cell carcinoma at the base of his
tongue and a new primary hepatocellular carcinoma
(hepatoma) with metastatic involvement (trans-
colemic spread). This man had a history of alcohol

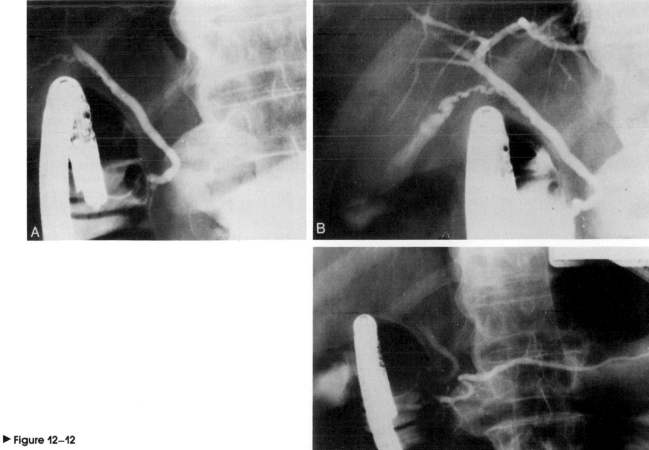

► Figure 12–12

A to C, Normal biliary and pancreatic anatomy via an
endoscopic retrograde chloangiopancreatography
(ERCP) procedure.

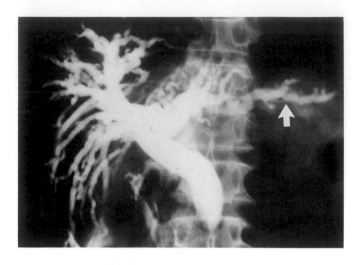

▶ **Figure 12–13**

Multifocal hepatobiliary obstructive disease and an abnormal pancreatic duct (*arrow*) suggesting fibrosis.

abuse and had smoked most of his adult life. A 23-gauge Chiba needle was inserted into the right axillary region. A No. 7 French catheter was passed over the appropriate guidewire.

Calculi usually appear as persistent filling defects on multiple films and often present irregular or faceted shapes. The presence of polypoid tumors and blood clots can make the diagnosis more difficult.

Figure 12–19 shows a PTHC, spot-film series revealing the presence of several large, radiolucent gallstones in an occluded common bile duct. This male patient is 57 years old.

▶ PERCUTANEOUS MANAGEMENT OF URINARY DISEASE

Percutaneous nephrostomy was first performed in 1954 by Wickblom, who utilized percutaneous puncture of the renal pelvis for antegrade pyelography. In 1955, Goodwin and Casey performed the first therapeutic procedure when they drained obstructed kidneys and gained access to the renal collecting system.

Percutaneous nephrostomy is indicated for most pathologies that result in obstructive hydronephrosis. In response to ureteral strictures, stents may be placed within the ureter on a temporary or permanent basis. Stricture dilatation and stent placement have added a new dimension to urologic treatment.

The large percentage of kidney stones (nephrolithiasis) are passed by way of the urinary tract. Approximately 40% require additional intervention, which until now indicated surgery (pyelolithotomy). Nephrostomy for stone removal was first performed in 1976. Since then, extracorporeal shock-wave lithotripsy and nephrostomy have replaced surgery as the primary treatment for kidney stones that are not passed.

Indications, Contraindications, and Complications

Table 12–4 lists the indications, contraindications, and complications of percutaneous management of urinary disease. Figure 12–20 is representative of a patient who has been prepared for a nephrostomy procedure. A nephrostomy tube placement with rotating disk is shown. Figures 12–21 and 12–22 are two examples of ureteral stent sets.

Stone extraction is another important function of

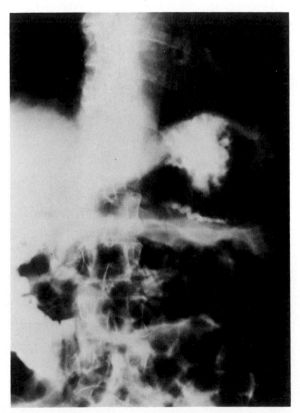

▶ **Figure 12–14**

Acute pancreatitis demonstrated on this endoscopic retrograde cholangiopancreatography (ERCP) study.

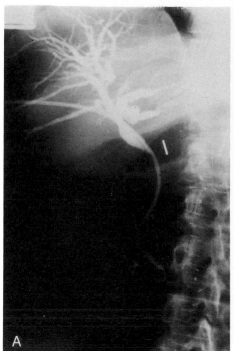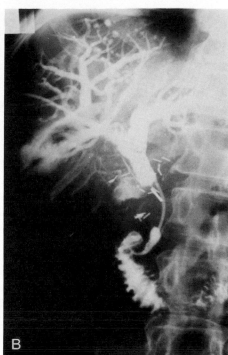

A

B

► **Figure 12–15**

A common bile duct obstruction. *A,* Early filling of the biliary tree via percutaneous transhepatic cholangiography. *B,* Later filming of the biliary tree.

the percutaneous nephrostomy technique. Stones are removed percutaneously using direct vision by endoscopy or by fluoroscopy. Figure 12–23*A* illustrates one type of retrieval catheter. This is a basket stone retrieval catheter with a three-prong grasping forceps. Baskets and flexible forceps are available in various formats and sizes for stone extraction. The basket must be large enough to accommodate the stone easily yet must be small enough to fully open when placed in the region of the stone. The advantage of baskets is that they are relatively atraumatic and can

be used for removal of stones both in the collecting system and in the entire ureter.

In Figure 12–23*B*, note the configuration of the distal end of the grasping forceps. The catheter is advanced to the location of the stone. The grasping forceps is advanced over the stone. The wire is then retracted back into the catheter. As this takes place, the wire basket closes over and captures the stone. The forceps is then retracted further so that the captured stone is held in place while the catheter is being removed. After the stone has been extracted, a ureteral stent is often inserted to assist in the drainage of fluid from the kidney.

Stones and ureteral strictures often produce obstruction and subsequent hydronephrosis. The following examples attempt to further illustrate the uses of percutaneous nephrostomy. Figure 12–24 is an example of percutaneous antegrade nephrostomy. This is a study of a 57-year-old man with an obstructing lesion in the proximal one third of the right ureter. The renal pelvis is hydronephrotic, and an obstructing calculus was removed via cystoscopy. A stent was inserted until the ureter was able to function normally.

Figure 12–25 shows a 62-year-old man with a history of liver cancer. A percutaneous nephrostomy was performed on the right kidney. Note the presence of a stent tube in the common bile duct. Ductal metastases were also present.

Figure 12–26*A* shows a 66-year-old man with an obstructive disease of the right ureter. Spot views reveal the presence of a contrast medium filling the renal pelvis and proximal ureter via a right percu-

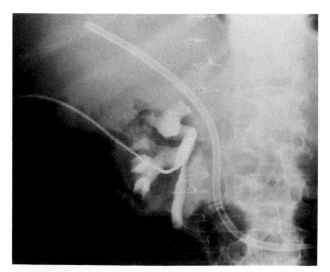

► **Figure 12–16**

Metastatic disease of the common bile duct with stent placement.

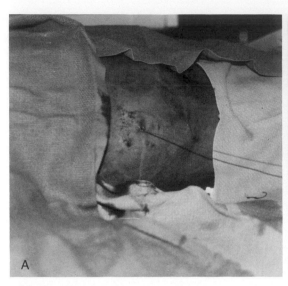
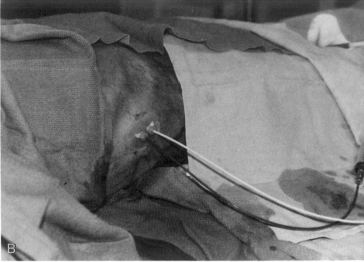

▶ **Figure 12–17**

A commmon bile duct occlusion in two separate areas of the duct. *A,* Catheter position. *B,* Position of the second catheter.

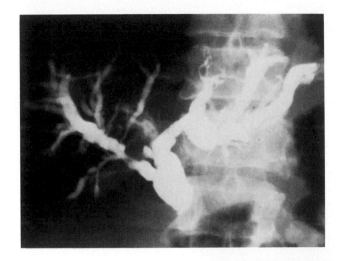

▶ **Figure 12–18**

A complete occlusion of the common bile duct.

▶ **Figure 12–19**

A spot film image of a percutaneous transhepatic cholangiogram revealing the presence of several large filling defects that represent radiolucent gallstones in an occluded common bile duct.

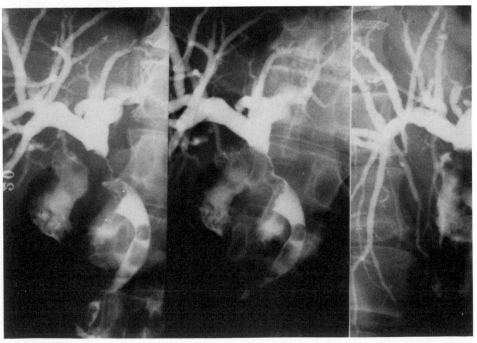

► **Table 12–4**

INDICATIONS, CONTRAINDICATIONS, AND COMPLICATIONS OF PERCUTANEOUS MANAGMENT OF URINARY DISEASE

Indications	Contraindications	Complications
Obstructive disease	Contrast media sensitivity	General anesthesia
Nephrolithiasis	Hypertension	Surgical intervention
Ureteral stricture	Vascular malformation	Hemorrhage
Renal drainage	Hemorrhagic disorders	Infection
Renal cyst aspiration	Endotoxic shock (septicemia with highly viscous pus)	Contrast media sensitivity
Ureteral fistulas and urinomas		
Male infertility studies		

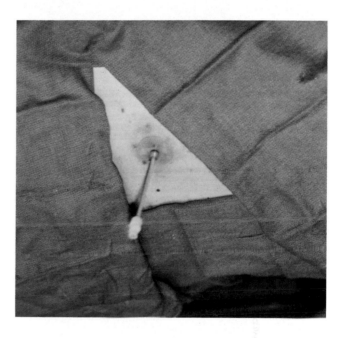

► **Figure 12–20**
A patient prepared for percutaneous nephrostomy.

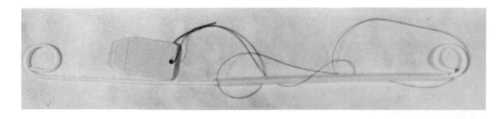

► **Figure 12–21**
A ureteral stent set.

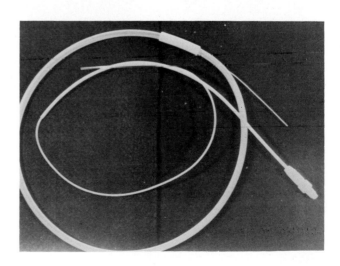

► **Figure 12–22**
A ureteral stent introducer.

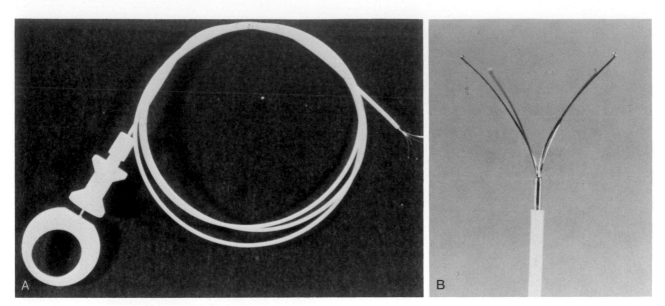

▶ **Figure 12–23**

Stone extraction. *A,* Basket stone retrieval catheter. *B,* The distal end of a grasping forceps.

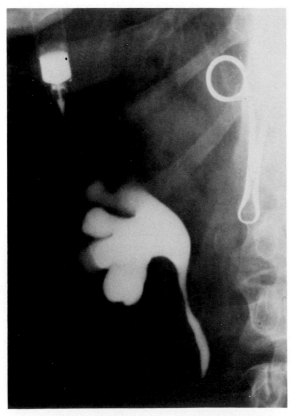

▶ **Figure 12–24**

Percutaneous antegrade nephrostomy.

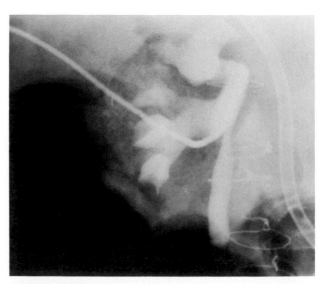

▶ **Figure 12–25**

Antegrade nephrostomy. Note the common bile duct stent.

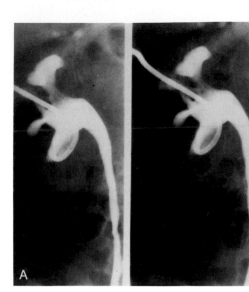
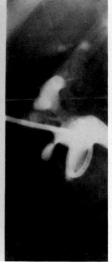
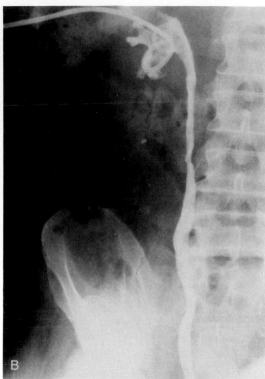

▶ **Figure 12–26**

A, Obstructive disease of the right ureter. B, A stent placed within the right ureter.

taneous nephrostomy. Figure 12–26B reveals the presence of a stent placed within the right ureter.

▶ BIBLIOGRAPHY

Bret PM et al: Abdominal lesions: A prospective study of clinical efficacy of percutaneous fine-needle biopsy. Radiology 159:345, 1986.

Casamassima F, Dilollo S, Arganini L, et al: Percutaneous needle biopsy guided by ultrasound in the diagnosis of intra-abdominal masses. Roentgen Ray 12:53, 1987.

Caturelli E, Rapacchini G, Anti M, et al: Malignant seeding after fine needle aspiration biopsy of the pancreas. Diagn Imaging 54:88, 1985.

Dondelinger RF, Rossi P, et al: Interventional Radiology. New York, Thieme Medical Publishers, 1990.

Goldberg HI and Gordon R: Diagnostic and interventional procedures for the biliary tract. Curr Opin Radiol 3:453, 1991.

Gothlin J and Gadenhold G: Percutaneous fine needle biopsy of abdominal pelvic lesions: passes necessary for secure diagnosis with fluoroscopy and CT guidance. Eur J Radiol 6:288, 1986.

Hunter DW, Castaneda-Zuniga W, Young AT, et al: Percutaneous removal of ureteral calculi: Clinical and experimental results. Radiology 156:341, 1985.

Kandarpa K: Handbook of Cardiovascular and Interventional Radiologic Procedures. Boston, Little, Brown, 1989.

Klein JS: Percutaneous drainage of intrathoracic collections. Appl Radiol 14:39, 1990.

Livraghi T, Damascelli B, Lombardi C, et al: Risk in fine-needle abdominal biopsy. J Clin Ultrasound 11:77, 1983.

Mankin H, Lang TA, and Spanier SS: The hazards of biopsy in patients with malignancy and primary bone and soft tissue tumors. J Bone Joint Surg [Br] 64A:1121, 1982.

Moss A: Interventional computed tomography. In Moss AA, Gamsu G, and Genant HK (eds): Computed Tomography of the Body. Philadelphia, WB Saunders, 1983, pp 1087–1129.

Onik G: Percutaneous biopsy: A practical approach. Postgrad Radiol 9:153–156, 1989.

Ring EJ and McClean GK: Interventional Radiology. Boston, Little, Brown, 1981.

Willis DA, Harbit-Drake M, and Julius LM: Gallstones: Alternatives to surgery. RN 6:70, 1990.

Wojtowycz M: Interventional Radiology and Angiography: Handbooks in Radiology. Chicago, Year Book Medical Publishers, 1990.

Wunschik F, George I, and Pastyr O: Stereotaxic biopsy using computed tomography. J Comput Assist Tomogr 8:32, 1984.

▶ SELF-ASSESSMENT QUIZ

1. What forms of guidance are available for lung biopsy?
   1. fluoroscopy
   2. computed tomography
   3. ultrasound
   4. angiography
      a. 1 only
      b. 1 and 2
      c. 1, 2, and 3
      d. 1, 2, 3, and 4

2. Which method of guidance is quick and inexpensive when doing a bone biopsy?
   a. fluoroscopy

   b. ultrasound
   c. computed tomography

3. What is the major disadvantage of fluoroscopic guidance?
   a. poor image resolution
   b. expensive
   c. takes too long
   d. radiation dose to the patient

4. Which guidance procedure is preferred for needle localization?
   a. ultrasound
   b. fluoroscopy
   c. computed tomography

5. A biopsy can be done with a needle on almost any site on the body.
   a. true
   b. false

6. Why is a biopsy of a hemangioma not usually done?
   a. too painful for patient
   b. not cost effective
   c. high risk of infection
   d. high risk of hemorrhage

7. Patients with severe pulmonary hypertension have an increased risk of _____ with needle biopsy.
   a. hemorrhage
   b. infection
   c. tumor seeding

8. The mortality rate for needle biopsy is
   a. very low
   b. moderate
   c. high

9. Hemoptysis may be defined as

   a. vomiting blood from the stomach
   b. blood in the feces
   c. spitting up blood from the lungs
   d. painful urination

10. An overpenetrated chest x-ray may be ordered for what purpose?
   a. to make the lungs darker
   b. to better demonstrate the apex
   c. to evaluate the diaphragm
   d. to better demonstrate mediastinal lymph nodes

▶ STUDY QUESTIONS

1. Why should a biopsy not be done in the case of lesions with malignant potential?

2. What are the two principal complications of a chest biopsy?

3. What is the relationship of needle size to the relative complication rate in needle biopsy?

4. What is the usual cause of death from needle biopsy?

5. What procedure could be helpful in determining fluid collections in the abdomen?

6. What radioisotope can be used to locate abscess cavities?

7. What is meant by the term "coagulopathy"?

8. What is one advantage of a basket stone retrieval catheter?

9. Under what conditions is a stent employed as a device for treatment?

► CHAPTER THIRTEEN

► THE FUTURE OF CARDIOVASCULAR/ INTERVENTIONAL TECHNOLOGY

► CHAPTER OUTLINE

Contrast Agents
Equipment
Cardiovascular/Interventional Technology
  Education and the Technologist
Vascular Interventional Procedures
  Intravascular Stents
  Atherectomy
  Laser Angioplasty

Angioscopy
Thrombolytic Therapy
Nonvascular Interventional Procedures
  Percutaneous Needle Biopsy
  Percutaneous Biliary Decompression
  Percutaneous Drainage of Abdominal
    Abscesses and Fluid Collections
  Percutaneous Nephrostomy

► CHAPTER OBJECTIVES

Upon completion of Chapter 13 the technologist will be able to:

1. Describe the emergence of cardiovascular and interventional procedures
2. Explain how new equipment design will have an impact on interventional procedures
3. Describe the controversies surrounding the use of ionic and nonionic contrast agents
4. Explain the role of "education" in the emergence of the profession and the technologist in cardiovascular and interventional technology
5. List and describe the vascular interventional procedures of the 1990s
6. List and describe the nonvascular interventional procedures of the 1990s

During this decade of the 90s we will celebrate the centennial of Roentgen's discovery of the x-ray beam. From the discovery of x-ray to the mid-1970s, diagnostic imaging depended on the radiologist's interpretation of the image produced on conventional x-ray film.

In the mid-1970s, revolutionary imaging modalities such as computed tomography (CT) and ultrasound emerged. This technology completely changed the role of diagnostic radiology.

During the 1980s, magnetic resonance imaging (MRI) emerged as the latest clinical imaging modality. Initially, MRI was seen as an adjunct to CT, and the research on MRI was somewhat slower to be utilized than research on CT until the medical community realized the unique advantages of diagnoses using MRI.

The uses of MRI seem to be expanding at regular intervals, usually monthly. New examinations, surface coil packages, and designs are continually proliferating to include contrast images and angiography.

The 1980s also ushered in the new specialty of interventional radiology. Since the appearance of angioplasty in the late 1970s, its progress has greatly increased both peripherally and cardiovascularly in the 1980s and early 1990s.

Interventional radiology has seen the radiologist's role shift from diagnostic film interpretation to full-time patient contact.

The arrival of interventional products and procedures, such as thrombolysis, embolization, percutaneous biopsy and drainage, angioplasty, and new catheters and guidewires, has created new relationships among radiologists, patients, and clinicians.

Interventional radiology essentially eliminates general anesthesia and some surgical procedures such as laparotomy and substantially decreases patient mortality.

Digital imaging has become an important diagnostic technology in CT scanning, digital subtraction angiography (DSA), MRI, and potentially angiography.

Digital angiography found a home in radiology in the early 1980s. DSA by way of venous injection is performed sparingly in some institutions, yet arterial studies are utilized extensively in arterial and interventional angiographic procedures.

Research and utilization are currently being directed at DSA with high-resolution cathode-ray tubes (2048 × 2048 pixels), providing outstanding gray-scale and diagnostic accuracy.

We expect a great deal of research into digital luminescence radiography. This could potentially replace the conventional film/screen radiography with digitization of the conventional x-ray latent image, allowing for instant quality processing for density, contrast, and fine-edge enhancement.

The continual upgrading of existing equipment and techniques and the emergence of new interventional procedures have helped to improve health care dramatically. Controversies regarding cost versus benefit continue to be discussed as new procedures evolve in diagnostic and therapeutic vascular and nonvascular radiology. Radiologists maintain that new technologies are necessary for improvements in medicine. Many politicians, on the other hand, believe that the new technologies substantially increase health care costs. Technology has become a primary target for curbing health care costs, but considerable evidence exists that new procedures are more accurate and cost-effective than other options.

▶ CONTRAST AGENTS

Iohexol, iopamidol, and hexabrix were approved for use in 1985. These three nonionic contrast agents have an osmolality of about one half that of conventional ionic agents, yet these agents could be 10 to 18 times more expensive.

The major questions today seem to revolve around cost and safety. How much safer are low osmolar agents; who would best benefit from their use; and are the increased costs justified?

Data examined from numerous studies tend to indicate that there may be a difference in the incidence of minor reactions but not in the mortality rate. Additional research has been directed at contrast-related renal failure (nephrotoxicity), and to date it appears that ionic and nonionic contrast agents have approximately the same effect on the kidneys.

Ongoing research is attempting to gauge the comparative thrombogenicity of ionic and nonionic contrast media.

Thus, to date, the results of past and present research have yet to substantiate conclusively the questions regarding cost efficacy, safety, and patient mortality. Because these questions persist, research continues; however, in response to these unanswered questions, radiology departments are now developing criteria for the selection and utilization of nonionic contrast agents. Some hospitals are now identifying patients in terms of "risk." High-risk patients may receive only nonionic agents. Other hospitals administer nonionic agents to patients for intravenous pyelography (IVP) and CT studies, regardless of potential risks.

▶ EQUIPMENT

In the 1990s, the working space for interventional procedures has undergone significant changes. Gone are the typical radiographic and fluoroscopic suites that used to be modified to accommodate special imaging equipment. Dedicated angiographic and nonvascular interventional suites are now the rule, rather than the exception. Angiographic suites are now spacious and are generously outfitted with C-arm fluoroscopy and digital imaging. High-efficiency generators, fractional focus x-ray tubes, serial changers, automatic contrast medium injectors, and a wide range of available disposable instruments and supplies are commonplace in most modern special procedure suites.

Improvements in room design and equipment utilization are expected to keep up as interventional procedures continue to evolve in the future.

Rapid serial film changers are undergoing continual refinement. The physical dimensions of this equipment are reduced, and more available floor space is being realized. Peripheral equipment is enhanced with the addition of programming devices and fluoroscopic-assisted positioning.

Film-screen science continues to improve, with faster film-screen combinations that yield increased contrast and image sharpness while reducing patient exposure to ionizing radiation.

The addition of electrocardiographic monitors and cardiac defibrillators makes possible the monitoring and recording of intra-arterial pressures.

► CARDIOVASCULAR/ INTERVENTIONAL TECHNOLOGY EDUCATION AND THE TECHNOLOGIST

The terms "special procedures" and "special procedures technologist" have been discarded and have been replaced by the terms "cardiovascular/ interventional technology" and "cardiovascular technologist." The American Registry of Radiologic Technologists (ARRT) has developed a certification examination in cardiovascular/interventional technology. Thus, a technologist (radiographer) has the opportunity to become registered in cardiovascular/ interventional technology, which is an advanced skill-imaging modality.

Several hospital-based and college-sponsored programs in cardiovascular/interventional technology have been developed. The American Society of Radiologic Technologists, House of Delegates, at their Annual Conference in 1992, ratified an *Educational Model Curriculum Guide for Cardiovascular/ Interventional Technology (CIT)*. Thus, educational guidelines are now established for institutions that wish to develop an advanced program in cardiovascular/interventional technology. Procedures for program recognition and evaluation are being studied. It is expected that a "formal" program, combined with a registry examination, will be the minimum requirement for technologists wishing to specialize in cardiovascular/interventional technology.

► VASCULAR INTERVENTIONAL PROCEDURES

At the 1990 meeting of the Radiological Society of North America (RSNA), 22 papers were presented concerning the use of vascular stents.

In an effort to solve the residual problems of restenosis and closure in percutaneous transluminal angioplasty (PTA), several new devices are being explored, such as intravascular stents, atherectomy devices, and lasers.

Intravascular Stents

Research is currently being conducted in both the clinical aspect and design of vascular stents. A requirement for stent material is that it be resistant to both thrombosis and corrosion in the vascular system. In addition, the placement depends on a system that has a high degree of flexibility. This means that the stent should be expandable so that it can be directed to the target area by way of a catheter system and, once installed, should be able to maintain a controlled position without the chance of injury to the vessel intima.

Atherectomy

Several atherectomy devices are being used in current and long-term clinical efficacy studies. The Simpson AtheroCath is currently being used in both peripheral and cardiovascular systems.

The Simpson catheter is propelled by a battery-powered motor-driven unit. The distal catheter tip houses a stainless-steel, small cylinder reservoir. This reservoir houses an adjustable cup-shaped cutter that can be controlled manually via the motor drive unit. The cutter, which rotates at 2500 rpm, is moved across and excises the plaque from the vessel intima.

Laser Angioplasty

Lasers are being commonly used today in ophthalmology, gynecology, urology, and dermatology. Over the years, several different amplified light sources such as ultraviolet, infrared, and visible light have been clinically tested for plaque angioplasty.

Research is focusing on the pulsed delivery of light in the ultraviolet and infrared range. Studies have shown that an intermittent pulsed beam minimizes the considerable heat build-up in the vessel lumen, thus reducing the chance of thermal intimal injury and vessel perforation.

Angioscopy

Miniaturized fiberoptic catheters (4/3 French) are designed for direct visualization of the intra-arterial lumen. The angioscopic technology will provide the ability to examine the patency of grafts and intimal conditions following angioplasty and atherectomy.

Thrombolytic Therapy

The use of streptokinase, urokinase, and tissue-type plasminogen activator will continue to be an exciting and effective treatment via the arterial, intracoronary, and intravenous routes. Other materials are currently being researched, and clinical trials will undoubtedly be underway upon publication of this text.

Selective regional thrombolysis, utilizing infusion wires, is currently being employed. These infusion wires provide a maximum distribution of the thrombolytic agent in either a slow drip infusion or a pulsatile high-pressure flow for rapid clot lysis.

▸ NONVASCULAR INTERVENTIONAL PROCEDURES

Percutaneous Needle Biopsy

Percutaneous needle biopsy provides the shortest, simplest, and least invasive approach to a cytologic or histologic diagnosis. The continuing improvements in needle science, the refinement of fine-needle biopsy procedures, and the improved resolution provided by ultrasound and CT guidance have made percutaneous needle biopsy a popular and relatively safe procedure. Needle intervention for diagnosis can be accomplished almost anywhere in the body. Lesions, for instance, are now being sampled in the lung, pleura, liver, bile ducts, lymph nodes, kidney, breast, and bone. The diagnosis and evaluation of primary and metastatic diseases can be accomplished via percutaneous needle biopsy with minor short-term complications.

Percutaneous Biliary Decompression

Patients with a history of obstructive jaundice and septic liver disease can benefit from percutaneous biliary compression. Only local anesthesia and a 22-gauge needle, which is passed via fluoroscopic guidance, are needed. A Cope biliary decompression and drainage system is one of the more popular systems utilized for biliary compression.

Percutaneous Drainage of Abdominal Abscesses and Fluid Collections

Percutaneous needle aspiration is another method of diagnosis and treatment of abdominal abscesses and fluid collections. Some of the types of lesions that are treated include abscess, hematoma, urinoma, biloma, and lymphocele. This procedure is responsible for lowering the mortality rate of patients with abdominal abscesses, who could not survive if this condition went untreated.

Percutaneous Nephrostomy

Percutaneous nephrostomy is a procedure used to facilitate external drainage of the renal collecting system. This procedure can also serve to decompress renal and perirenal fluid collections (infected cysts, abscesses, and urinomas). Percutaneous nephrostomy, using an antegrade approach, facilitates the insertion of devices for stone retrieval, biopsies, stricture dilatation, and antegrade ureteral stenting. Through an introduction catheter, drugs can be infused for the purpose of dissolving stones in order to administer antibiotics or antitumor agents.

▸ BIBLIOGRAPHY

Bettman M: Questions still plaguing low-osmolar contrast. Diagn Imaging 11:A72, 1990.

Tilkian A and Dailey E: Cardiovascular Procedures: Diagnostic Techniques and Therapeutic Procedures. St Louis, CV Mosby, 1986.

Wholey M: No end in sight for new interventional hardware. Diagn Imaging 11:A60, 1990.

▸ SELF-ASSESSMENT QUIZ

1. Which of the following procedures is/are interventional studies?
   1. thrombolysis
   2. embolization
   3. percutaneous biopsy and drainage
   4. angioplasty
      a. 1 only
      b. 1 and 2
      c. 1, 2, and 3
      d. 1, 2, 3, and 4

2. Which of the following is/are advantages of interventional procedures?
   1. general anesthesia not required
   2. decrease patient mortality
   3. eliminate some surgical procedures
   4. eliminate the need for asepsis
      a. 1 only
      b. 1 and 2
      c. 1, 2, and 3
      d. 1, 2, 3, and 4

3. Nonionic contrast media is/are
   a. more expensive than ionic media
   b. less expensive than ionic media
   c. as expensive as ionic media

4. It appears that ionic and nonionic contrast media have the same approximate effect on the kidneys.
   a. true
   b. false

5. Which of the following is/are requirements for stents?
   1. resistance to thrombosis
   2. resistance to corrosion
   3. high degree of flexibility
   4. thrombogenic effect
      a. 1 only
      b. 1 and 2

    c. 1, 2, and 3
    d. 1, 2, 3, and 4

6. The Simpson atherectomy cutter rotates at what rpm?
    a. 500
    b. 1000
    c. 2500
    d. 5000

7. Which light sources are used with lasers?
    1. ultraviolet
    2. infrared
    3. visible light
    4. cosmic rays
        a. 1 only
        b. 1 and 2
        c. 1, 2, and 3
        d. 1, 2, 3, and 4

8. Which instrument can determine the patency of a vascular graft?
    a. angioscope
    b. Simpson catheter
    c. stent
    d. balloon catheter

9. Pulsatile high-pressure and slow-drip infusion are terms associated with what procedure?
    a. angioscopy
    b. laser therapy
    c. angioplasty
    d. thrombolytic therapy

10. Tissue plasminogen activator is used
    a. in angioscopy
    b. with laser beams
    c. as a thrombolytic agent
    d. in conjunction with a stent

▶ STUDY QUESTIONS

1. Describe three areas of interventional imaging that are expected to flourish in the 1990s.
2. Explain the operation of a Simpson atherectomy catheter.
3. Explain the purpose of angioscopy.
4. List the medical specialties that currently utilize lasers.
5. What is the purpose of thrombolytics, and how are they administered?
6. List and describe the indications for percutaneous biopsy.
7. List and describe the purposes for percutaneous biliary compression.
8. List and describe the indications for percutaneous drainage of abdominal abscesses and fluid collections.
9. Describe the applications for percutaneous nephrostomy.

► SELF-ASSESSMENT QUIZZES

► ANSWER KEY

► CHAPTER ONE

1. b	4. b	7. a	10. b	13. d	16. c
2. d	5. b	8. d	11. d	14. a	17. d
3. a	6. a	9. c	12. a	15. c	18. a

► CHAPTER TWO

1. a	3. b	5. a	7. c	9. a	10. c
2. a	4. c	6. c	8. b		

► CHAPTER THREE

1. c	6. a	11. d	16. d	21. c	26. b
2. d	7. a	12. a	17. a	22. d	27. a
3. a	8. b	13. a	18. a	23. a	28. b
4. b	9. d	14. b	19. c	24. e	29. c
5. b	10. c	15. d	20. b	25. e	30. d

► CHAPTER FOUR

1. c	5. a	9. b	12. c	15. a	18. a
2. d	6. d	10. c	13. d	16. a	19. c
3. b	7. c	11. c	14. d	17. d	20. d
4. e	8. a				

► CHAPTER FIVE

1. d	6. b	10. b	14. b	18. d	22. d
2. a	7. d	11. c	15. c	19. a	23. a
3. c	8. b	12. c	16. b	20. d	24. d
4. d	9. a	13. a	17. b	21. b	25. a
5. c					

▶ CHAPTER SIX

1. b	6. a	11. b	15. c	19. a	23. b
2. b	7. b	12. a	16. c	20. a	24. d
3. a	8. d	13. b	17. c	21. c	25. d
4. a	9. a	14. c	18. d	22. a	26. d
5. a	10. d				

▶ CHAPTER SEVEN

1. b	6. d	11. d	16. a	21. a	26. c
2. c	7. a	12. c	17. c	22. b	27. c
3. a	8. b	13. d	18. d	23. c	28. c
4. b	9. c	14. c	19. d	24. d	29. c
5. a	10. b	15. a	20. a	25. a	30. a

▶ CHAPTER EIGHT

1. d	6. d	10. c	14. c	18. c	22. d
2. e	7. a	11. b	15. c	19. a	23. d
3. b	8. b	12. a	16. d	20. b	24. b
4. b	9. d	13. e	17. c	21. c	25. d
5. a					

▶ CHAPTER NINE

1. c	6. c	10. d	14. a	18. d	22. a
2. d	7. b	11. c	15. c	19. d	23. a
3. a	8. c	12. a	16. a	20. c	24. c
4. d	9. a	13. d	17. c	21. d	25. a
5. b					

▶ CHAPTER TEN

1. a	8. c	15. d	22. c	29. d	35. d
2. c	9. d	16. b	23. b	30. a	36. a
3. a	10. c	17. a	24. c	31. d	37. c
4. b	11. d	18. b	25. a	32. d	38. d
5. c	12. d	19. b	26. b	33. b	39. c
6. c	13. a	20. c	27. a	34. d	40. c
7. b	14. d	21. c	28. c		

▶ CHAPTER ELEVEN

1. c	5. d	9. b	12. a	15. c	18. a
2. a	6. d	10. b	13. d	16. d	19. c
3. b	7. d	11. c	14. c	17. d	20. b
4. c	8. c				

▶ CHAPTER TWELVE

1. c	3. c	5. a	7. a	9. c	10. d
2. a	4. c	6. a	8. a		

▶ CHAPTER THIRTEEN

1. d	3. a	5. c	7. c	9. d	10. c
2. c	4. a	6. c	8. a		

▶ INDEX

Note: Page numbers in *italics* refer to illustrations; page numbers followed by (t) refer to tables.

275

ISBN 0-7216-3283-1